TOOTH AND VEIL

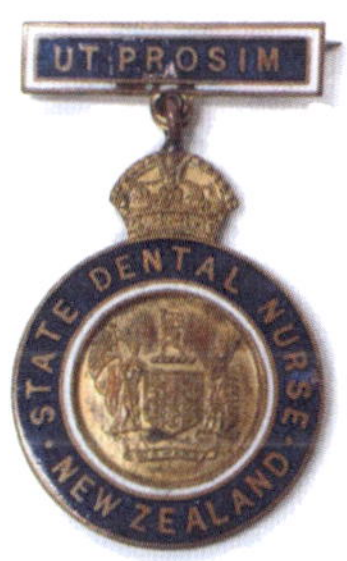

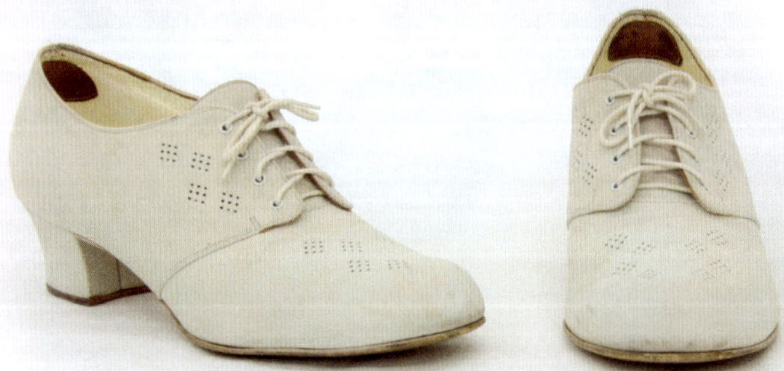

NOEL O'HARE

TOOTH AND VEIL

The life and times of the New Zealand dental nurse

MASSEY UNIVERSITY PRESS

To my sisters Patricia and Nuala,
who helped me more than I knew

CONTENTS

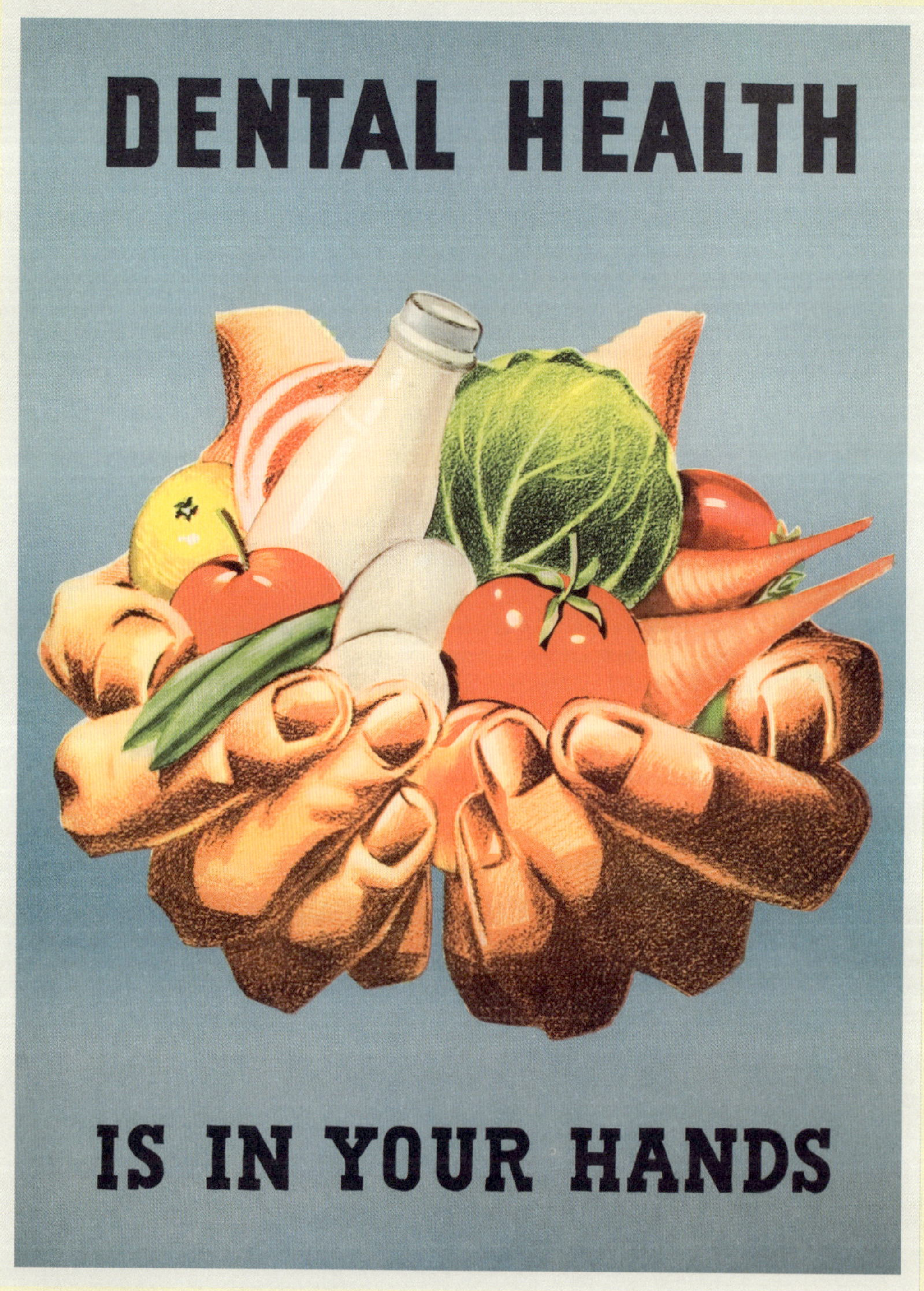
DENTAL HEALTH
IS IN YOUR HANDS

INTRODUCTION

Shop assistants working along the 'golden mile' in Wellington had witnessed many marches down Lambton Quay over the years: rowdy protestors against the Vietnam War, apartheid and nuclear testing in the Pacific; Jesus marches with Salvation Army bands; rallies for Māori and women's rights.

They waved flags, hoisted placards and banners, spilling onto the pavements and stopping traffic. The bullhorn-led chants, shouts and jeers, amplified in the narrow street by the tall buildings on both sides, made it impossible to attend to customers and there was nothing for it but to wait until the protestors had passed and the noise subsided.

The school dental nurses' march on a sunny autumn day in 1974 was different. It was, one observer noted, 'almost certainly the largest organised demonstration of women since the days of the suffragettes'. Shop assistants and passers-by had never seen anything like it: young women marching four abreast in starched white uniforms, veils and red cardigans. There were no placards protesting this or demanding that, just small signs held aloft at intervals stating which part of the country the women hailed from: Northland, Auckland, Waikato . . . a geographical spread that finished with Timaru, Dunedin and Invercargill. And most impressive of all was the silence. A powerful hush that made you strain to listen, to understand.

They were far from typical protestors. Most were middle-class, the daughters of farmers, accountants, businessmen and lawyers — conservative folk who deplored street politics and could be relied on to vote National. Many of the marchers had never been to the capital, and certainly never envisaged that on their first visit they'd be parading down the main shopping street while bystanders stared. It felt weird. Since the first day they'd reported for training, the rule had been stressed: *the wearing of the uniform in the street is not permitted*. This was disobedience, rebellion. Who knew the consequences when they returned to their clinics? It made some nervous, but there was comfort in numbers: 600 of their colleagues were marching with them.

They were the least militant group of workers. However, like a long-suffering partner in a relationship, there'd been some 'That's it!' moments when suddenly the hurts, slights and indifference had become too much to bear.

Pay was ostensibly why they were marching. For 30 years their wages were tied to those of public health nurses in a system of relativity. Any pay rise either group negotiated was passed on to the other. This had not always worked in the dental nurses' favour, as some pay claims were rejected because it would have put them ahead of public health nurses. However, in 1973 public health nurses negotiated a big backdated pay increase and dental nurses expected to receive a similar boost. Then, in an about-turn, the State Services Commission (SSC) declared that relativity was no longer relevant and it did not intend to break the wage freeze by passing on the increase to the dental nurses.

Much as they were upset by the State Services Commission's duplicity, pay relativity was not what many of the marchers cared about or even understood. It was merely the instrument that lanced the boil of anger and frustration that had been building for decades. For more than 50 years, dental nurses had endured a workplace milieu in which they'd been treated as inferior beings, discouraged from thinking for themselves and subjected to petty military-style discipline. 'You learned from an early stage that you were a dental nurse, slave of the dental profession,' remembers one nurse.

Previous generations of dental nurses had stoically accepted their lot, but times had changed. The marchers had grown up in the radical free-wheeling 1960s (though the subversive virus took a long time to reach New Zealand). The School Dental Service, on the other hand, had calcified in the late 1940s, and the military style of management grated with new intakes of dental nurses. They were tired of having to stand to attention with hands behind their backs when addressed by a superior, tired of the unscheduled inspections of their clinics to catch them out for petty failings like dust on a high ledge or a scuff mark on their white shoes, tired of the starched uniforms and veils that chafed their skin and made a mess of their hair, tired of being transferred on a week's notice from Auckland to Haast and discovering the caravan where they were to live was also occupied by four fisheries officers, tired of the antiquated equipment they had to use, tired of inflicting needless pain on children because the Health Department allowed the low-strength anaesthetic they supplied to be used for extractions only, not fillings. They were tired of the epithet 'murder house' and of being slagged off for doing 'unnecessary' work on patients.

As the marchers reached the end of Lambton Quay, they passed, on their right, the Old Government Buildings. It was there, in an annexe known as the Tomato House, that the first dental nurses had trained. Colonel Thomas Hunter had founded the

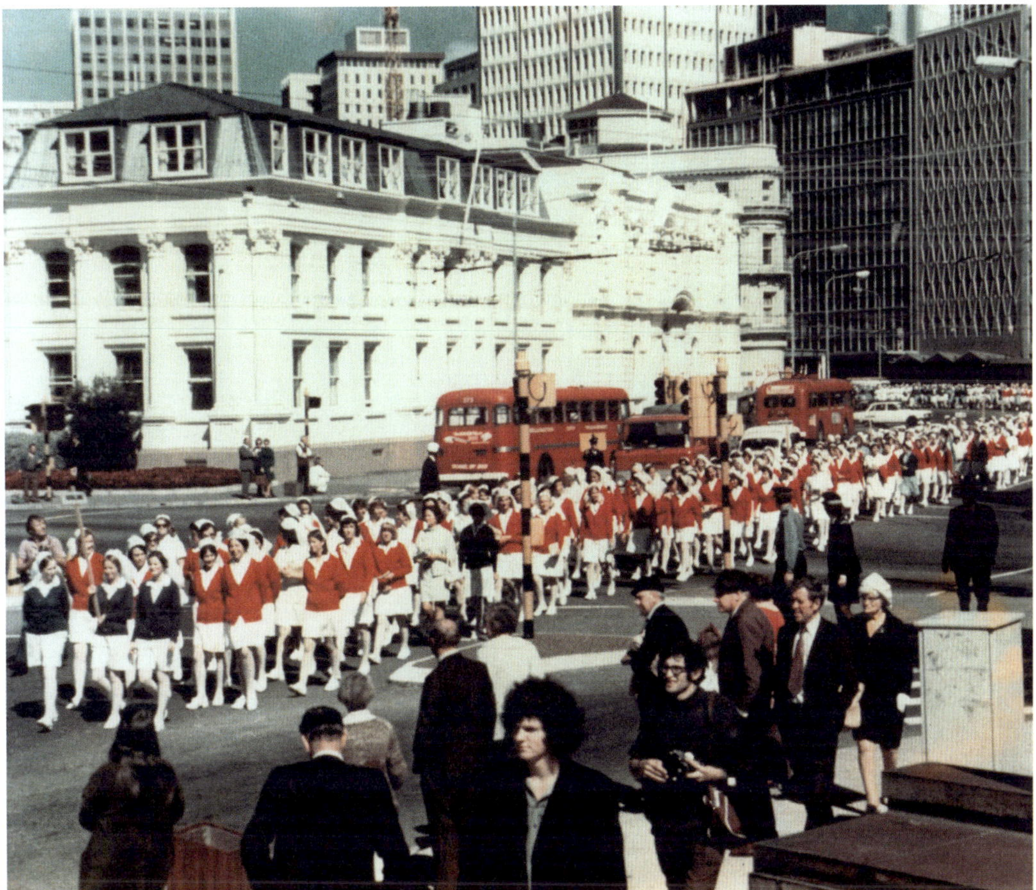

In 1974 more than 600 dental nurses marched down Wellington's Lambton Quay in one of the largest organised demonstrations of women since the days of the suffragettes.

School Dental Service in 1921. The colonel, who'd led the New Zealand Dental Corps in the First World War, was appalled at the state of children's teeth in New Zealand, a large percentage of whom needed extractions and/or fillings. As this book will show, despite opposition from many dentists and a lack of funding, the service thrived, a unique New Zealand social experiment that would be lauded around the world and modelled in 15 countries.

In 1940, 295 dental nurses were in training when the Dominion School for Dental Nurses and Children's Dental Clinic opened in Willis Street, Wellington. The new clinic was a wonder of the dental world. In a room the size of a rugby field, with six-metre-high windows, more than 50 children could be drilled and filled at the same time. Health experts, foreign delegations, even royalty visited regularly, escorted through the building by senior staff. 'We were never introduced to overseas guests; it was always the men,' one dental nurse recalled.

If they'd been asked what it was like being a dental nurse, what stories they could have told. Those first precarious years when the whole world seemed to be set against them: the press, the medical establishment, dentists, even parents. The loneliness of pioneering dental nurses sent to the backblocks to set up makeshift clinics. The

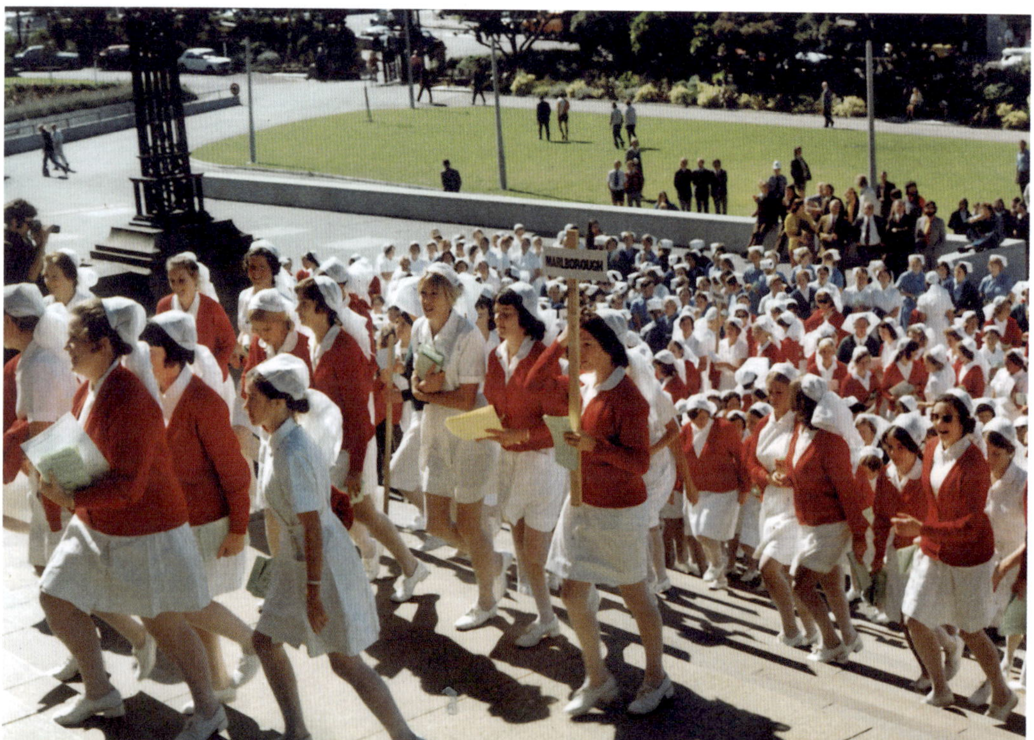

Dental nurses ascend the steps of Parliament. They were refused entry but these women were 'not for turning'.

privations of the Great Depression, and how once, after work, they'd picked their way through broken glass along Lambton Quay after the unemployed could curb their desperation no longer and had rioted. Then came the war and the move to the new Willis Street clinic, from the roof of which they'd watched excitedly as American troopships arrived at the Wellington docks. By then they were living in hostels around the city, one a former brothel. At night, drunken soldiers who hadn't caught up with the change in occupancy would come knocking.

Conformity had been the watchword of the uptight, strait-laced 1950s. Schools were bursting at the seams with the baby boom, and it was a hectic time with so many teeth to drill and so few dental nurses. Then there was the dizzy, turbulent, miniskirted 1960s, when training to be a dental nurse felt like stepping back in time. And now here they were, massed on the steps of Parliament while photographers and television news cameramen jockeyed for position to capture the drama. The prime minister, Norman Kirk, had agreed to meet them. 'Parliament Invaded by Dental Nurses' ran the headline in the *Evening Post*: 'The deputation moved into the building to go to the Prime Minister's suite. The nurses moved to follow them. Parliament messengers and police blocked their way. So the nurses went skirmishing. They found unguarded doors and surged in a white wave into the corridors.'[1]

As dental nurse Annette King reflected later: 'We were a bunch of women who had never done anything like that. We were nice girls — that was the sort of label we had.'[2]

How had it come to this?

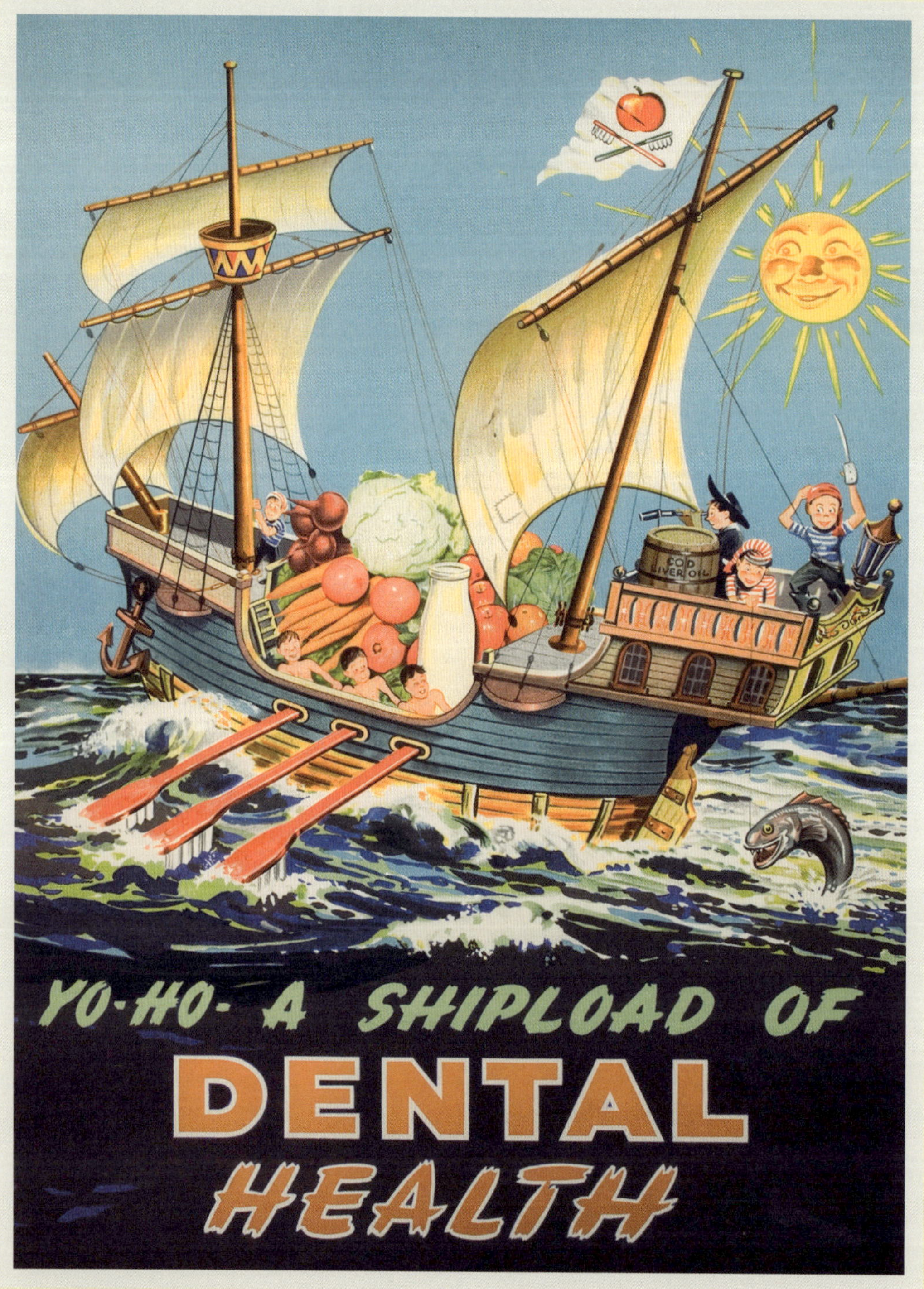
COD LIVER OIL
YO-HO- A SHIPLOAD OF
DENTAL
HEALTH

1

RAISED IN THE TOMATO HOUSE

May Falconer was the first person to apply to train as a dental nurse.[1] At 34, she just met the criteria. The education department had advertised for 'Probationer Dental Nurses', preferably registered nurses aged 25 to 35. May was not a registered nurse, but she had gained nursing experience serving in military hospitals in the last years of the First World War.

It was December 1920, and the proposed new state dental service, championed by the head of the Department of Health's new dental division, Colonel Thomas Hunter, was attracting a lot of adverse comment in the press. Many dentists, fearing competition, were opposed and the debate had become strident and bitter.

May's brother Alex, superintendent of Dunedin Hospital, encouraged her to apply; he'd become an advocate of a school dental service after meeting Hunter at a medical conference. In that era, her career options were limited and dental nursing seemed an attractive alternative to teaching in overcrowded classrooms or the regimented life of a hospital nurse. Still, she remained cautious: there were no guarantees that the service would succeed with the strong opposition from the medical, dental and trained nurses associations. She travelled from Dunedin to Wellington, where the training course was based, and had a long talk with Hunter himself before applying. Even after being accepted for the course, she was still in two minds. She approached Richmond Dunn, the newly appointed supervisor of the service, to withdraw her application. After some dithering Dunn retrieved her file from the bundle of successful applications and May had second thoughts again. 'I caught a glimpse of it and decided on the spot to leave things as they were as I might not get in another year.'

The scene that greeted her when she turned up for training on the morning of 4 April 1921 would have done little to confirm that she'd made the right decision. The training school was in the annexe of the Government Buildings in Whitmore Street, across the road from Parliament House. Unlike its majestic parent, the annexe was a nondescript structure originally erected to house First World War records. A long two-storey building with a surfeit of large windows and unlined rooms, it had earned the nickname 'Tomato House' because of its sweltering temperatures in summer; with no heating system, it was fridge-cold in winter. May could see little evidence of a dental facility. In one large, empty room workmen were putting up long benches. There was a small furnished room and another small windowless one, with two offices leading off it bearing the name plates *Colonel T. A. Hunter* and *Dr Truby King*. (King had founded the Plunket Society in 1907, and was the Health Department's director of child welfare.)

Confusion reigned as the 30 trainee dental nurses milled about the rooms. 'We all felt strange, all meeting for the first time and taking up work that was so different,' recalled Meba Armstrong, who had given up her office job in Auckland.[2] The trainees ranged in age from 18 to 36, and had left behind home towns from Auckland to Invercargill. Some, like May, had worked in military hospitals, others had been dentists' assistants, and about a third were making the jump from office work. Hunter had hoped to recruit experienced nurses, but opposition from the Trained Nurses Association had stymied that plan because it was felt that nurses' years of training and experience would be wasted on such specialisation.

The recruits' first-day-at-school anxiety may not have been eased by the trio who greeted them. Hunter, Dunn and King were all men not far off retirement. Hunter, lean, dapper and moustachioed, was every inch the stereotypical colonel, except in height. A 'physically . . . insignificant little fellow' was Wellington trainee Elsie Haines' first impression.[3] But he made up for his lack of height with an energy and sense of purpose that bordered on the fanatical. He'd fought for years to set up a school dental service and was now staking his reputation on its success. Until he ran into a blizzard of criticism for promoting the scheme, he'd led a charmed life, smoothly riding to the top of his profession. The third son of Scottish emigrants who settled in Dunedin, he was 58 — a comparatively late age in those days to be embarking on such a controversial venture.

Hunter had already devoted 44 years to dentistry. At 14 he was apprenticed to Dunedin dentist Alfred Boot. It was his first stroke of good luck: Boot was not only a very successful dentist but also a progressive one. Dentistry then was a trade, not a profession. 'Dentists were scarcely distinguishable from other artisans. Some dentists were in fact much less skilled than many artisans, in terms of both overall technical ability and manual dexterity,' writes Tom Brooking in his history of dentistry in

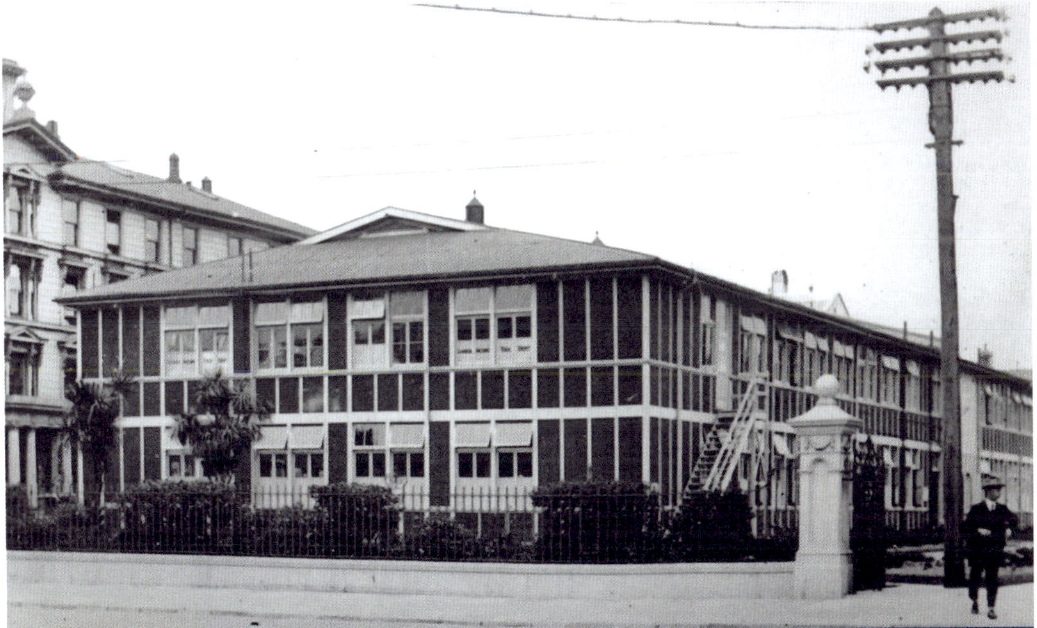

The Tomato House, Whitmore Street, Wellington, where the first school dental nurses trained.

New Zealand.[4] 'Essentially dentists extracted teeth, a service also provided by chemists, doctors, blacksmiths, quacks, and anyone with strong wrists.'

Boot was an exception in believing people should hold on to their teeth. To promote his unusual idea, he published a monograph, *The Preservation of Teeth*, in which he advocated prevention, identified tartar build-up as a cause of tooth decay and stressed the importance of brushing and a sound diet. It was a message the young Tommy Hunter absorbed and would never tire of repeating.

Boot travelled to Invercargill to try to increase his clientele, but nothing came of it. Instead, he sent his young apprentice round the Otago gold fields, 'either to give me more confidence in myself or in the hope it would increase the practice', Hunter wrote later. 'My first stop was at Milton, then on to Lawrence and by coach the rest of the way.' The roads were so bad, he added, that at times 'the dust completely hid the leading horses'. He set up shop in the parlour of a hotel. 'This arrangement did not afford a great deal of privacy and of course my equipment was limited.'[5]

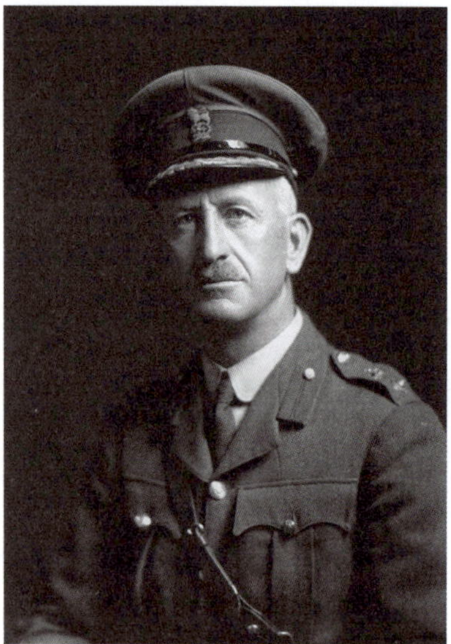

Colonel Thomas Hunter, the dentist who overcame fierce opposition from his colleagues to set up the School Dental Service.

Nevertheless, he gained a reputation as an excellent tooth puller, such that by 17 he'd completed his apprenticeship and set up his own dental practice.[6] It probably says a lot about dentistry in those days that people were willing to entrust the care of their teeth to a callow youth. Hunter seems, however, to have been able to inspire confidence at a young age. By all accounts he was a born leader. Away from the surgery, he played rugby and was the popular captain of the Otago team. (He was also recruited to make up the numbers in local cricket and football games and was praised for his prowess as a piano player and singer in the hotel.) By his forties he was a wealthy man with a flourishing dental practice in the Octagon, a residence in the elite Heriot Row, and membership of the exclusive Dunedin Club.

Hunter was instrumental in setting up the New Zealand Dental Association, to raise the status of the profession and reduce competition by squeezing out the quacks and charlatans who promised painless dentistry at low prices. As the association's second president he oversaw the establishment of Otago University's Dental School, guaranteeing £1000 (about $160,000 today) of his own money to ensure it was built in 1907.

He had a hand, too, in appointing the first dean of the Dental School, an ambitious 28-year-old from England called Dr Henry Percival Pickerill. Pickerill proved to be an outstanding choice, and his dental research earned the fledgling school international recognition. However, Hunter was to rue the day Pickerill ever landed in New Zealand, for the prickly Englishman was to become a trenchant and influential critic of the state dental nurses scheme and would do everything in his power to scuttle it.

For now, though, the two men got on well enough, sharing a deep concern for the state of the nation's teeth. Both were appalled when war broke out in 1914 and large numbers of recruits had to be rejected for poor dental health or because their teeth and gums needed remedial work. In 1915 the New Zealand Dental Corps was formed and Hunter was appointed director with the rank of colonel; Pickerill became an assistant director with the rank of major.

Poor dental health might have seemed the least of recruits' worries, given they risked having their head blown off by an enemy shell. Certainly that was how the humour magazine *Punch* saw it at the time. In one cartoon a medical officer says to a potential recruit, 'Sorry, I must reject you on account of your teeth.' To this the man replies, 'Man, ye're making a gran' mistake. I'm no wanting to bite the Germans. I'm wanting to shoot 'em.'[7] Nonetheless, the Dental Corps proved invaluable, working under fire on the shores of Gallipoli and at the Battle of the Somme. On top of everything else, the notoriously hard biscuits in the soldiers' rations were capable of cracking teeth if they were not first soaked in tea or water.

After his success with the Dental Corps, in 1919 Hunter became head of the Division of Dental Health and turned his attention to the long-standing issue of the dental health of children, an estimated 90 per cent of whom needed treatment. As the Dental School was unable to turn out enough dentists to treat the children, he proposed a scheme to recruit young women who, after two years' intensive training, would be deployed in schools. He won the support of the minister of health and education, the pugnacious James Parr, but he knew he would have to tread carefully to win over the dental profession. To mollify opposition, he argued that women were more suited to treating children, that any work they did would be supervised by dentists, and that, in any case, most would be in the job for only a short time before fulfilling their destinies as wives and mothers.

That proved enough to win over most members of the Dental Association, but not all. Pickerill lambasted Hunter's scheme at every turn and became the nucleus for opposition to it. Why, he asked, should children not have the same dental care as adults, i.e. from fully trained dentists? 'Why then should they be subjected to being operated upon (as is proposed) by half-trained women, and if these women are good enough for the children why are they not good enough for their parents?' he wrote in the press.[8] The Otago branch of the Dental Association predicted that the scheme would lower the standard of dentistry in New Zealand and no less 'degrade the profession for all time'.[9]

Richmond Dunn, as supervisor of the training school, also came under fire, even before he had taken up the role. The white-haired 59-year-old was 'a man who, whatever his capabilities in his profession, belongs distinctly to the old order of dentists and who can scarcely be conversant with the modern methods so essential on the part of a dentistry instructor', claimed the *Otago Daily Times*.[10]

In fact Dunn was a scholarly convert to dentistry who was far from old school. A former science teacher at the exclusive Wanganui Collegiate boarding school, he had switched to dentistry and set up a successful practice in the town (teaching thermodynamics to farmers' sons was perhaps like pulling teeth). Dunn shared Hunter's passion for children's dental care, 'but such was his single-mindedness that his very zeal and enthusiasm sometimes brought him into sharp conflict with others', the dental nurses' journal *Niho Pai* later noted in an obituary; 'It is a tribute to his character, however, that none could long remain at variance with him.'[11]

Zeal and enthusiasm also knew no bounds when it came to the 63-year-old Truby King, the last of the trio who welcomed the trainee nurses that day in 1921. King was a gifted polymath who, as superintendent of Seacliff Lunatic Asylum, the country's largest such institution, had not only transformed the care of the mentally ill inmates but also turned the asylum into a productive farm. He published pamphlets on plant and animal husbandry and many other subjects that attracted his interest. In a 1917 pamphlet *The Story of the Teeth and How to Save Them*, he wrote: 'No race or family can remain great or even perpetuate itself, if it fails to develop properly and give due exercise to jaws and teeth. Every function of body and mind is ultimately dependent not only on what the mouth delivers to the stomach, but [also] on the complete grinding and mixing with saliva of every morsel of food before it is swallowed.'[12]

King himself chewed every mouthful 35 times, which must have discouraged colleagues from arranging lunchtime meetings with him. Not that they were likely to. When he died in 1938 an obituary observed: 'Many of his friends and professional contemporaries would run round corners rather than meet him in the street, for fear he would draw them into interminable discussions, and then force them to do something against their will.'[13]

'Looking back I realise it was fortunate we did have Truby King so near, and very interested in our welfare,' said Elsie Haines. 'One of his theories was that nobody should be asked to, nor could they, concentrate for more than 40 minutes at a time, so our day was planned to vary the lectures as much as possible.'[14] In 1906 King had published a pamphlet, *The Evils of Cram*, stressing the dangers of mental overexertion in children. The strain, he warned, quoting the English philosopher Herbert Spencer, would cause girls to become 'flat-chested and unfit for maternity'.[15]

All three men — Hunter, the fanatical colonel; Dunn, the absent-minded professor; King, the kindly zealot — had enough hobby horses between them to run a herd. Like all right-thinking people of their time, they were racists. Racism then was not only

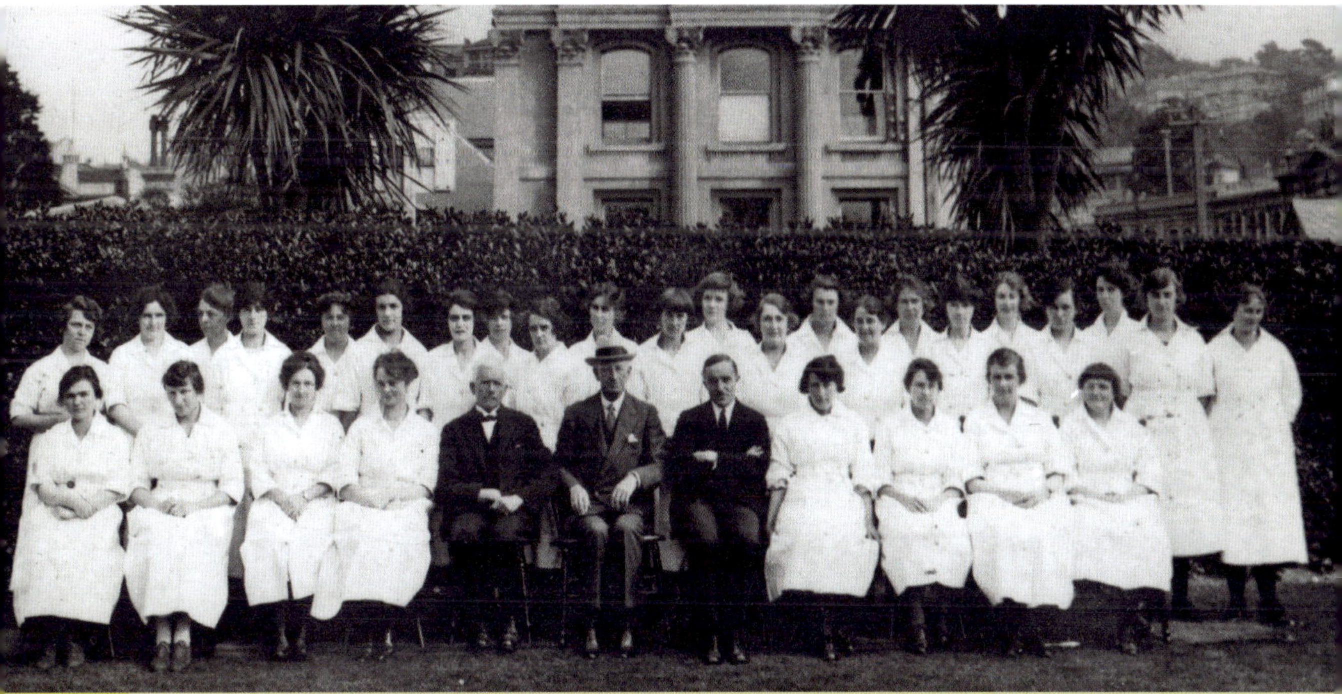

The first draft of student dental nurses in 1922, pictured with (from left) Richmond Dunn, director of the training school; Colonel Thomas Hunter, head of the Department of Health's dental division; and James Parr, Minister of Public Health.

socially acceptable but downright patriotic. A nation's greatness depended on the quality of its racial stock and to preserve the British Empire, of which New Zealand was a proud outpost, it was imperative to maintain the superiority of the Anglo-Saxon stock. Dentists naturally saw the country's rampant dental decay as a sign of national decay. In his presidential address to the Dental Association in 1906 Hunter proclaimed that defective and unclean teeth were signs of the 'physical and moral degeneration of the race'. (Another dentist gave the conference attendees pause for thought, however, when he observed that Chinese, Indians and other non-Anglo-Saxons had perfect teeth.)

Hunter advocated dental care as a way to reinvigorate the race, but his friend Dunn, in an 'oh why do we bother?' Darwinian moment, wrote 'we spend our lives in great measure in bolstering up the unfit . . . Only the dentally well provided should survive in the struggle for existence . . . Dentists, doctors and nurses are all at the same game to some extent, diluting the vigour of future generations by nullifying Nature's attempts to weed out the weaklings.'[16]

King agreed that the empire was in dangerous decline, and that its children had become soft and weak, but he was not going to stand aside and let nature take its course. Self-indulgence, decadence and selfishness had led to the decline of ancient Greece and Rome, and it all started in the home. The 'preposterous farce' of giving boys and girls an identical education was leading to a decline in the birth rate and degeneracy in the 'white race'. Only by training girls for motherhood and boys for mental and martial pursuits could decline be arrested. His famous solution, the Plunket Society, which Hunter hoped would be a model for the School Dental Service, was a system of infant care that was efficient, scientific and character-building. It was ignored by the medical profession but found favour with mother-of-eight Lady Victoria Plunket, wife of the then governor-general. Her endorsement was echoed by the wealthy upper classes. As historian Erik Olssen has observed, 'For the ladies and gentlemen compulsory courses in domestic science promised a supply of well-trained servants and a method of outflanking the feminists and restoring some sense of social order.'[17]

In addressing his neophytes that morning Hunter would have stressed that what they had signed up to was not just a job but a mission. They would go forth as missionaries preaching the gospel of dental health, waging war against tooth decay, doing their bit to reinvigorate the children of the empire. The colonel knew how to rally the troops and they responded to his passion and vision. 'Oh, I remember we all wanted to please that man,' Haines said. Looking back, Miss J. R. Robbins, a trainee from Timaru, wrote: 'Mr Hunter was our guide and inspiration . . . He filled us with a spirit of enthusiasm and loyalty to our cause which has prevailed through the years.'[18]

In the teeth of fierce and very public opposition to the new venture, Hunter's sense of mission was probably vital. In the press his old nemesis Pickerill had resorted to personal abuse, sneering at Hunter's lack of formal qualifications: 'The whole scheme is the product of an untrained mind. If the chief dental officer had been fortunate enough himself to have received any systematic dental training, if he possessed any degree, diploma, or certificate showing that he had been trained at all, he would be, I feel sure, the very last man to deprive others of the benefits of a proper training.'[19]

From day one there was a circling of the wagons. Attacks from the tabloid *Truth* were unremitting, referring to the trainees as 'Parr's Pretty Pets', 'Hunter's Harem' and 'Dunn's Duds'. The name-calling drew the women together. 'We rather liked the term "Dunn's Duds" and often referred to ourselves as this,' recalled May Falconer. The *esprit de corps* helped them overlook the shortcomings of the job.

The most obvious shortcoming was equipment — there wasn't any. Still officially director of the army Dental Corps, Hunter managed to obtain a few ancient dental chairs and discarded instruments that had been mothballed after the war. 'What a collection,' remembered Falconer: 'no two the same but very comfortable for the patient. Mine worked by winding up at the back — hurdy gurdy [style].'

First, however, came months of lectures. Each trainee was given a copy of *Grey's Anatomy* and told to buy notebooks, for all instruction would be dictated or written on the blackboard. Chemistry, physics, biology, anatomy, physiology, pathology, dental surgery and *materia medica* (pharmacology) made for a demanding curriculum — especially for some, like Elsie Haines, who had left school at 13. (Lectures included instruction on spotting mouth sores caused by syphilis, common after the First World War and a risk to dental nurses.)

The lecture room was makeshift, furnished with swivel chairs salvaged from the saloon of an old ship. A blackboard ran the length of the wall and to one side stood bony Annabelle, the model skeleton; it would be 1940 before she got her own cupboard. Things did not start well. The noise of lorries and trams clattering past outside, the clip-clop of dray horses on the cobblestones as goods carts plied the docks, and the hubbub from Inland Revenue clerks in adjoining rooms made it impossible to hear the lectures. The trainees were given 10 days' holiday while the room was lined.

Another interruption occurred when Hunter decided that the trainees needed uniforms to look the part. Dunn's wife, Isabel, turned up with bolts of white calico and sewing machines, and those with stitchery and dressmaking skills were duly put to task. Mrs Dunn 'offered to help us but as she wanted the uniforms to be ankle length and one nurse suggested to cover the calf of the leg only, she refused to help us and we were left to our own devices', recalled Falconer. 'At this time it was considered rude to contradict an older person but we managed to make very presentable uniforms.'

Though their own doctors had examined them as part of the application process, they were now required to get a medical certificate from a government-appointed doctor. The experience so rankled that half a century later the name 'Dr Platts-Mills' was still etched in Meba Armstrong's memory. The formidable and opinionated Daisy Platts-Mills was one of the first women to qualify as a doctor in New Zealand and had

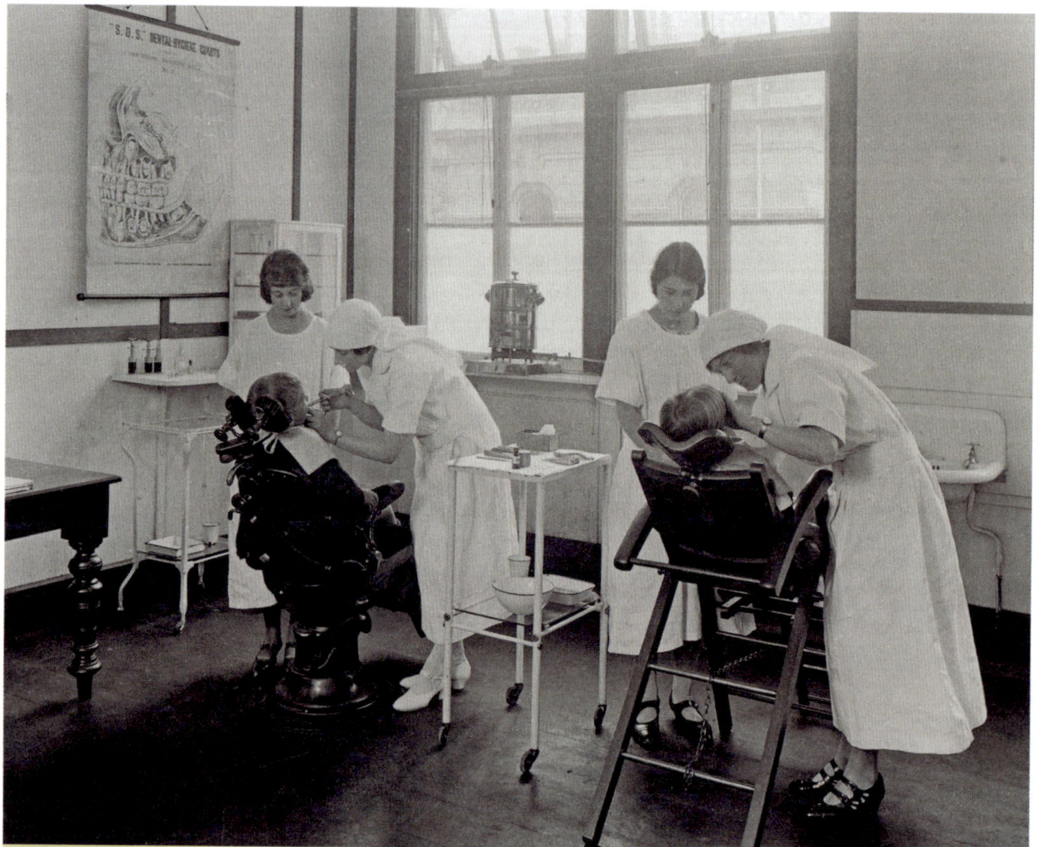

The extraction room in the Wellington clinic. It was bloody work, with more than 100 teeth removed each day.

a distinguished career in public health. An opponent of the school dental scheme, she gave every trainee a bad report, and most emerged from her office in tears. May Falconer remembered her, too: 'She considered my short hair unprofessional and she held my certificate over till I grew mine to a suitable length — until then I was medically unfit.' When the extent of the doctor's obstruction became clear, her reports were ignored by the health department.

The trainees saw little of Hunter, who was often travelling the country, arranging the setting up of dental clinics and countering the bad publicity the service was getting in the press. It was left to Dunn to deliver all the lectures in his own eccentric way. Trainee nurse Robbins recalled one incident:

> Mr Dunn has just completed an outstanding drawing of the nervous system on the board in readiness for the next lecture. Before this could take place, a party, headed by the Minister of Health, arrived on a visit to see how the girls were progressing. On being shown the drawing, they beheld numerous mice of diminutive proportions creeping along the main branches of the nerves, mesmerised by the beady glances from the owls on the branches above.[20]

Sometimes Dunn forgot he was no longer a science teacher. 'He was mad on chemistry,' Meba Armstrong said. 'We needed a certain amount of chemistry because of the drugs we used but we were stuffed with all kinds of chemistry we didn't need at all.'

Mid-morning recess was bedlam with the 30 trainees chatting and laughing in the small space outside Hunter's and King's offices. 'This so annoyed these two gentlemen that in desperation Mr Dunn allowed us 15 minutes to go for a walk around Parliament Buildings provided we did not have morning tea anywhere,' May Falconer wrote. Tea breaks were strictly forbidden for the effect it would have on dental health. 'So we chewed an apple and soon became known as the "Apple Brigade". This did not add to our popularity.'

Sweets were taboo — dental nurses would be required to set an example for children and parents. However, illicit indulgence was not unknown. Meba recalled one incident when during an exam 'somebody dropped a bag of blackballs and they rolled all over the floor. There was silence. We carried on with the paper and the blackballs were picked up afterwards. Mr Dunn, a very tactful man, never said a word. We were, of course, all very amused.'

The months of intensive study — lectures by day, swotting by night — passed quickly, with little time left for any kind of social life. Soon it was time for the practical work. Every day reluctant children from schools and orphanages all around the Wellington region trooped through the training school to be treated. As J. L. Saunders wrote in his history of the School Dental Service, published in 1964,

> In the mind of the general public, dental treatment was regarded with extreme apprehension and was pictured as being associated with ruthless extraction, a barbarous drill, and excruciating pain. This . . . was well exemplified by an experience at one of the main hospitals, where the

> establishing of a dental department was deferred because it was objected that the 'continuous screams from the dental department' would seriously disturb the staff and patients in the vicinity.[21]

Mr Peacock, a young dentist newly arrived from England, was employed to oversee the practical work. 'Mr Peacock showed us how to work the drills, how to drill a tooth,' said Meba. 'He marked the spot and you drilled it then we mixed silver amalgam with mortar and pestle and filled the tooth.'

'It was expected of us that it should not be necessary to show us twice how to do anything. We were not allowed to mix for our next neighbour but had to be absolutely independent,' recalled May. '"Did I expect a little black boy at my elbow when I went out [in the field]?" I was once asked when helping another.'

Many of the children's teeth were so decayed that they had to be pulled out. For the nurses on extraction duty, it was a full day without breaks. May: 'An extraction day started at 8.30 a.m. — both nurses on duty then. The instruments were sterilised — everything was made ready — a lecture from 9 a.m. to 9.30 and then to work. Lucky to have finished, cleaned up and away by 5.30 or later.' It was bloody work in the extraction room, with more than 100 teeth removed a day. The children spat blood, pus and saliva into an enamel bowl, inevitably splattering the nurses' uniforms.

The health department reluctantly agreed to provide two uniforms a week, but the blue uniforms of the juniors were changed only twice a term despite the dirty manual chores they had to do. One monotonous ritual was to shine the large copper vessels in the surgery. 'Every day the urns and sterilisers were polished by four juniors, this duty being more known as being "on copper",' recalled nurse Elsie Hitchcock. 'We got to the clinic early, spread paper on a long table in the surgery, went through tins of Brasso and raised some beautiful shines. With uniforms infrequently changed we all acquired a subtle "eau de Brasso" aroma around the surgery.'[22] While the copper gleamed, however, nothing was done about the showers of dust that descended from the open-beam ceiling when the clerks moved about upstairs.

Another chore for junior nurses that continued right up to the 1960s was collecting teeth from local dentists for students to practise on. (There was to be no practising on patients.) The teeth were then inserted into metal dummy jaws. The reuse of human teeth has a long history in dentistry.[23] In the sixteenth century poor people could sell their teeth to the wealthy — the teeth were yanked out and riveted into ivory dentures. Supply was limited, given that only the truly desperate were prepared to make such a painful trade, so grave robbers were employed to meet market demand.

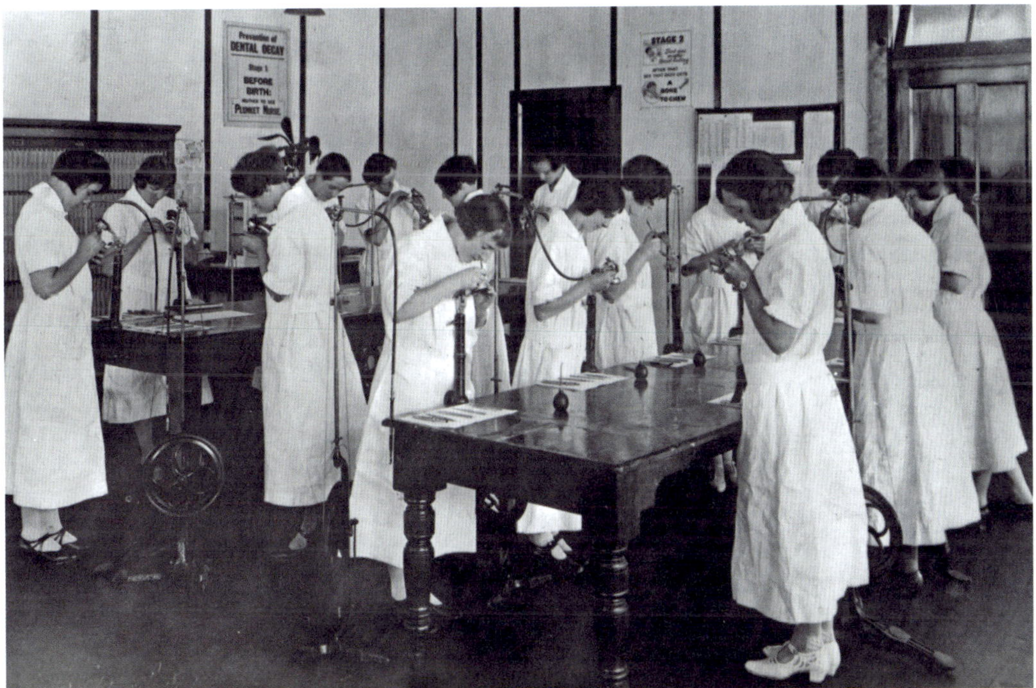

Dental nurses practise drilling on extracted teeth collected from local dentists. Contrary to popular belief, children were not practised on.

The Battle of Waterloo proved a godsend for denture-makers. In one grisly day in June 1815, tens of thousands of soldiers, many with good teeth, lay dead on the battlefield. Looters were quick to see the potential and the market was flooded with 'Waterloo teeth'. Though collected randomly, when sorted into upper and lower they looked like they came from a single mouth.

The same sorting took place when the junior nurses brought their collections back to the clinic. 'Miss Haines boiled them to sterilise them, [I] remember the smell!', recalled nurse Flora Morris.[24] A perk of this Saturday chore was morning tea at Kirkcaldie and Stains' department store. Once, a 'nurse forgot to pick up the jar which had been put under the table and had to go back to the lost property office to claim a jar of teeth'. It was the first of many mishaps with tooth collecting over the years.

As well as extracting and filling teeth, the nurses were expected to be dental evangelists. Dunn was a believer in spreading the word; as he once mused to colleagues, 'Wonderful propaganda work had been accomplished in Germany in connection with the military and also in other countries. Was not such a propaganda scheme possible for New Zealand in dental and general health matters?'[25]

'We were saturated with propaganda,' wrote May Falconer. 'The worst ordeal of all was suddenly being told by Mr Dunn to collect the mothers in the Lecture Room, knowing all the time that Mr Dunn was probably listening at the door, murmuring under his breath "imbecile", his favourite expression to himself — but sometimes overheard — when he thought one could do better.'

Suddenly it was 1923 and their two years of training were over. But the future of the scheme was no more certain than when it began. With the economy in the doldrums, the government had slashed public servants' pay by 10 per cent. The new service suffered a temporary setback when the 1922 draft of trainee dental nurses was reduced by half, to 15. After all the hard work, May and her fellow graduates were dismayed that not only was there to be no graduation ceremony, but they were also not going to receive any certificate (for fear nurses might use this to as an aid to leaving the service). 'However,' wrote May, 'after standing firm and saying we did not wish to leave Wellington without some sort of reference for our two years' work . . . it was decided to issue us with a certificate.'

Though Hunter had sold the scheme to dentists by arguing that dental nurses posed no competitive threat because most would leave and get married, that was, in fact, the last thing he wanted. It was rumoured he had hand-picked the successful applicants to minimise that risk. The education department, perhaps at Hunter's instigation, sought to impose a five-year bond. Dental nurses would be required to pay £200 (over $16,000 today) if they left before the five years were up for whatever reason, including getting married. 'This put the breeze up everybody,' Meba Armstrong recalled. 'No one was keen about it. They couldn't make up their minds what to do and in the end we didn't have to sign anything.'

As pioneering dental nurses, they were despatched with trunks of equipment to the four corners of the country, often to makeshift and rudimentary premises: a room behind a shop, a cloakroom in the town hall or the classroom of a country school. Always keen to save money, Hunter had persuaded school committees or local councils to pay the transport costs of the nurse by rail or boat and to arrange board and lodging.

The storm of criticism that had accompanied the setting up of the service had not abated and some parents were openly hostile about having their children treated by 'half-trained girls', a sentiment encouraged by local dentists.

'We had been told to get in touch with our previous employers as the scheme might not be able to carry on as a depression was coming,' May wrote. In 1923 the government ordered recruitment of trainees to be put on hold and no new appointments made. To add to Hunter's worries, Richmond Dunn suddenly resigned, citing unhappiness with the workload and his own lack of temperament for the job. Hunter found himself alone, director of a training school without a tutor. But worse was to come.

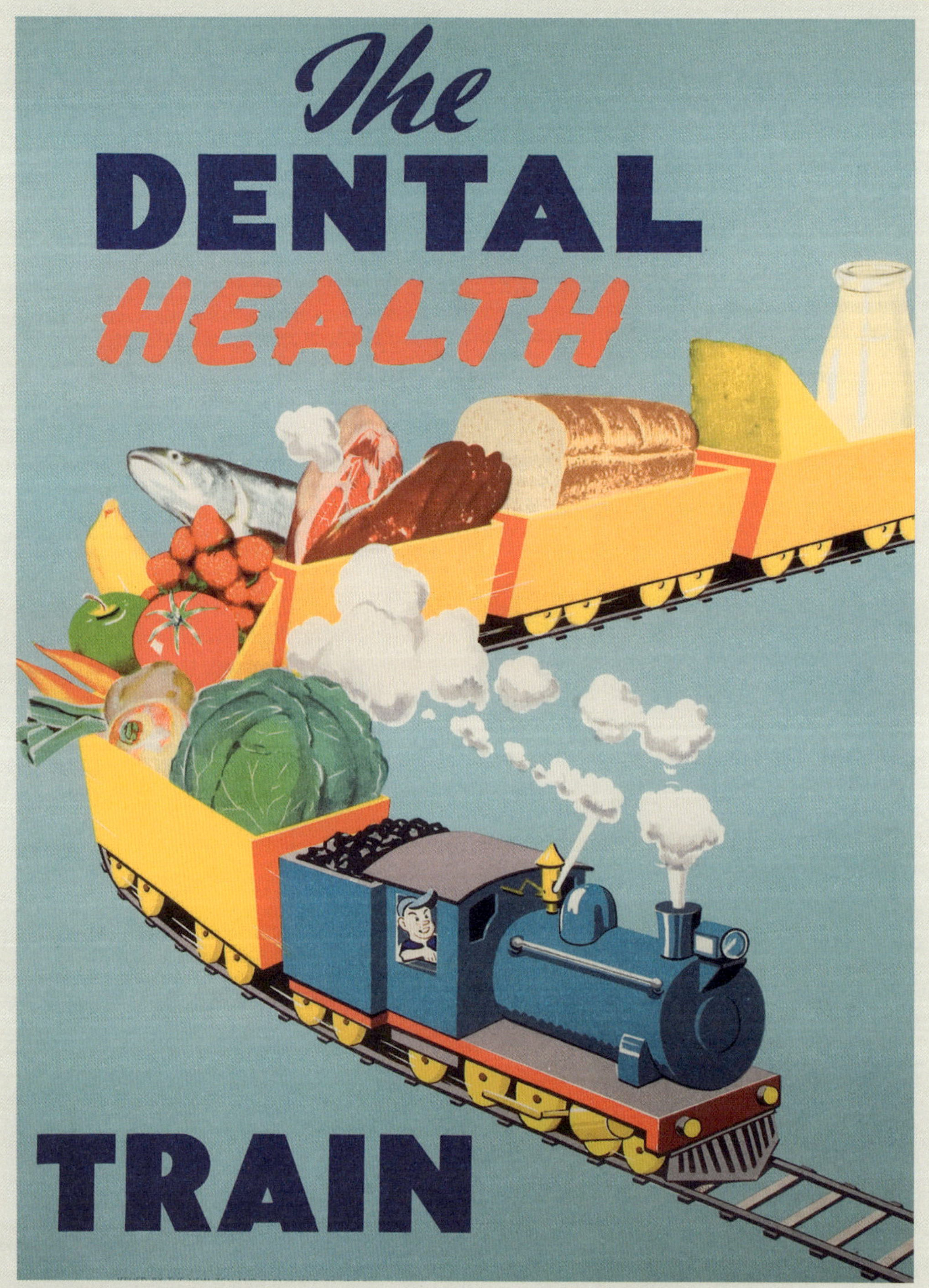
The
DENTAL
HEALTH
TRAIN

2

THE COLONELS TAKE CHARGE

The sudden departure of Richmond Dunn was more than an inconvenience: it left Colonel Hunter without supervisor or teachers. Once again he put on his Dental Corps colonel's hat, pulled rank, and diverted a young dentist, Major R. D. Elliott, from his work in an ex-servicemen's hospital to take over as acting supervisor and lecturer.

Finding a permanent replacement, he knew, would be more difficult. Most experienced dentists were either opposed to the School Dental Service or wary of taking up the post amid the controversy and uncertainty about its future. It took eight months, but he finally had his man: John Llewellyn Saunders. A Christchurch dentist who'd shared his colleagues' misgivings about the service, Saunders initially turned down Hunter's offer. But when Hunter approached him again with the offer of deputy director and the promise of a free hand, he accepted. Like Hunter, Saunders was a colonel who had served in the First World War, but as a regular soldier, not as a dentist. Perhaps the prospect of a lifetime of peering into the mouths of Christchurch burghers was losing its appeal after years of commanding men in battle, and a new challenge to lead, however risky, proved too tempting.

Whatever the motivation, Saunders quickly put his stamp on the fledgling service, creating a military culture of strict discipline and unquestioning obedience that lasted for decades, well beyond what was in tune with the times.

Tall, ramrod straight, with the *de rigueur* moustache, Colonel Saunders DSO had a lifelong love and respect for all things military. 'Quite early I developed an interest in military activities and my immediate ambition was to be in the school cadet corps and handle a rifle. This was duly achieved and my great joy and satisfaction was to take part in live ammunition practice,' he wrote later.[1] Commissioned in 1912, he was soon to get plenty of practice, serving as an infantry officer on Gallipoli and at the Somme. Twice wounded, he was one of the few who could boast that smoking had

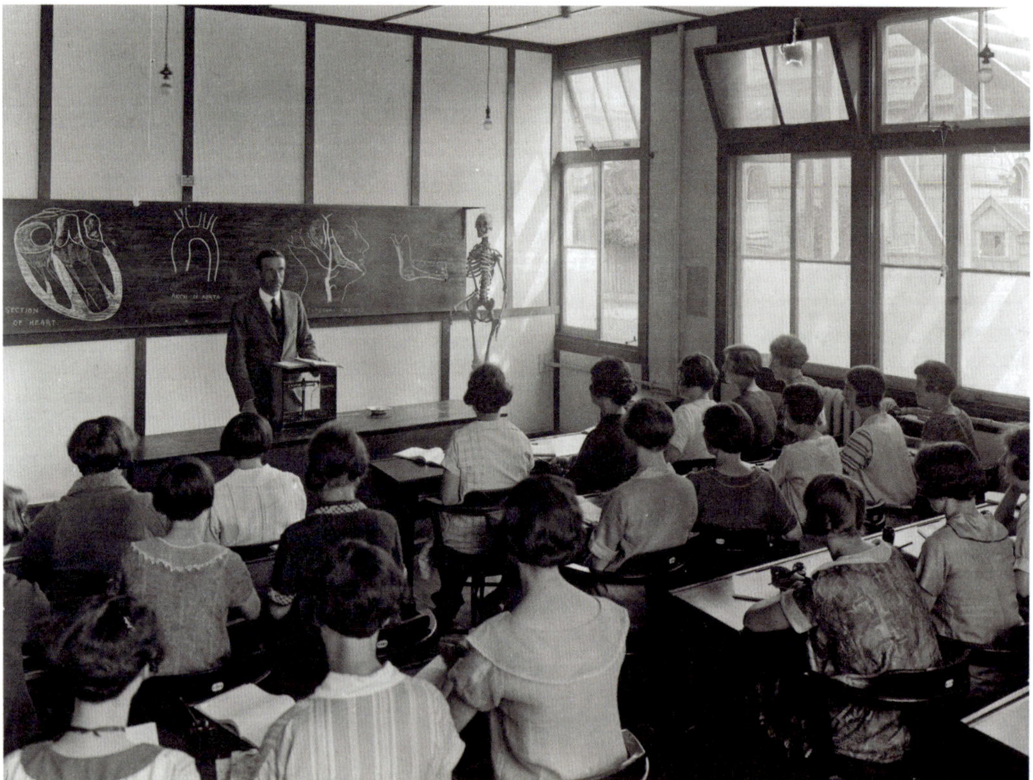

Colonel John Llewellyn Saunders lectures dental nurse students in 1925. By the window stands bony Annabelle, the skeleton without a closet.

saved their life. Wading through the mud in France, he was hit by a bullet. 'I subsided into a shell hole and looking down saw jagged strips of my cigarette case protruding from my left breast pocket.' The bullet had passed cleanly between his ribs, emerging one inch below the heart. He was soon back in action. Saunders never lost his taste for soldiering. In 1956 he reluctantly relinquished his last military appointment as honorary colonel of the Wellington Regiment 'on attaining the maximum age'.

It was inevitable that his love affair with the army, his passion for order, efficiency and discipline would shape his leadership of the School Dental Service, much to the chagrin of the nurses who were subject to the petty rules and regulations he imposed.

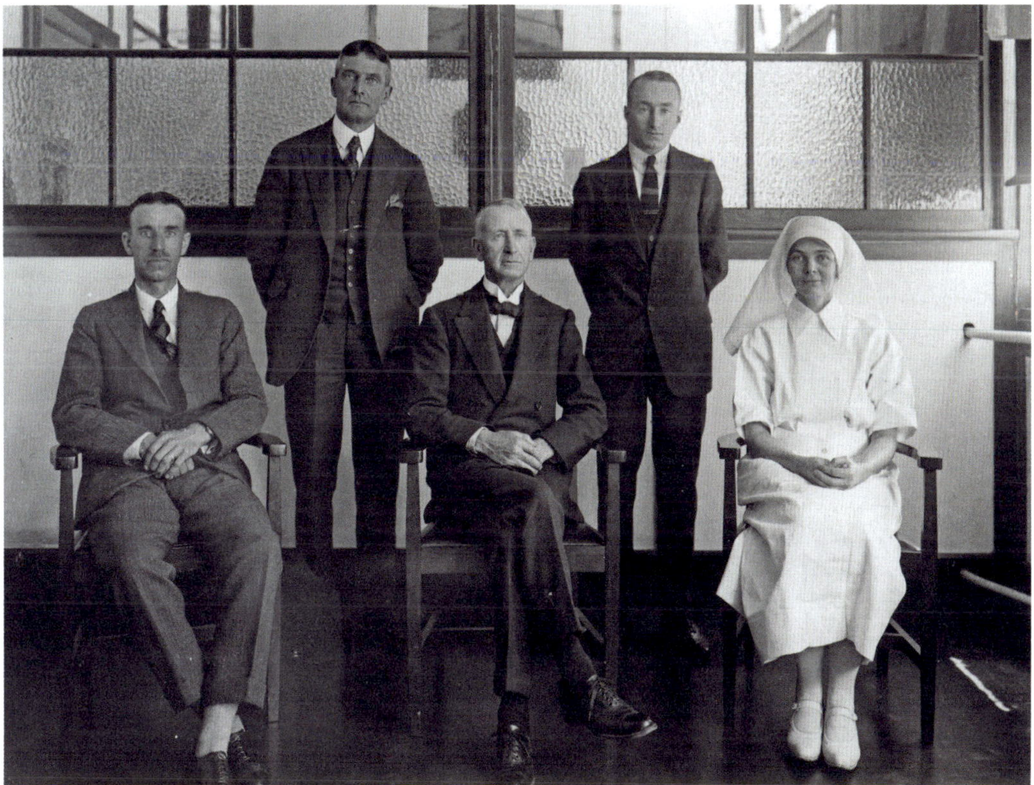

The training school's staff in 1926. From left: Colonel John Llewellyn Saunders, J. B. Bibby, Colonel Thomas Hunter, Major R. D. Elliott, Matron Elsie Haines.

Saunders was not so much a director as a commanding officer. In a 1949 *Dental Gazette* editorial about staff shortages he urged dental nurses to

> hold the line . . . until such time as we have gathered sufficient strength to renew a full-scale offensive against the enemy of child health which is our particular concern. Face to face with unprecedented difficulties, let us remember those inspiring words with which Mr. Churchill concluded one of his famous wartime speeches: 'So far we have not failed. We shall not fail now. Let us move steadfastly into the storm — and through the storm.'[2]

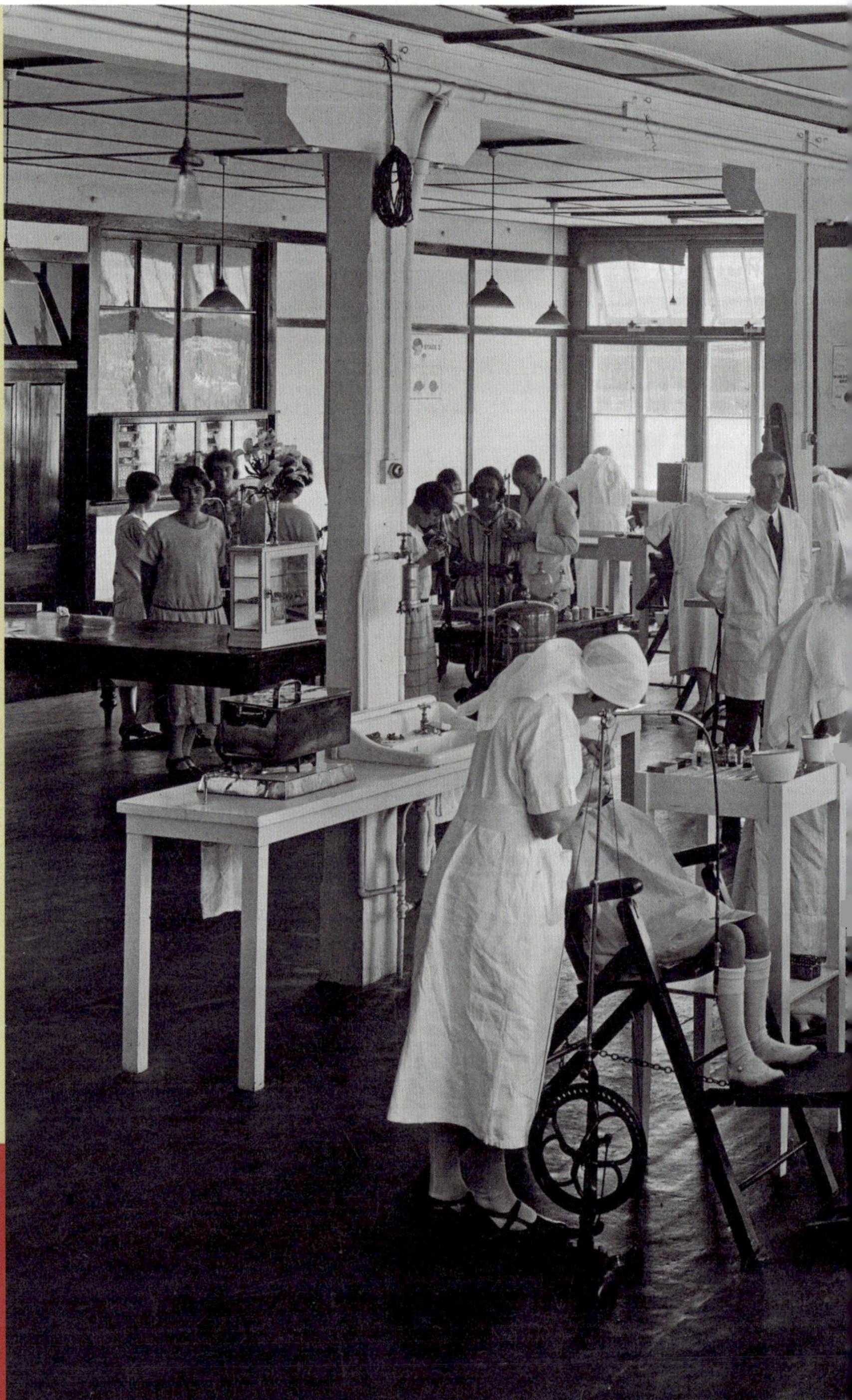

Colonel Saunders supervises a busy session in the clinic. Dental nurses had to rely on natural light when inspecting children's mouths, a problem in the shorter days of winter.

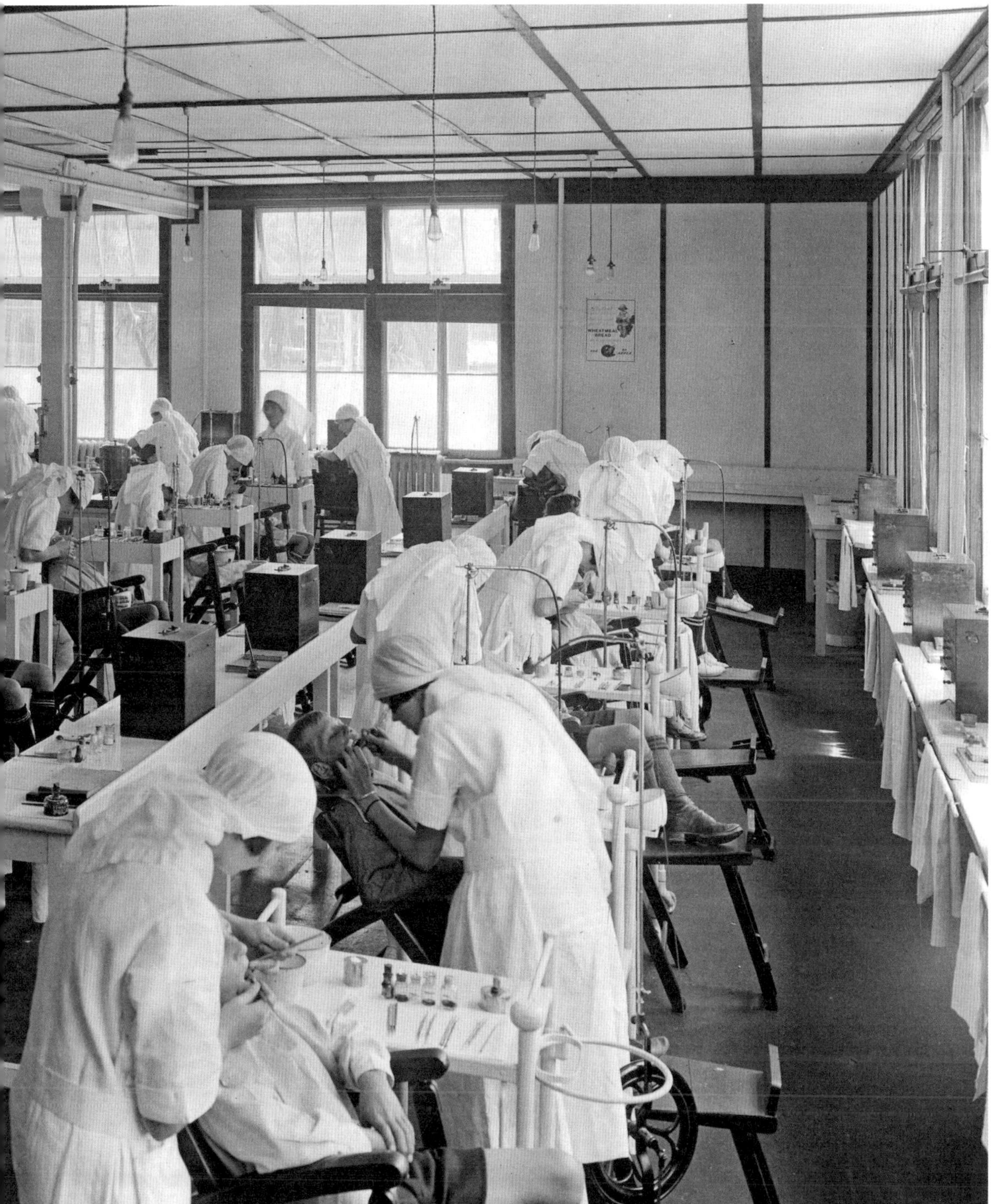
WHEATMEAL
BREAD

Commanding a school of young women nurses, however, was different from barking orders at army subordinates, and Saunders never quite got the hang of it. He fell back on a technique he'd used as a young dentist in Christchurch Hospital: 'I was soon to learn that the advent of a young dental surgeon on the staff was giving rise to much giggling and curiosity among the nurses. Being rather shy I was inclined to put up a defence by adopting an air of aloofness. At all events the nurses gave me up as a bad job.'[3]

After the patriarchal Hunter and the mild-mannered Dunn, the aloof Saunders did not go down well. Elsie Haines thought 'he was a very stingy sort of man. He walked round as if he owned the place. I think we were all a bit afraid of him.'[4] Saunders set about establishing 'a new order', introducing a new curriculum and timetable, creating, as he wrote later, 'a distinctive "dental clinic" atmosphere based broadly on hospital atmosphere and discipline'.

As the oldest and most experienced in handling patients, Elsie was appointed matron. Saunders sent her for a month to Wellington Hospital to be schooled in the dark arts of matronly control: instilling blind obedience, sniffing out and punishing insolence and ruling by fear. Though she learned to be a 'fair disciplinarian', in Saunders' words, Elsie failed to morph into the traditional battle-axe; instead, 'Hainesy' became a widely liked house mother to the trainees.

As matron, though, she was not afraid to take Saunders to task for his brusque manner. You never say anything good about the work, she once told him. Well, if you didn't do it well, he replied, I'd tell you to do it again. That's not the way Mr Hunter would have wanted us trained, Elsie replied. 'It wasn't fair,' she said later. 'Some nurses had put their heart and soul into it and he'd just pass it as if it was nothing at all.'[5]

Hunter had indeed always been effusive in his praise; so fulsome were his tributes in annual reports to Parliament that in the House dental nurses were dubbed 'Tommy Hunter's Angels'. But Hunter was now seldom around. At 64, the 'old bachelor',[6] as nurse Cecily Montefiore referred to him, married Greta Ewen, a banker's daughter 24 years his junior, and he toured the country's dental clinics introducing his new wife. Truby King, too, was gone, having returned to his old stamping ground as inspector general of mental hospitals. In that role he sat on the Committee of Inquiry into Mental Defectives and Sexual Offenders, which proposed (among other things) the compulsory segregation and sterilisation of 'incurable' mental defectives. He was knighted in 1925.

Under Saunders' reorganisation the service was flourishing. Val Clarkson arrived in 1927 and found the clinic buzzing with activity:

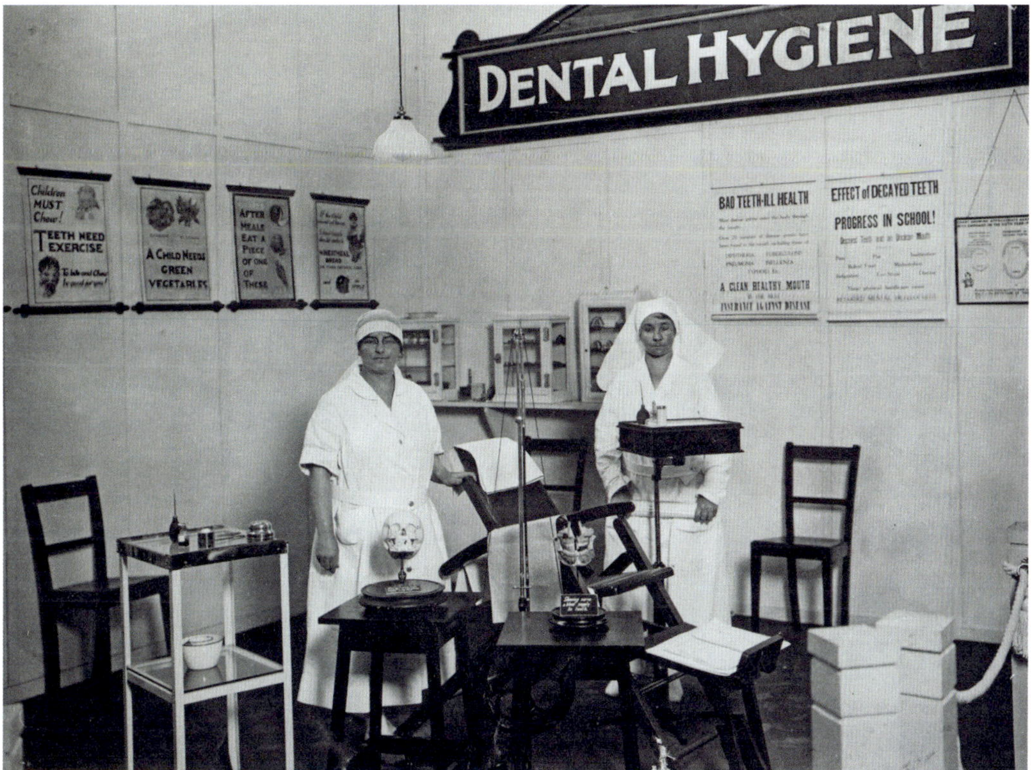

Nurses May Falconer and M. M. Anderson promoting the work of the School Dental Service at the New Zealand South Seas International Exhibition in Dunedin in 1926.

I found myself in a large L-shaped room with — to me — the rather alarming sight of 30 nurses all in white uniforms busy with their patients. I seized on the only nurse who looked different because of her floating veil, Miss Haines, the matron. She ushered me into the lecture room and introduced me to the 30 new juniors all in their blue uniforms, 'Nurses dismiss — you all know your duties!' I followed them all into the surgery where they disappeared in various directions, polishing the copper sterilisers and urns — or polishing chairs etc for the senior nurses. I stood out like a sore toe in my little home-made frock. Miss Haines was in full flight — she had 30 senior nurses who we only learned later had just started treating live patients plus the new draft

> of junior nurses to cope with. I finally caught her eye and asked 'What should I do?' And she said, 'Oh I don't know, just walk about!' So I did just that for several days until I had a uniform and merged into the general scene.[7]

Val was one of 200 who applied that year, in 'a desperate bid to escape from two soul-destroying years in a country place with a dearth of young people'. It was the days before hostels, and her parents had arranged for her to stay with two elderly spinsters, where 'a gas caliphont provided hot water over the bath, and after a few days I was told I could not have a daily bath — twice a week being considered adequate. So each morning winter and summer I filled the bath with cold water, soaped myself all over and dived in. I was paying them 35 shillings per week and . . . there was little left over for tram fares etc and none for luxuries like pure silk Corticelli stockings at 10 shillings and eleven pence a pair. I left at the end of the year for more congenial surroundings and cheaper board.'

After her year as student and skivvy, she arrived at her first 'exciting and terrifying day as a senior', gaping into a child's mouth and 'the dreaded days on extractions every three weeks, abscesses, roots at all angles, inflamed tissues, not to mention the huge cavities dealt with in the surgery. It was not unusual to find oneself extracting six-year molars [permanent teeth] in children aged eight or nine. The syringes were truly antique and were forever leaking and proving too stiff to operate. This necessitated re-packing with asbestos — a tricky job and not always successful.'

Aside from the alarming effect of injecting children with syringes big enough to tranquillise a horse, the asbestos packing seems to have raised no concerns, though its dangers had been known for decades. In his *Mechanics of Surgery*, published in 1899, instrument-maker Charles Truax had warned: 'Asbestos fibre was for a time advocated as a suitable material for hypodermic syringe packing. Extended experiments, however, revealed the fact that the friability of this substance rendered its use exceedingly dangerous, as detached fragments were continuously being loosened from the packing and either occluding the needle or being injected subcutaneously.'[8]

There were now long waiting lists for children to be treated in Wellington and elsewhere, and press coverage was becoming more positive. A visiting *Evening Post* reporter wrote a glowing report of his visit to the training school under the heading 'NO ONE CRIES':

> In connection with the treatment of the children, there is one very striking feature of the work being performed by the training school in Government Buildings.

> When a *Post* representative paid a visit to the clinic recently there were 30 children receiving attention. Not one was crying. The reassuring manner which the staff of 34 has with the small patients is very noticeable, and in most cases the youngsters respond with complete trust. It has been found that a walk round the clinic, the explanation of one or two of the instruments, and a few gentle words of encouragement will serve to quiet the most difficult of children.'[9]

Elsie Haines believed the docility of some children was due to other factors. She observed that Chinese children frequently fell asleep in the chair and concluded that they 'had been given opium by their parents'.[10] This may have reflected a common prejudice towards Chinese people at the time. Tales of Wellington opium and gambling dens, not entirely unfounded, often appeared in the press.

Dentists and government officials visited regularly. Nurse Kath Rowden recalled the time when a 'beautifully tailored and very good-looking representative from de Trey's [a Swiss dental supplier] was being escorted round the surgery by the director. At my chair, and within hearing of the nurses on either side, they reached the point in the conversation when he mentioned the great advantage of breast feeding for infants. In those days any part of the human anatomy was not mentioned in polite conversation so we three nurses found it quite impossible to hide our scarlet faces and acute embarrassment.'[11]

Meanwhile, the pioneer dental nurses posted to the far corners of New Zealand were having to cope alone with conditions very different from Saunders' efficient operation in Wellington. Local school committees or councils provided the clinics and often arranged accommodation and transport to schools in the area, but situations varied widely. Val Clarkson was posted to a clinic in Geraldine in South Canterbury, which turned out to be a big empty classroom to which alterations had yet to be made. 'A huge fire at one end — no cardigans allowed and getting into my starched uniform on frosty mornings was a nightmare.'[12] May Falconer found she had to work out of a room in Dunedin Hospital. An official, with perhaps a wry sense of humour, assigned her a room previously occupied by Dr Pickerill during the war, and with his name still on the door.

Some committees took great pride in the facilities they were providing. Nurse K. N. McCormick arrived at her clinic in Cromwell to find two men laying new

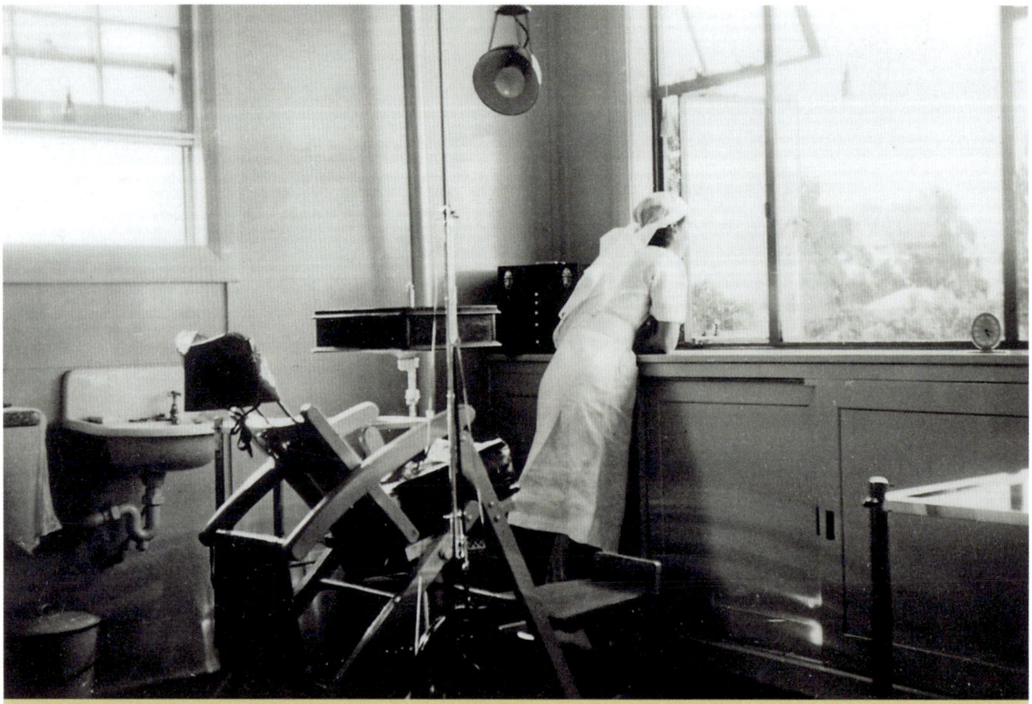

For a dental nurse posted to a rural area, it could be a lonely existence, most keenly felt when the day's work was done.

linoleum, and she never heard the end of it: 'I walked into the post office, said to the man at the counter, "Any letters for me?" "No — no letters. What do you think of the lino we put down? Quite decent, isn't it. Is it lying flat alright?" In any shop, grocer's, or draper's, someone seemed to be interested in the linoleum. I felt like asking the editor of the local paper to make an announcement to the effect that I was overjoyed with the floorcovering.'[13]

Nothing could be done until the consent forms permitting treatment were returned from parents; one simply had to wait. For one nurse, this was when the reality of life in the backblocks sank in. 'My window looks straight down a side street, which joins the main road and there I stood watching for hours the traffic. Sometimes a housewife would pass along the main road on the way to the store, sometimes a cow, sometimes a man with a wheelbarrow. Once I saw a dog come up the side street. The motor traffic is always interesting. I have seen as many as five cars pass in a week.'[14]

By 1928, the School Dental Service had set up clinics right across the country.

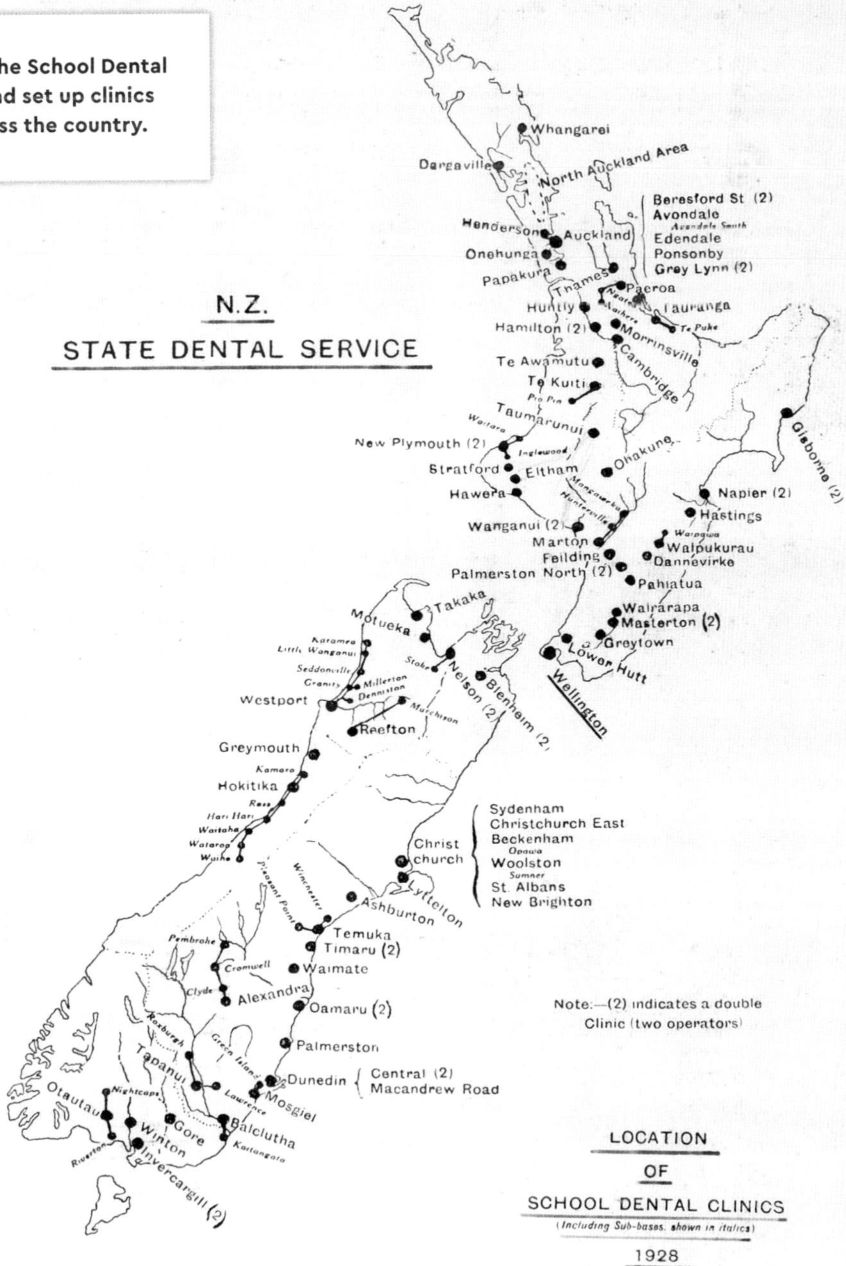

When the consent forms came back, it became clear the nurse's work would not always be appreciated. One parent wrote:

> To Dentist, — I absolutely refuse to have either of my children's teeth interfered with, if so you take the law into your own hand, as I consider interfering with children's teeth at the age of five years an unnatural act and liable to affect their interest in school work. My children detest having their mouths probed, and do not wish to attend school. It seems to me that nature is being overridden as nature provides the second teeth with the ejecting force, and it is only of late that the drawing of infants' teeth has come into force; yet in the olden days people outlived our age, though tampering with the effects of nature.[15]

Nurse Isabel Hesselyn found only confusion when she was posted to the small settlement of Ōtautau in Southland:

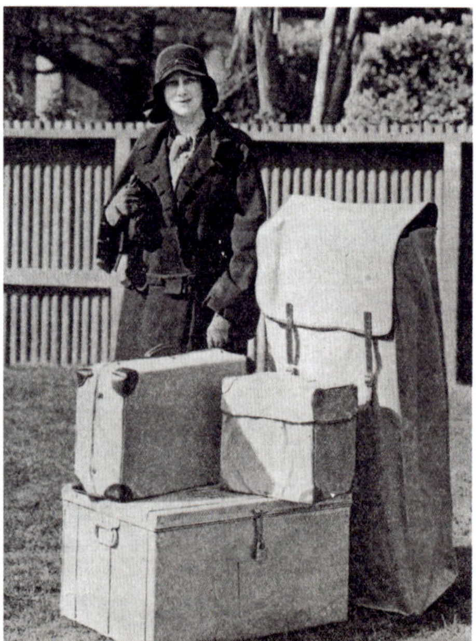

School dental nurses did not travel light; they had a lot of equipment to lug around and had to rely on local transport.

> No one in the township knew just what a dental nurse was expected to do and as there was no resident dentist I soon had people knocking on my doors with dentures to be mended, gold inlays to be replaced and many extractions needed, etc. Looking back it is amazing the amount of ignorance and opposition we had to face up to. Quite a lot was due to the dental profession who had always opposed the setting up of the School Dental Service . . . Quite a few parents were upset when they found we only worked on primers instead of treating the older ones in Form 1 and 2, who they considered were more in need of it . . . There was much argument with parents at first, some didn't want fillings or other extractions and even when we had consent and extracted teeth that hadn't ached [we] were due for a good telling off. I remember, too, rows over six-year molars,

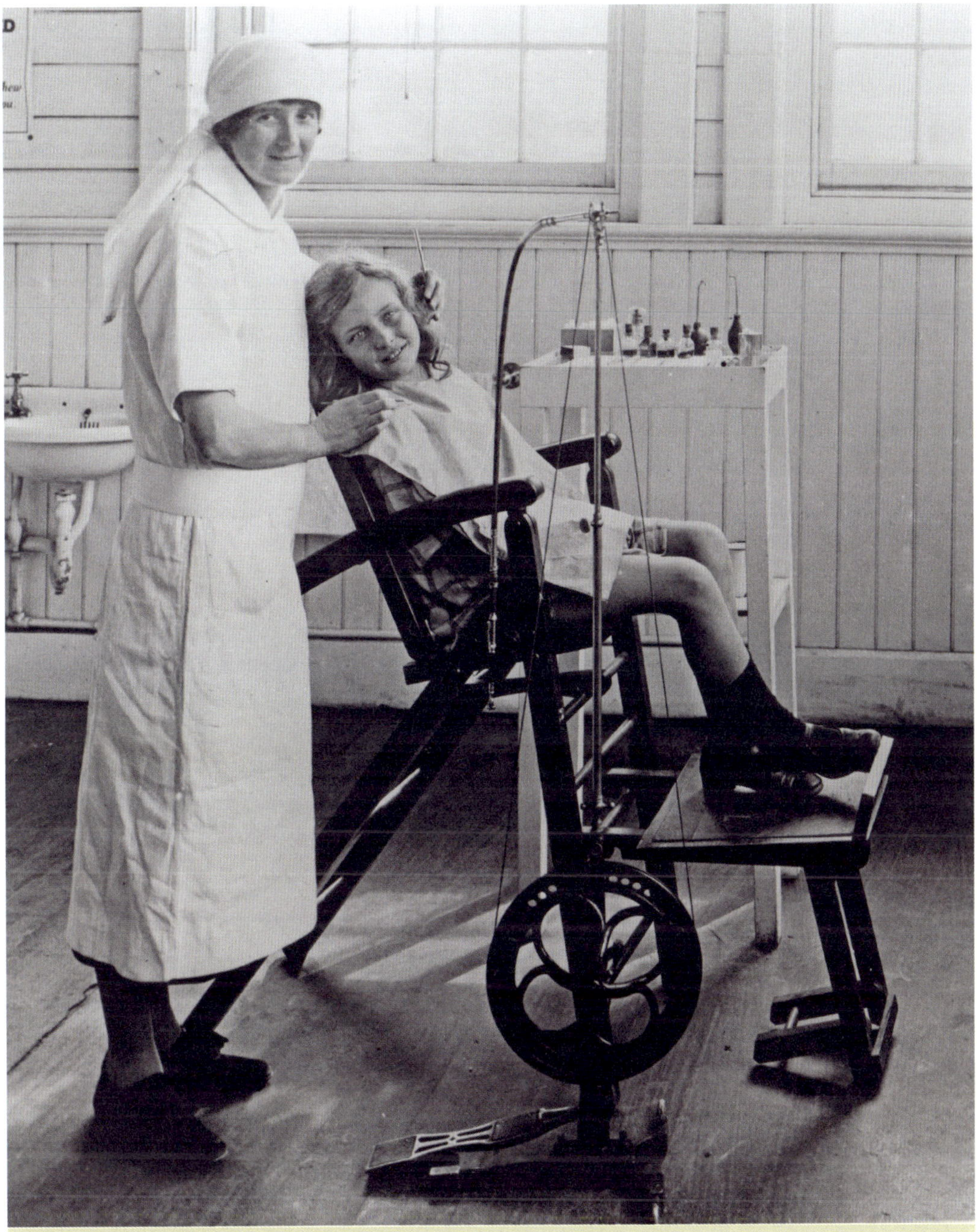

A dental nurse at work in a 1920s clinic, treadle drill at hand. It was an instrument of torture but there was no alternative.

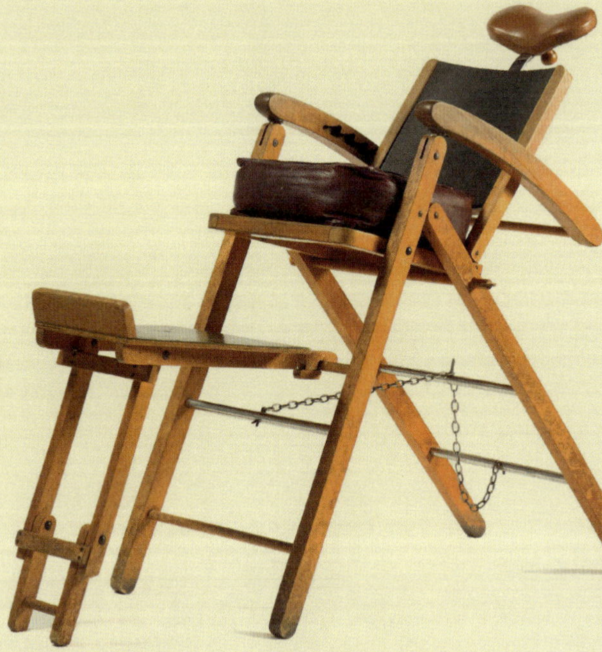

The school dental clinic chair, described as 'the best portable dental chair in the world', was designed by an anonymous public servant in Wellington.

> mothers 'knew' it wasn't a permanent tooth. After all, what would I know about it, I hadn't any children but only spent my days looking at the mouths of 750. Looking back I wonder how I had the patience and tact to deal with all that.[16]

The things they carted. Each clinic had sub-bases that the nurses had to visit several times a year. If the clinics were often make-do, the sub-bases were literally makeshift. Equipment had to be packed up for travel: chair, drill, handpiece, burs (grinding pieces), forceps, excavator, probe, pliers, bucket, spittoon, steriliser, drugs, gauze, cotton wool, disinfectant, carbolic acid, charts, etc. The infrequency of transport — a train a day, the daily milk truck or weekly boat — meant that forgetting an essential item rendered the whole trip futile. The picture on page 40 shows a dental nurse at this time setting off to visit a sub-base. By her side is a shoulder-high canvas bag, at her feet a metal trunk on which sits another canvas bag the size of a wine case, and a small suitcase. 'The galvanised iron box . . . when packed, took two strong men to shift. How the carriers groaned when they saw it!' wrote nurse Flora McDonald. 'Then when one arrived at the base quite often something had not arrived.'[17]

The treadle drill and the chair were the two biggest items in the dental nurse's armoury. The treadle drill with a cast-iron pedal base was state of the art in 1871. Capable of speeds of more than 1000 rpm, it was a huge advance on the standard hand drills, which could manage no more than 15 rpm. But it was still far from the ideal tool to cut through tooth enamel, which is as hard as steel.

Though the treadle was almost silent in operation, the patient experienced unpleasant and noisy jarring as the drilling put pressure on sensitive dentine, and as the bone around the tooth roots transmitted vibrations through the skull and to the ears. One source of pain — the heat build-up caused by cutting and grinding — could have been eliminated by handpieces delivering jets of water, but that technology only became possible with the later electric-powered drills. While the treadle got the job of removing tooth decay and relieving toothache done, it was an instrument of torture a Spanish inquisitor might have given his eye teeth for. Though electric drills came into use in the 1920s, some dental nurses were still having to use treadles until the 1950s and beyond.

The chair, at least, was comfortable. Described by Michael Smythe, author of *New Zealand By Design*, as 'the best portable dental chair in the world', it had been invented by an anonymous public servant in Wellington. 'The chair design achieves structural strength, stability, significant adjustability and collapsibility as well as being light enough for the nurse to carry in a canvas bag. Stable but light kauri was the ideal timber. The geometry of the adjustable backrest led to an elegantly curved arm rest, and the bull-nosed ends to the leg frames accommodated all angles. While the variable footrest was a little clunky in its resolution, the no-nonsense use of the chain to hold the whole structure in place was a vote of confidence in its tensile strength.'[18]

As Nurse Ngaire Mune recalled, 'The chair certainly was very comfortable. I remember after a long day on our feet, when the last patients of the day had been treated, we would sit and relax in our chairs with a very welcome cup of coffee and chat. Of course, we were not permitted to eat or drink (and definitely no smoking) anywhere in the clinic, but the school staffroom was usually across the playground, and often locked as we worked much longer hours than the teachers and most would have gone home.'[19]

Comfortable it may have been, but its childhood occupants grew up with other associations. Ngaire tells the story of a chair and its dental legacy in the 1990s:

> The organisers of a school fair decided to auction off surplus bits and pieces from around the school, including a wooden dental chair that had been in the store-cupboard for years. The school had no dental clinic, and unfortunately, unbeknown to the fair organisers who were new to the school, the chair was used by the dental nurse when she periodically visited the school to examine

> the children's teeth. The dental people were rather cross about it being sold; and asked the organisers to see if they could get if back, which they willingly agreed to do. They ultimately tracked it down to a B&D parlour, in a nefarious part of town, repossessed it, refunded the purchase cost, and triumphantly returned it to the dental nurse. Maybe the chair had not been the exotic drawcard for the business the purchasers had anticipated, and they were happy to return it anyway![20]

As the decade wound to a close, Colonel Saunders had cause to feel cheerful. The training school was now fully staffed and school dental nursing was gaining recognition as a profession, with its own institute and journal, *Niho Pai* (Māori for 'good teeth'). Despite the disapproval of trained nurses, dental nurses also had their

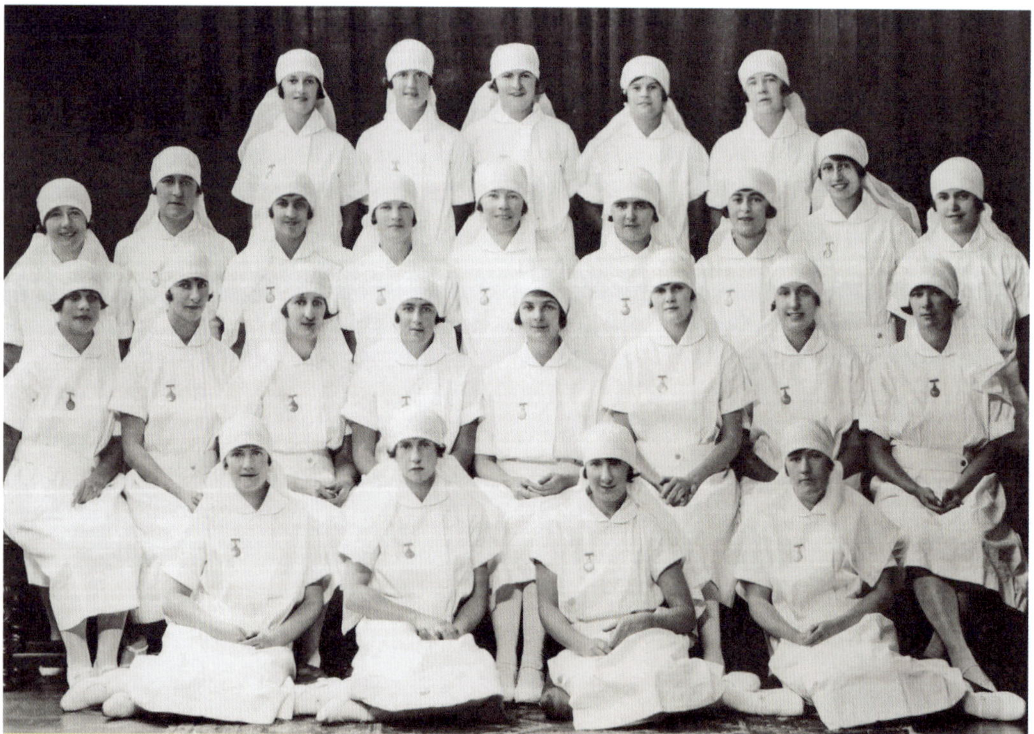

A graduation class of dental nurses in the 1920s. Their future careers were far from certain.

own medallion, with the motto *Ut Prosim* — 'that I may do good' (though they had to pay six shillings for it). The service was expanding, even extending to Rarotonga. In 1928, Minister of Health J. A. Young, himself a dentist, had announced publicly that 300 dental nurses would be needed to cope with the growing demand for the service. As well, Hunter was soon to retire, clearing the way for Saunders to take over as director.

On 30 October 1929, as he settled down after dinner to read the *Evening Post*, Saunders could have been confident that bad press was now a thing of the past. After a final blistering attack on the School Dental Service in the London *Spectator* magazine,[21] which outraged the New Zealand dental fraternity, Pickerill had given up dentistry. During the First World War he had gained an international reputation, along with New Zealanders Harold Gillies and John McIndoe, as a pioneering surgeon in facial reconstruction and plastic surgery. In 1927 he returned to that speciality and moved to Sydney to practise plastic surgery (in an ironic twist three of his granddaughters were to become school dental nurses). The *Post* that evening made no mention of the School Dental Service, though it did contain disturbing news that was to cast a cloud over the entire country for years to come. As Saunders flicked through the paper, however, it was not immediately apparent.

As usual, the front page was filled with classified ads: 'Will the sneak thief who stole a Beautiful Shrub from my garden last night return same this evening?' There was petty crime ('The trial of Norris Frank Davey, a clerk, on a charge of indecent assault on a male . . . was concluded to-day. The accused was found guilty, with a strong recommendation to mercy, and was remanded until to-morrow morning for sentence.'[22] The young clerk later changed his name to Frank Sargeson) and a picture of Lord Moynihan, 'who predicts that cancer will soon be curable'. And on page 11: 'WALL STREET PANIC — WORST APPEARS OVER — RALLY IN MARKET (Received 30th October, 1 p.m.) NEW YORK, 29th October. The worst flood of selling which has wiped out approximately twenty-five billion dollars' of "values" in the past week appeared over later in the afternoon when a brisk rally left losses on a number of market leaders ranging from two to twenty-five dollars. Sales totalled approximately sixteen million shares.'

The worst was not over. A year later New Zealand exports plummeted, tens of thousands were thrown out of work and the country joined the rest of the world in what became known as the Great Depression. Dental nurses were not immune from the shake-up — nor was it the only tremor they would have to contend with.

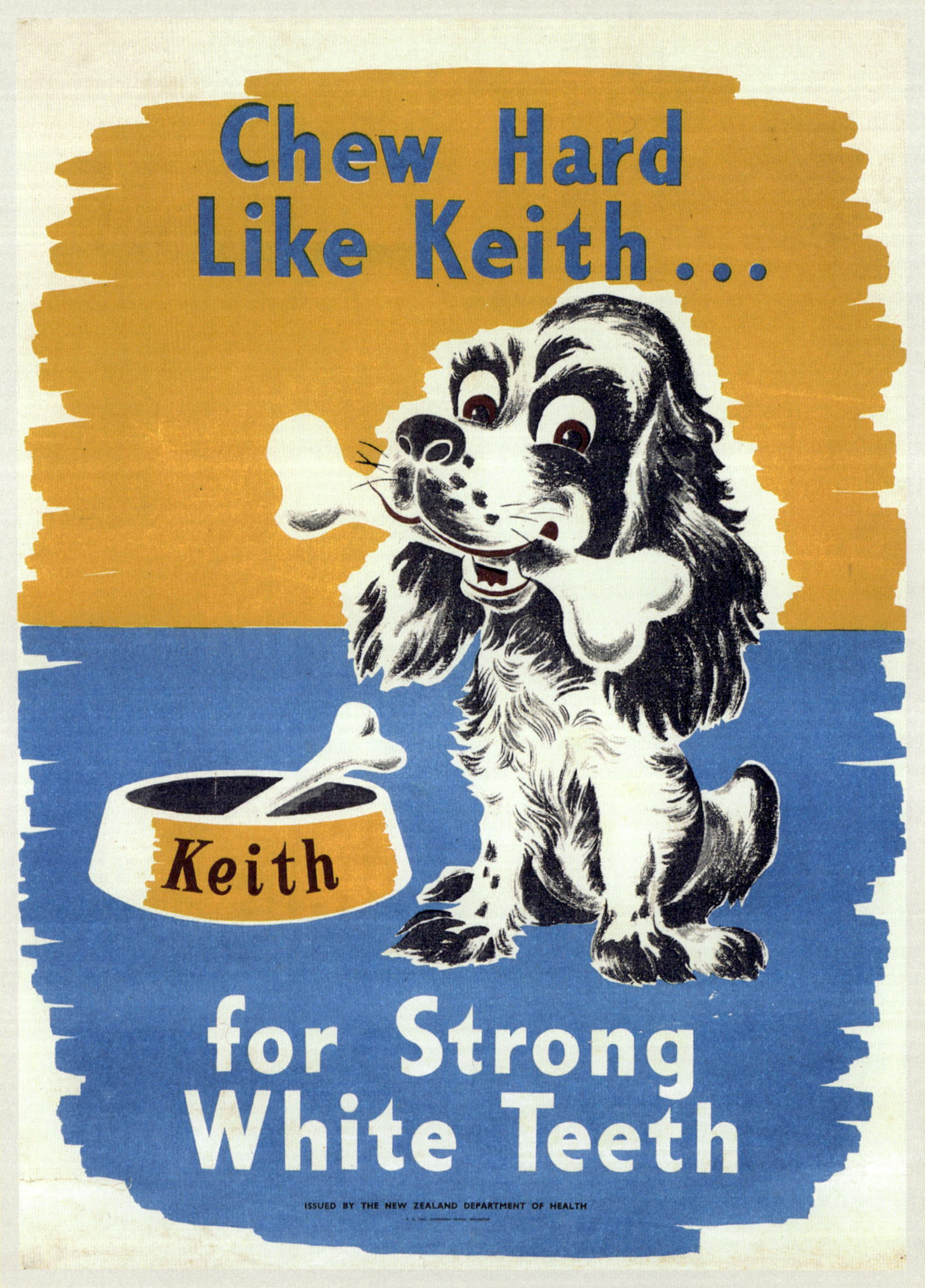
Chew Hard
Like Keith . . .
Keith
for Strong
White Teeth
ISSUED BY THE NEW ZEALAND DEPARTMENT OF HEALTH

3

SURVIVING THE DEPRESSION

It was a lovely warm day in Wellington on 3 February 1931 and Nurse Irene Taylor was looking forward to getting out in the sun at lunchtime. The junior nurse assisting her at the chair commented on the light swaying. They agreed it was probably a minor earth tremor.

Irene thought no more about it, and at lunchtime went for a swim at Thorndon Baths. 'Some girls who had been up the town came back with the horrifying news of the Napier earthquake. I truly felt my hair stand up.'[1]

Irene was worried about her family in Napier, but there was no way to contact them and no public transport to get her there. 'By the end of the next day I decided to get home somehow . . . the only hope was the A.A. whose members were offering their services.' She was told she needed to get a permit from the transport department. 'Many of the long queues came out of the office weeping and by eavesdropping I learned that only those who had received notice of a dead relative were given a permit. When I went home to my digs, the landlady had just heard that one of her boarders who had gone to Napier on business had been killed. So I told a little white lie and got the green light . . . It was 10.30 p.m. when we left Wellington in a draughty car with side curtains and the night was very cold after the hot summer day.'

When they reached Napier, the ruined city centre was ablaze. Fire had started within minutes of the earthquake in three chemists' shops with their stocks of chemicals and oils and gutted 11 blocks of the city. The water supply failed and the fires continued for 36 hours. By nightfall more than a hundred separate fires were illuminating the devastated city. Irene was relieved to find her family safe and well in their battered home. 'After some breakfast and a short sleep for the driver (my dust and horror-filled eyes wouldn't shut) we went to Nelson Park where army tents [had been erected] and queues of dusty, tired and bewildered people waited to be evacuated.' Irene and the driver were able to take a family back to Wellington.

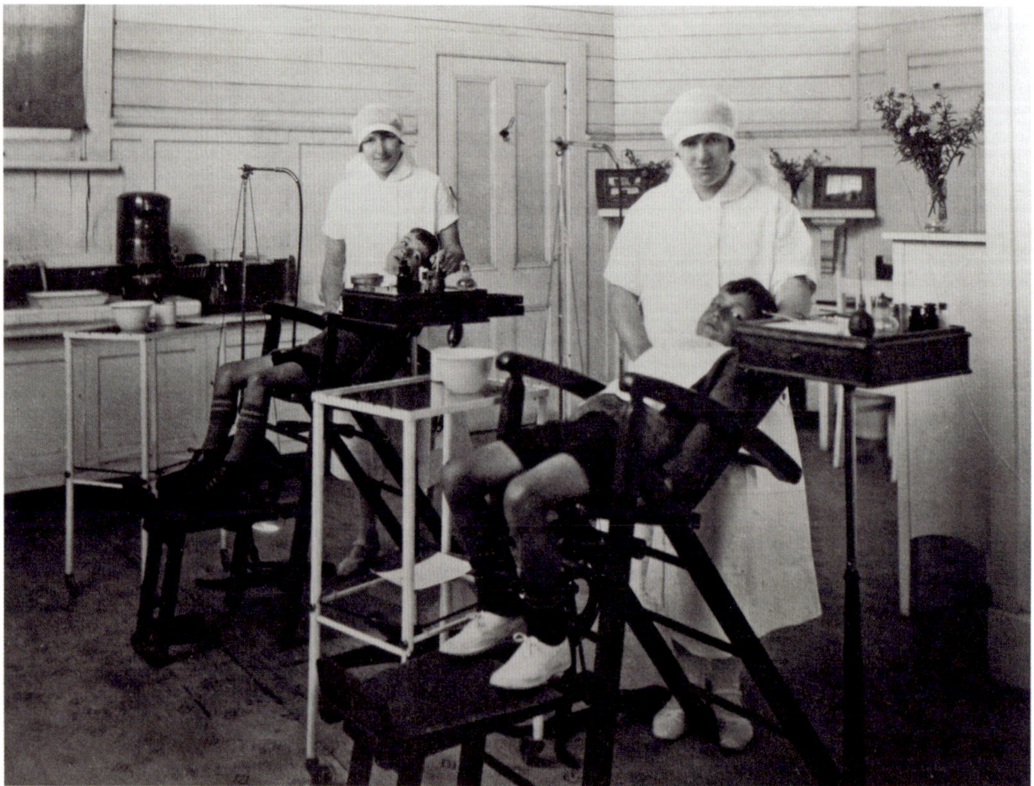

Nurses at work in the Napier dental clinic before it was destroyed in the 1931 Hawke's Bay earthquake.

In an emergency such as an earthquake a dental nurse was required to take instructions from the head teacher or other local controlling officer. If no such officer was available, she should take action to ensure her patients and her own safety. For nurses working in Hawke's Bay that day there was no time for chain of command niceties. A Nurse Whittington, who later recounted her experiences in the journal *Niho Pai*, was working in the Napier clinic with colleagues Mullan and Oliver when 'without the slightest warning we felt a terrific jerk and things began to fly in every direction. We knew in an instant that it was serious and our first thought was to get the children out safely.'[2] However, the door was jammed and it was difficult to stand as the floor heaved. 'We eventually got out to the street and were absolutely dazed at

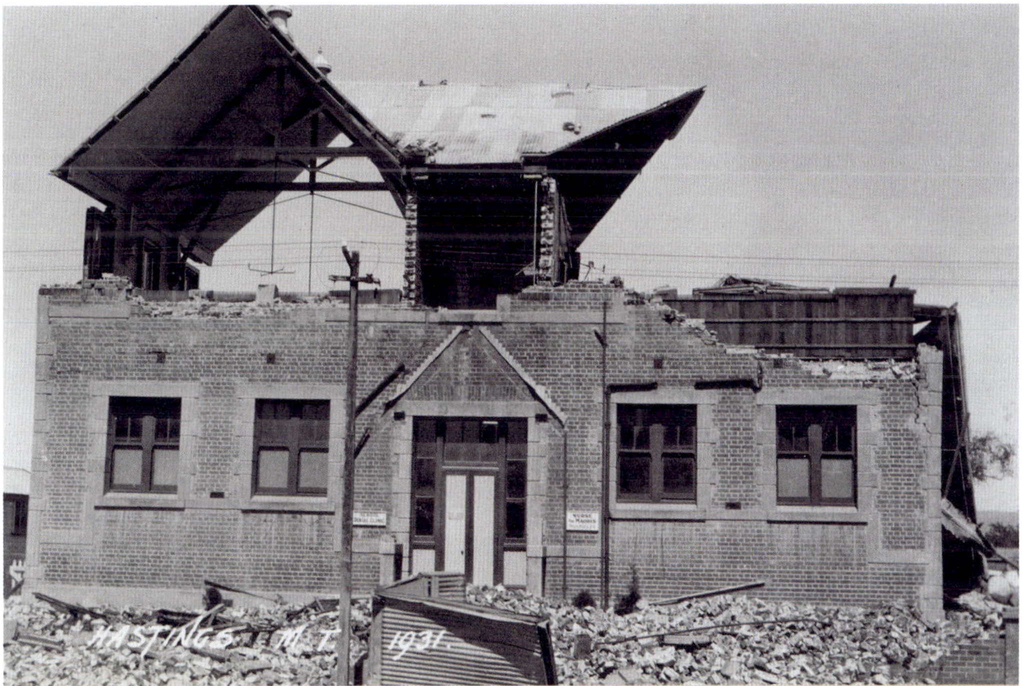

Earthquake damage to the exterior of the Hastings school dental clinic. Nurse Johnson and Nurse McPhee were working inside at the time of the quake. Despite being 'hurled from wall to wall', they got the children out safely, the group escaping with only minor injuries.

the sight of buildings down all around us. This apparently upset the children too and they began to cry piteously so we took them over to the Square, where all except three were safely delivered to their parents.'

The nurses turned their attention to injured children from the nearby technical school, which had been reduced to rubble. Returning to the clinic they retrieved gauze, cotton wool, towels and a couple of unbroken bottles of iodine and Lysol to treat the injured. 'By this time,' wrote Whittington, 'night was falling rapidly, so we went to the clinic, but found we could not shut the doors. As the building was still shaking violently, we did not consider it safe to remain there.' They slept in the open at Civic Square. 'I say slept, but very few people closed their eyes that night, as the earth shook continuously and the fires were raging fiercely, to say nothing of the poor broken-hearted men and women who were constantly enquiring for some lost relative.'

They had been trained to follow orders and so they were at a loss what to do the next day. 'We called several times at the temporary post office, as we were expecting a message from headquarters advising us what to do. In the meantime, however, Nurse Mullan happened to see the Public Service Commissioner who gave us permission to leave.'

Instead of leaving, however, they returned to the clinic. 'When an officer takes charge of a clinic she becomes responsible for all equipment, furnishings and materials therein.' The strict instruction seems to have weighed heavily on their minds, above concerns for their own safety:

> We found the instruments and equipment scattered all over the floor and charts lying in water everywhere. Things were in a terrible state, so we just gathered up the instruments etc, put them in a big tin and locked them up in a cupboard. As there was no water we were unable to clean the instruments. We managed to sweep the clinic and gather up the broken glass, and some of the men from HMS *Dunedin* closed the windows for us. The doors, however, would not shut so we had to leave them open. During these operations we had to rush outside a dozen times, as the shakes were quite violent and very frequent.

They endured another night of aftershocks outdoors in the rain. 'Next morning I decided to leave for Wellington, to report and receive instructions,' recounted Whittington. 'Nurse Mullan left the same afternoon for Pahiatua, and Nurse Oliver on Saturday for Otane. After leaving Napier we experienced the same sensation as coming off a boat — everything seemed to come up to meet us!'

Nurse Johnson, along with her colleague Nurse McPhee, was busy in the Hastings clinic when the earthquake struck.

> Nurse McPhee was the first to realise that this was no ordinary earthquake, and made a hasty exit with her patient. Things began to fall and I decided to follow, but custom was strong and I stopped to take off my patient's bib. Progress to the front door was very slow: we were hurled from wall to wall. In the passage I found a little girl in the waiting room so I collected her and tried to get the children through the door.
>
> Bricks were falling around us thick and fast. I pushed the children through the half closed gate but there was no time to follow them so I decided to climb

> over the brick fence. Just as I was on the top, a mighty shake brought down the top storey, which crashed on the fence and flung me into the street. It was impossible to stand but I eventually gained my feet. Bricks were still being hurled right across the street, so I got the children away from the falling debris. One little girl had received a nasty gash on the base of her skull and her arms and legs were scratched and bruised.[3]

Nurse Johnson calmed the panic-stricken children until their parents arrived, then found Nurse McPhee, who was having her arm dressed. 'In escaping from the clinic she had received a nasty wound on her left forearm from a broken window.'

They wandered aimlessly along the rubble-strewn main street. The entire front of the five-storey Grand Hotel where they lived had fallen into the street, killing eight people. 'Then I realised my left elbow was getting more painful as time went on. Soon I was obliged to see a doctor who was treating casualties on his front lawn. Somewhat puzzled, he asked me what I had in my hand. Why, of course, the mirror and explorer [dental instruments] I was using when the shake came.'

After getting her arm in a splint, they decided to make for Havelock North where Nurse McPhee lived:

> First we went to have a look at the clinic. I made up my mind to go in and secure my purse and my frock, now my only worldly possessions. While I hesitated another shake came, bringing down more debris. There was now a chance of getting in before the next one, so I climbed over bricks and through the back door, and tiptoed along the passage, terrified that at any minute the wall would come tumbling down. The clinic was in a state of chaos. I collected my personal effects and crept out again. We then proceeded to Havelock. The bridge was down, but we were able to scramble across. We surely looked like refugees — still in uniform, caps gone, shoe straps broken, and each with an arm in a sling.
>
> That night we spent under the stars with a rug. At nine o'clock there was another terrific shake. We could hear the rest of Hastings falling, and soon the sky was lighted up with the fires that followed.

Like their counterparts in Napier, the clinic was never far from their thoughts. 'On Thursday I made up my mind to leave,' recalled Nurse Johnson, 'but had to see the clinic again and try to leave things secure. This I found impossible as the doors were jammed and would not shut. I felt I must save something from the wreck, so collected the official stamps and a once-discarded coat. Nurse McPhee and her family were leaving for Masterton. So at 4pm we stole away, leaving a very sad and desolate Hastings.'

The Hawke's Bay earthquake, with the loss of 251 lives, was another blow to morale in a country already struggling through the Great Depression. But life carried on. At 5 p.m. on 6 April 1931 Elsie Hitchcock boarded the train at Matamata for Frankton Junction, outside Hamilton. She was setting off for Wellington to train as a dental nurse. 'It was Easter Monday and the booking I got was "fourth relief — leaving 11pm". I sat on that station surrounded by the alien crowds and wanted to go back home. Our train had antiquated carriages and I got a seat third behind the engine and the soot came in. We made Wellington at 2pm the next day. No more forlorn material ever arrived to be moulded. I was a cross between a zombie and a chimney sweep.'[4]

Elsie and her fellow trainees could not have picked a worse time to enrol. The country was in the throes of the slump: wool and dairy exports were plummeting and unemployment was surging like a Rotorua geyser. The staggering economy had been held down and sedated by a government intent on slashing public spending. It set up a razor gang, the National Expenditure Commission, to expend as little as possible. Nothing escaped the commission's attention. Cats officially employed by government departments to keep mice at bay had their milk allowance cut by half.[5] It was no surprise, then, that dental nurses had money extracted from their pay packets. Their meagre pay was cut by 10 per cent in 1931 and a further 10 per cent in 1932.

Many dental nurses feared for their jobs because women, like Asians, were not entitled to state help, or 'sustenance', as it was quaintly termed. The chances of landing another job were slim: the few jobs on offer went to men supporting a family. Unemployed women were told to seek work in domestic service. But as journalist Robin Hyde wrote at the time: 'A country with a population of less than one and a half million would make itself look both snobbish and silly by the creation of a large servant class. It is idiotic to think that our womenfolk can live by taking in another's washing.'[6]

The commission decided that children's teeth were not a priority: 'We are definitely of the opinion that this Service should not be allowed to expand . . . we recommend that no new trainees be enrolled and that every effort be made to reduce the cost of the Service.'[7]

The streets were filled with unemployed men in shabby suits, heads bowed with shame and humiliation. The government introduced relief schemes in which men worked, often doing pointless tasks, but the intolerable conditions and poor pay fuelled resentment, and on 16 April 1932 their frustration and anger boiled over. 'Riots in Auckland' read the newspaper billboard as Elsie made her way back to the YWCA after Saturday morning duties at the clinic. Describing the riots as unforeseen as the Hawke's Bay earthquake, the *Evening Post* opined that 'the human earthquake that shook the city of Auckland' had 'stained the honour of the Dominion'.[8]

The Auckland riot erupted after police barred a crowd of unemployed relief workers from attending an already jam-packed town hall protest meeting. Anger turned to violence when a march leader, Jim Edwards, rose to appeal for calm and was batoned by a police sergeant. Hundreds of people were injured and over 40 arrested. Some rioters smashed shop windows and looted. The New Zealand History website notes: 'One chemist shop was cleaned out of contraceptives; a man was seen staggering off with a grandfather clock on his back, and the department store Milne & Choyce "grieved over the spoliation of their very costly wax dummies".'[9]

A month later Wellington's unemployed added a fresh stain. Working in the Tomato House, Elsie and her colleagues heard the commotion as thousands of the unemployed gathered at the Cenotaph. The protestors waited for hours as a deputation went up the hill to Parliament to meet with Gordon Coates, the minister responsible for employment. A false rumour circulated that a drunken Coates had dismissed their protest with the remark, 'Let them eat grass!' The marchers became incensed. Someone shouted, 'Let's smash the bloody town up!' The angry crowd charged up Lambton Quay and Willis and Manners streets, and the sound of crashing glass filled the air. There was some looting. Elsie remembered walking down Cuba Street 'after the big riot — the broken and boarded shop windows and the quietness of shock and fury spent'.[10] The department store Kirkcaldie & Stains, on Lambton Quay, a favourite haunt of dental nurses, had 11 plate-glass windows smashed. In all 193 windows had been broken between Bowen and Cuba streets.

The government responded by granting police draconian powers to detain people, and violence around the country ceased. Anger gave way to quiet desperation. It was a grey make-do-and-mend era that historian Tony Simpson called 'the sugarbag years': families bought sugar in bulk in jute bags, which were then made into aprons, oven cloths and embroidered cushions; the Women's Division of Federated Farmers ran a competition for the most attractive article made from a sugarbag. In 1934 a young Englishwoman, Margaret Jepson, who had arrived in New Zealand in 1930 (the mother of novelist Fay Weldon, she was pregnant with Fay in Napier when the earthquake struck), caused a storm with her novel *Via Panama* by portraying New Zealand as a dull-witted country where industrious housewives 'embroidered the curtains, the cushions, the napkins, the duchess sets, the tablecloths, and even the oven cloths; but they seldom embroidered their underwear. Every house had its tea trolley. Two perambulating shelves on which the housewife loaded the six or more varieties of cakes of her own baking, which convention compelled her to offer her guests at supper, afternoon tea or morning tea — a species of tea party at which these incredible women found time to congregate at 11 o'clock in the morning.'[11]

They were also serving up tooth decay. One character in Jepson's novel was 'fair and slight, with blue eyes, and she had the false teeth of a New Zealander'. Dental nurses were fighting a losing battle. At the same time, the government introduced a fee of two shillings and sixpence for dental treatment per child per year. (Up to that point, there had been no charge.) 'So many, many people could not afford that amount and filled out exemption forms and the facts in those forms [were] truly pitiful,' remembered Elsie.

Some nurses — most of whom came from middle-class backgrounds — may not have appreciated how far some families had slipped into poverty. Journalist Ted Reynolds recalled one nurse 'publicly berating a boy who had grown a line of bright viridian-green scum along his upper gumline. We seven-year-olds knew how close to destitute was the boy's family. So we understood when he told the nurse his mother said toothbrushes wore away teeth that the real message was: "We can't afford toothbrushes." The nurse, though, raged. In front of the class, she instructed the boy to make his mother buy a brush.'[12]

Dental nurses themselves were not far off the breadline. After paying board, there was little left to live on, and the public service practice of paying salaries by the calendar month meant that every so often five weeks' board came out of the 'fragile pay packet'.[13] With little money for trams, they did a lot of walking. To make her shoes last until she could afford new ones, Elsie made cardboard inners to cover the holes in the soles.

Singalongs helped keep the grimness at bay. 'There was free community singing twice weekly in the Town Hall from 12 to 2pm. The Town Hall would be packed and these gatherings helped so much to keep up people's spirits and for a short time to leave cares behind. It was not far from the clinic and we often went along an hour.'[14] One day, however, the organiser happened to bump into Saunders and remarked how nice it was to see them there with their blue uniforms under their coats. Dental nurses were immediately banned from taking part in any more community singing; the wearing of uniforms outside the building was strictly forbidden.

Elsie remained in Wellington for a year after graduation.

> We had all grown up a lot and acquired a tissue of pseudo-sophistication — or liked to think so. I had moved a little away from the sooty girl on the station platform. That year George Bernard Shaw visited Wellington. I heard Peter Dawson [the renowned bass baritone] sing, and Rear-Admiral Byrd took a second expedition to Antarctica. On his return, I was taken to a reception given him — the Mayor had a slip of the tongue and called him Admirable Bird.
>
> A long way away Hitler became Chancellor of Germany and the next year Fuhrer. On looking back it amazes me how little we thought of or discussed any world event. It must have been because there were no transistors, TV or much radio to bring it home . . . our horizon was no further than where we were going to be sent.

Belle Lindsay was one of those with eyes set on that horizon. As she stood on the platform at Wellington railway station, one evening in 1933, 'ready to catch the express to my first clinic, I felt excited, healthy and exhilarated. On my head was my beret, as fashion dictated, on my feet my new snakeskin shoes (35/- per pair!) and in my purse my beautiful new medallion, with the cut-out crown, and my name on the reverse side. All night, to the hiss of steam and the smell of smoke and the clank of rails, I thought about it, and early next morning there it was. My new world, hills looming out of the fog, roosters crowing, and fresh inland air in my lungs.'[15]

The enormity of the task ahead of her soon became clear. 'In the early 30s, caries [dental decay] were rampant. In shops, banks, post offices, on the streets, in schools, one saw them. Caries obvious in anteriors [front teeth], ruining smiles, tainting breaths, making nights and days a misery of pain. And so many were poor, and so many knew so little, and in the end forceps were victorious and dentures were the order of the day. School dental nurses did not treat anteriors, these were the patients' responsibility, and we battled with posterior teeth, saddened by the futility of it all, knowing few could afford to have anteriors treated.'

She visited the smaller outlying schools by train.

> At 6am, it would hoot and puff into the station, with its one or two wooden-seated carriages. The bread and other goods would be unloaded and we would hop on board. I shall never forget the smell of that wonderful bread on the morning air. After a series of stops and jerks and grinds we would arrive at our little station.

> There a committee member affluent enough to own a car would be waiting. After a magnificent morning tea at his home, it would be around three or four tiny schools, usually a solo teacher establishment. A chair would be produced and placed in the porch among the school bags, gumboots and raincoats, the mugs would be filled with water and lysol, the mirrors and probes dunked therein, the charts produced, and everyone checked out, later to come to the big clinic in carloads by appointment for treatment, and big days they would be, as nobody could leave the hay or the shearing or the docking or whatever for long.[16]

In Feilding in 1929 schoolgirl Kath Salter was dreaming of becoming a dental nurse. At choir practice she'd met a dental nurse named Madge Grocott, who was 'one of the second draft to graduate. Madge said, "You'd make a wonderful dental nurse" and that was it. From the age of 14 I wanted to be a dental nurse.'[17] But the goal nearly proved elusive. The Salters had emigrated to Feilding from England, where Kath's father, Hubert, had been a gentleman's tailor who had employed journeymen and apprentices. But there was little demand for tailored clothes in Feilding, and even less as the Great Depression deepened. The tailoring business died 'a sudden death . . . we were harder up than people on relief but too proud to admit it', recalled Kath.

In small-town Feilding, the Salters' English accents set them apart. 'I was chased all around the playground at school because I had a bit of an accent. This was a spur to me,' Kath remembered. She excelled at sports and became dux at primary school. Her mother Edith found it less easy to adapt. 'She had abandoned all her friends and heritage and came out to make a better life for her children. She thought she was coming to another part of Britain.' To add to the alienation, the Salters found themselves scapegoats for the growing unemployment. 'As soon as the depression came we struck all this terrible senseless ignorant attitude to pommies. One afternoon, we went to afternoon tea and a woman picked up the paper and said 'No pommies need apply — that's what I like to see.' I can still see the tears streaming down mother's face to this day.'

There weren't many afternoon teas. Edith Salter was busy trying to keep the family afloat on what little money they could scrape together. She encouraged Kath to stay on at school, even though friends had left and were earning 7/6 doing housework. One day she found her mother preparing sanitary towels for her first periods: '"You'll need these now you're growing into a woman," she said, and sat on the bed and got the Bible out and we talked about the women with issue, meaning she was bleeding.'

Then Edith became ill and Kath had to drop out of school to nurse her. 'I felt very bitter about it at the time. I was just about to sit UE.' Her mother had Bright's disease, a chronic inflammation of the kidneys. 'When mother died it was a relief, she was slowly poisoning to death. After she died I went back to school. We had no money and lived pretty rough. Father liked a drink and standing drinks for his mates, playing the big man. We lived on the shelves of gooseberry jam mother had made before she died.'

Kath counted herself lucky at first to land a job as an assistant to a local dentist. But it turned out to be a misery. 'I went home in tears and humiliation for two and a half years.' Though it was to prove useful experience for her later career as a dental nurse, she had to endure the petty tyranny of her employer. 'His daughter and two other women had walked out enraged. He was a very clever man but he had a terrible temper. His wife would sit in the surgery for two hours, eyes downcast before he'd fling the housekeeping cheque which was very small at her feet.'

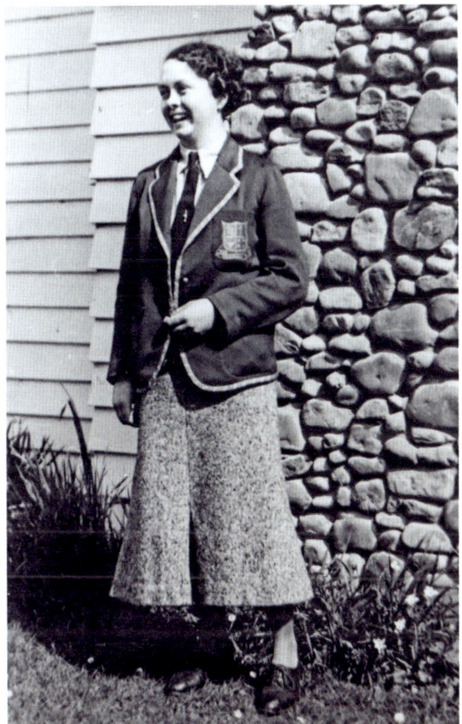

Kath Salter had dreamed of becoming a dental nurse since she was 14 years old. When the interviewer questioned Kath's height, 'I stood up very straight and said I was a good athlete, a muscular little girl and very fit.'

On frosty mornings Kath had to arrive early 'and build a great coke fire for him to sit at because often he had no work until market day on Friday. Occasionally one of the well-to-do farmer, polo-playing clientele who'd hung on to their land by living on credit at the town people's expense for years would turn up. He'd make me go out and chat to the elderly lady and he'd rush out, have a shave, hold his feet up and make me polish his shoes and get into a clean jacket and then it was "Oh Mrs so and so, how are you" and he'd hover over her. He was a terrible snob. And yet I'd seen him when a boy came in and only had a shilling, he would have to have a six-year-old molar out without anaesthetic. It was a shilling without anaesthetic.'

When she asked him for a reference for her dental nurse training application, he refused. 'Just tell them you don't drink or smoke and they'll have to take you, he said.' Nonetheless, she was confident her dental experience would get her in. 'At the interview I was so cocky but they said, "You're only five foot two". I stood up very straight and said I was a good athlete, a muscular little girl and very fit.'

While she did her training Kath lived in a student teachers' hostel (Wellington Teachers' College closed for several years during the depression). 'At the hostel we had huge breakfasts and dinners which some of the girls sneered at and moved around their plate because they'd been spoilt. But to me it was great to have two solid meals.' It was hard to survive, though, for those like her who did not receive cheques from home. The grimness of those years stayed with her. 'Dreadful lighting, dirty little cloakroom with 30 people on a wet day crowded round a small table with wet coats, trying to eat Weet-Bix and jam which was all we could afford. We used to steal sugar from the hostel and make our own jam.'

There was no money or time for drinking or other social activities. 'If we could have a nine penny double header ice cream on pay day we looked at each other with smug satisfaction.' Many girls had led sheltered lives and were dangerously naive about sex. 'There was one girl who got very ratty with me and swore that babies came out of the belly button. She was 22.' Kath had been told by her brothers that if a boy tried anything, she was to slap his face. 'We didn't know anything about birth control so if the temptation was there I just kept my legs crossed. I thought about my job, my career and my pension and I wasn't going to jeopardise that.'

Like many trainees, Kath took up smoking. 'It was the thing to do, you were sophisticated if you smoked cigarettes.' She was earning 10 shillings a week — 'we had to buy lunch, clothes and fares out of that but it was security'. And more security was on the way. Previous drafts of nurses had feared for their jobs because of the constant criticism, opposition from dentists and government cutbacks, but the election of the Labour government in 1935 would put an end to that worry.

The new government promised social security from cradle to grave, and within two weeks of being elected it was making plans to expand the School Dental Service. It wanted dental services available to all primary school children within five years. In a 1938 Labour Party film replete with old-fashioned boosterism, the narrator enthused: 'Care of the teeth is the first thing in health! The Labour government has extended

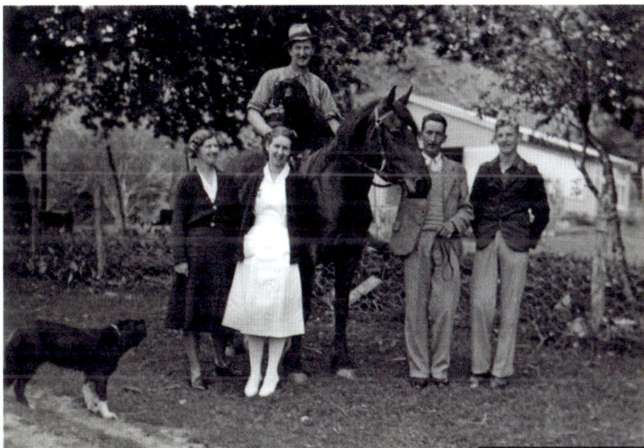

Beryl Dickson graduated as a dental nurse in 1938 and was a real pioneer. She was the first dental nurse to be sent to Pelorus Sound.

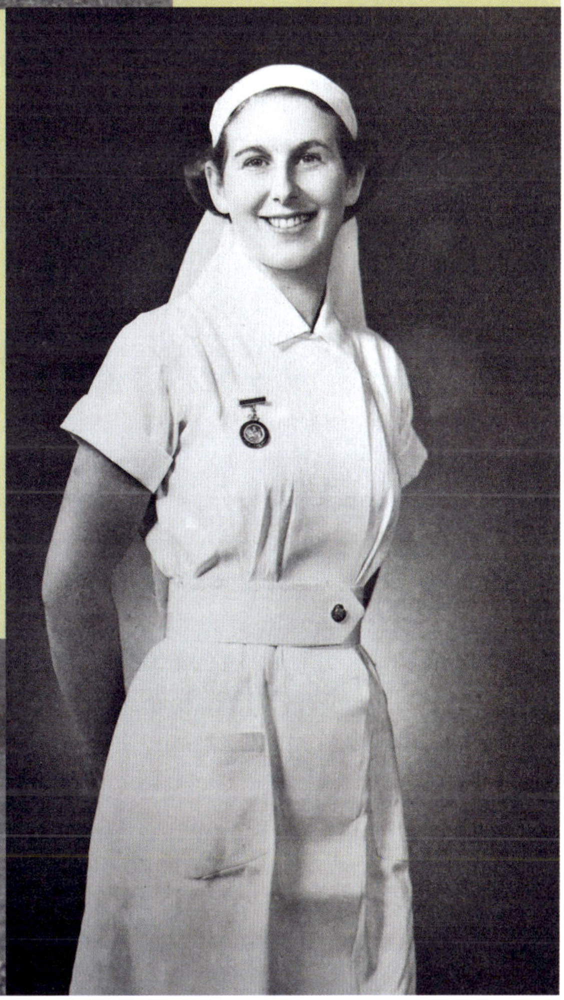

Taking the Wellington-Nelson ferry, she disembarked at French Pass, climbing down a rope ladder on the side of the ship at midnight to board a rocking and pitching launch, along with her equipment. The next day her equipment was dragged along the beach on a sledge by a horse. There were no roads, so she followed the walking tracks, setting up clinics in people's kitchens and boiling her instruments on a wood stove.

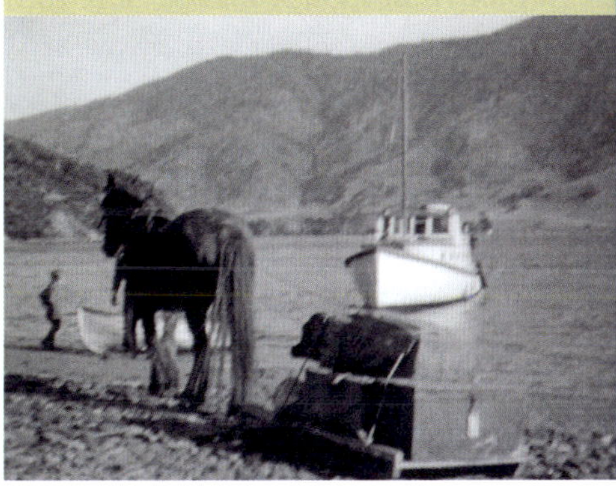

useful and valuable dental clinics. Good teeth mean good citizens! Watch how the youngsters almost enjoy it. Can they take it? I'll say!'[18]

In 1939 the number of trainee dental nurses had increased to 156, forcing the service to find additional space. The minister of health, Peter Fraser, generously offered Premier House at 260 Tinakori Road, which had been the prime minister's official residence since 1864. (The 'temporary' arrangement would continue until 1976.) Saunders took the opportunity to shunt Matron Elsie Haines sideways to supervise the Tinakori Road annexe and appointed Challis Hooper, a former Karitane nurse, midwife and general nurse, as matron.[19] The change did not sit well with Elsie, according to whom Challis Hooper was stuck up and widely disliked. 'Matron Hooper couldn't trust people. Someone opened the door rather quickly and she was listening at the keyhole.'[20]

Saunders, however, wanted someone with experience in 'institutional management and experience' and, no doubt, a matron who, unlike 'Hainesy', would keep a proper distance from the recruits.[21] The matron would be in charge of a new, ultra-modern training school and clinic to be built in Willis Street. Dr Bruce Bibby, the superintendent of the training school, was to oversee the project, a task he was well suited to. He had joined the service as a shy young dental instructor and earned a reputation as a 'supreme perfectionist' who drove the trainees crazy with his persnicketiness.

In the meantime, Saunders sought to modernise equipment by adding a foot-controlled electric motor to the treadle drills. It was a Heath Robinson solution that spat sparks and elicited curses as it kept breaking down; Cecily Montefiore 'felt like throwing it out of the window at times'.[22] And not everywhere had electricity. Reefton could boast that it was the first town in the southern hemisphere to have electric street lighting in 1888 but it did not switch to AC power until 1945. Freda Patterson, working on the West Coast, took up the offer of a local electrician to fit a Singer sewing machine engine to her treadle. Freda was delighted as the thing 'went like a bomb'.[23] However, when the principal dental officer turned up at the clinic, he was aghast. Did she not think about the risk to herself and her patient of using mains power without a transformer? Metal drill, wet mouth, 220 volts. Freda got it.

With larger numbers of trainees flocking to Wellington, the health department decided to invest in hostel accommodation. Whether through naivety or the desire to save money, it leased a private hotel called The Mansions to provide living quarters for 56 trainee nurses. Formerly a brothel, The Mansions was in Ghuznee Street, then, as now, the heart of Wellington's red light district. The hotel was one of many properties owned by Wellington entrepreneur Clara 'Ma' Hallam, who specialised in doss-houses, rent-by-the hour hotel rooms, sly grog and brothel-keeping.[24] For young dental trainees from the provinces, a stay at The Mansions surely added an extra dimension to their education.

Like all public servants, dental nurses also benefited personally from the change of government, which on assuming office restored their cut pay. In 1936 a 40-hour week was introduced and they no longer had to work on Saturday mornings. That year George V died. 'God Save our Gracious King' was the anthem they had stood for every time they went to the cinema because he was 'King of the British Dominions beyond the Seas'. At the Berlin Olympics, Hitler's extravaganza, Jack Lovelock won gold in the 1500 metres, setting a world record. The global events that seemed so distant to Elsie Hitchcock when she began her training in 1931 were no longer so. Radio, which had advanced from crystal sets with headphones to mantel radios that the whole family gathered round, was bringing the world closer. The Labour government set up the National Broadcasting Service and there was a new national magazine free to all radio licence holders, the *New Zealand Listener*.

The news from the other side of the world, however, was growing alarming. On 1 September 1939, Germany invaded Poland. Two days later, New Zealand followed Britain's lead and declared war on Germany. Dental nursing in wartime was to bring new challenges and adventures.

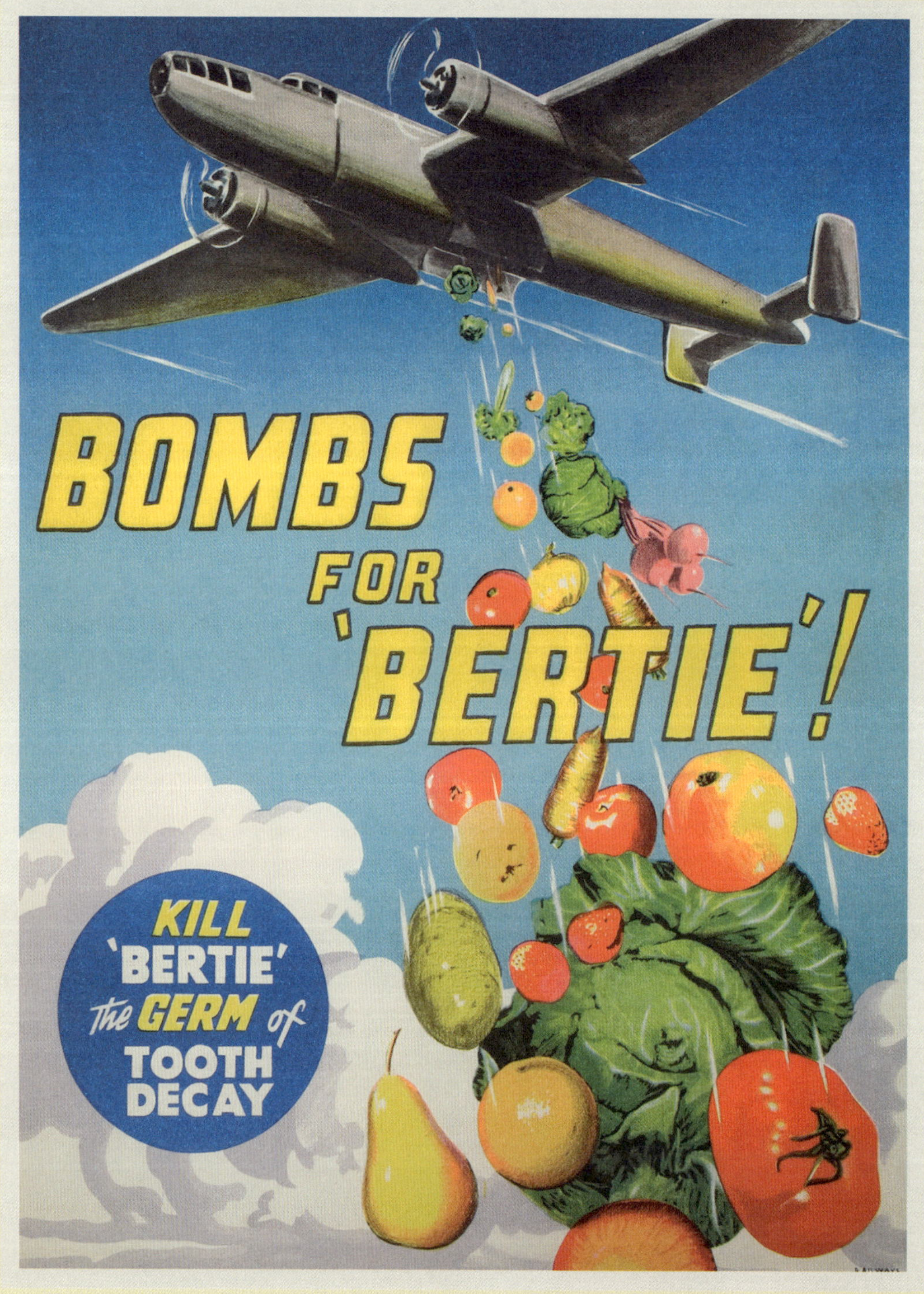
BOMBS
FOR
'BERTIE'!
KILL
'BERTIE'
the GERM of
TOOTH
DECAY

4

KEEP DRILLING AND CARRY ON

On 14 May 1940 German forces were on the rampage in Europe, attacking the Netherlands and France. The RAF launched a counter-offensive with 70 bombers, 40 of which were blown out of the skies over Rotterdam.

Half a world away, the new Dominion School for Dental Nurses and Children's Dental Clinic, a wonder of the dental world, was officially opened in Wellington. An imposing building, it loomed over Upper Willis Street. Inside, the spaces and floors coalesced into a machine for industrial-scale dentistry, with its vast, high-ceilinged room where dozens of children, their mouths open like baby birds, could be treated at the same time.

Dr Bibby, visionary and principal of the new school, conducted a tour of the building for *School Dental Service Gazette* readers with the pride of a first homeowner: 'Walking up the wide entrance steps and passing through swinging glass doors, one enters the ground-floor foyer, or waiting-hall. The first glance shows a spacious hall, colourful and light. To the right, on a pedestal, the bust of Thomas Anderson Hunter, the founder and first Director of the School Dental Service — opposite, 40 ft. away, the lift-doors with diamond-shaped windows and touches of red; to the right again a broad stairway leading to the floor above, and on the left, bronze grille windows opening to the Records Office beyond.'[1]

Turning first to the records office, Bibby notes that 'the counter has been lowered so that the smallest of children may hand in cards and be given charts without standing on tiptoe to see'. Down a wide corridor he pauses at the clerical office with its little interview alcove: 'It is here that the Records Officer talks quietly to the mother and child as she fills in cards and chart and gives that personal touch, so important on their first visit to the clinic.'

In the waiting room is a big indicator board of colour-coded lights, which come on when a chair is vacant in either the main clinic, the auxiliary clinic, or the orthodontic or extraction room. Bibby enthuses: 'a scene of animation meets the eye. Parents sit in

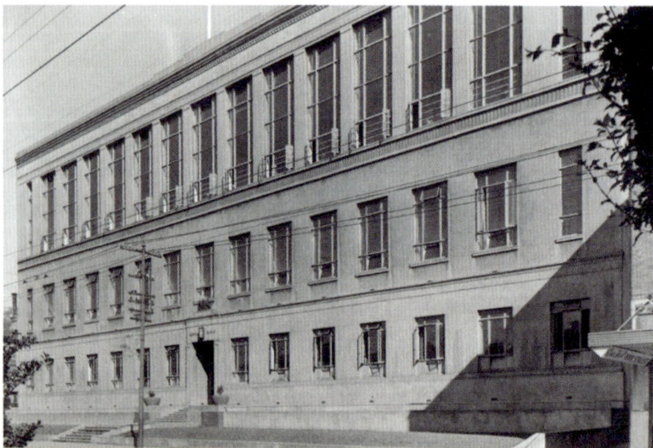

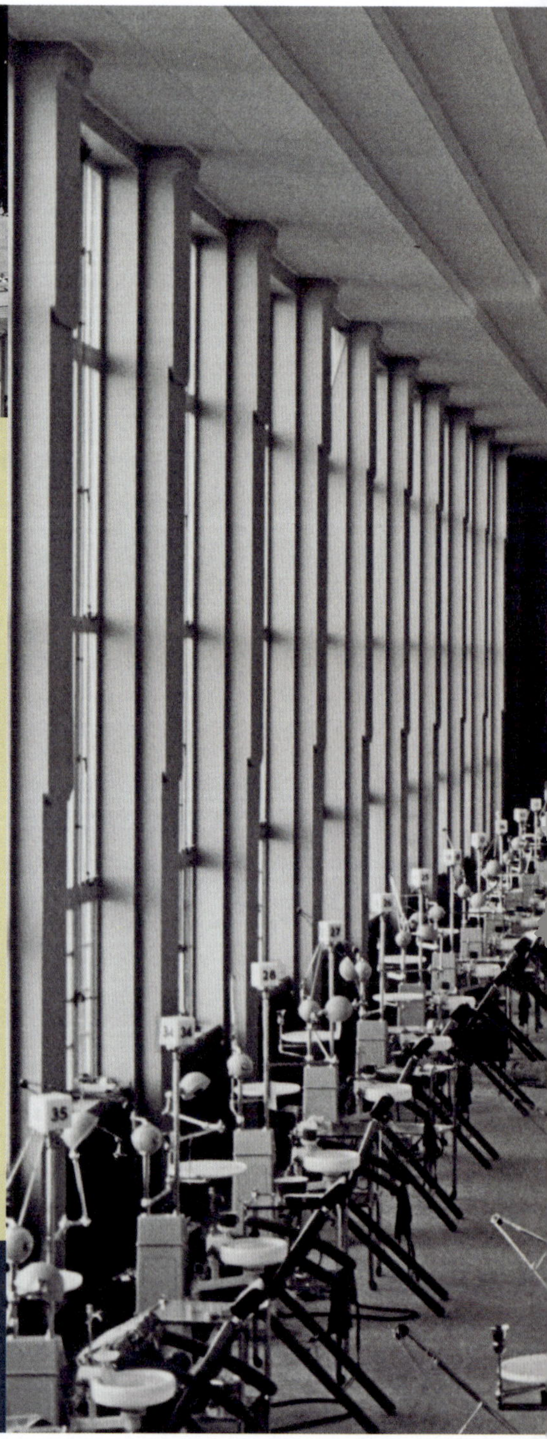

Above: The new Dominion School for Dental Nurses and Children's Dental Clinic loomed over Willis Street. As they climbed the wide entrance steps, children may well have felt apprehensive about what lay ahead.

Right: The new clinic was a wonder of the dental world when it opened its doors in 1940. It was dentistry on an almost industrial scale. By the clock is the small balcony where visiting dignitaries could observe the busy scene.

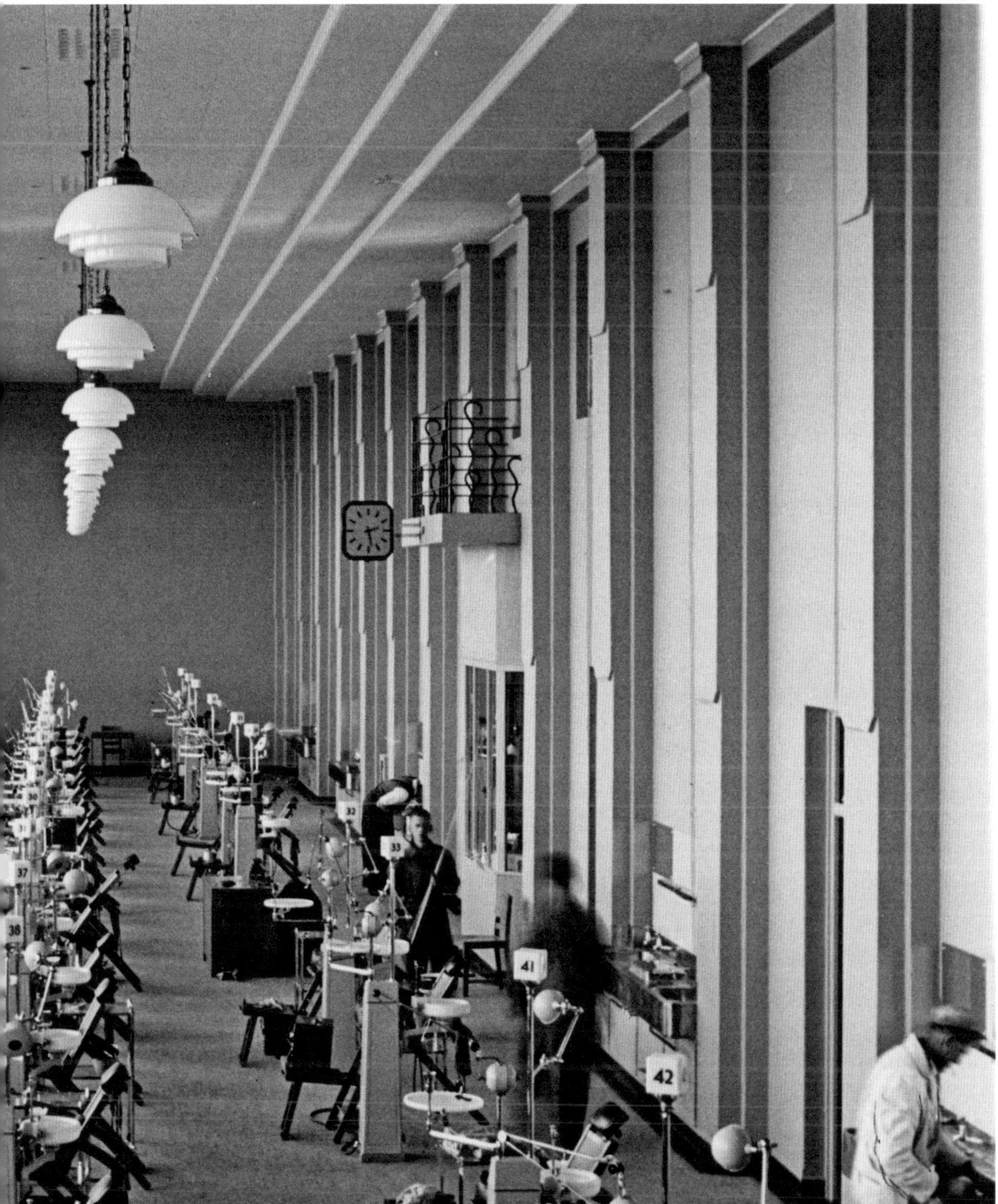
37
38
33
41
42

easy chairs in the glazed loggia, reading or listening to the radio programme. Young children play with the toys, or sit in miniature chairs at miniature tables; older children read the inevitable "Comic Cuts" at a large, low, centre table.'

Up a wide stairway to the floor above is the training school, a far cry from the Tomato House. 'In place of the old familiar ink-stained benches and swivel seats are fifty individual desks and chairs, while the lecture bench, dark stained and chrome edged, is complete with lectern and light, laboratory sink, and Fonomatic call system to floors above and below. Even bony Annabelle has a cupboard of her own in which to hide her bareness. Yes, one almost forgets the days when lights were dim, benches rocked, and the lecturer's voice was drowned in the rattle of nearby trams.' Across the corridor from this section a canteen serves lunches 'attractive and yet light on the student purse'.

The second floor, where the children are treated, is the heart of the building. The big room is wide enough to take three rows of chairs. 'Each chair has an electric unit with light, bracket table, and spittoon, and a little table with cabinet, cupboard, and writing bracket.' Though construction of the building had begun before the outbreak of war, Bibby catered for that eventuality, for 'even a dental clinic is not free of air-raid fear, and "down below" is housed our air-raid shelter where, in time of alarm, parents, patients, and staff may be free of bomb blast and splinter'.

Nineteen-year-old Margaret Sybil McLean from Westport was one of the first drafts to train in the new clinic. The Teutonic efficiency of the building was mirrored in the exacting attitude of staff. Regimentation and standardisation were the touchstones. (Left-handed people, for example, were not initially accepted for training because equipment was in a fixed position.) 'Everybody had to be alphabetical, it was an alphabetical life,' Margaret recalled.[2] 'Stand and open the door for any dental officer to walk through, hands behind your back. You never spoke to a dental officer or tutor unless they spoke to you. Praise was very scarce, you were ruled by fear that you wouldn't come up to the mark.' Demerit points were imposed for minor slip-ups and a report on each nurse's demerits published each month.

Besides studying, she was rostered on to 24 different duties. 'Nurses had to do all the cleaning, polish the floors, dusting, cafeteria, works, making sandwiches, sewing duty, mend all the laundry and uniforms. You had to prepare matron's lunch and take it to her. You hated that because no matter how good you were, she always found something wrong with you.'

Like servants in an English country house, nurses were never permitted to use the main entrance to the clinic. The clinic attracted streams of visitors, from overseas dentists to foreign dignitaries, but dental nurses were all but invisible to them. Young dental officers fresh out of university had to be treated like authorities. 'They were just so uppity, they had no practical experience and we could run rings round them. It did cause quite a bit of friction at the time. But a lot ended up marrying dental students.'

Margaret quickly found that dissent was not tolerated. 'You were pushed back in the bottle until you learned your place. You learned from an early stage that you were a dental nurse, slave of the dental profession.'

Every week nurses were lined up for doses of cod-liver oil, and had weekly exercise sessions on the roof. 'You were weighed every month to see if you were putting on too much weight.' Or perhaps to find out if any were pregnant: 'The innocence of people was unbelievable, one girl couldn't believe she was putting on so much weight.' Pregnancy was grounds for instant dismissal.

Margaret's ignorance was of a different kind. She'd been placed in The Mansions hostel in Ghuznee Street and arrived to find the girl in the room opposite was Māori. 'I was terrified that she was a cannibal. I locked my door. I was really frightened of her.' Margaret had never encountered Māori in Westport. 'There were very few Maori on the Coast. I first saw a Maori when I was six or seven but never had anything to do with them.' It turned out Kahu Metekingi didn't bite; in fact, she became her best friend.

Margaret enjoyed the hostel camaraderie, where everything was shared — 'first up, best dressed' — but it was not a home from home. The rickety building, with its lingering odour of boiled cabbage, shook in the wind. At night drunken soldiers were apt to rap on the door, asking for Elsie or Joan, former residents who had a reputation for comforting the lonely. There were stickered admonitions everywhere: 'DO NOT USE THE LIGHTS AFTER MIDNIGHT; PLEASE TURN THE IRON OFF AFTER USE', and so on. A 7 p.m. curfew was extended to 9.30 p.m. one night a week, with one weekend off a term, approved by the matron. Seven to nine in the evening were 'silence hours', with no phone calls allowed.

The matron, Miss Pengelly, a retired army nurse, was not to be crossed. Writer Lauris Edmond, who had encountered her as the warden of a Victoria University hostel, described her as 'a big ugly woman with a booming voice — she wasn't just bossy, she was savage', a tyrant who wanted 'noisy disobedient girls dismissed after a warning'.[3] Margaret McLean discovered the matron 'would open our mail and stick it down again'. In the evenings, meals would go cold while they waited for matron to show up. Nurses who got sick were never referred to a doctor; instead, Miss Pengelly would brandish her favourite remedy, Friars' Balsam; 'Then she'd bring in skeins of wool to work on because you couldn't be sitting doing nothing all day. You realised you'd be better off going to work,'[4] another hostel inmate recalled.

The day arrived when Margaret was confronted with her first live patient. 'I was scared stiff and my hands were shaking.' The sight of a child spitting blood in the next chair unnerved her. She got through it, but never got used to the pain she had to inflict. 'It was cruel dentistry in those days but you had to get the work done to relieve the patient. I can see how it built up a tremendous fear in children.' The drawn-out supervision process didn't help. 'You had to wait until an inspector would look at your work at every stage and a child could be in the chair for two hours. You had some very difficult children because of the state of their mouths. You had to fight with them and hold them down. Sometimes you had other people holding them down and they'd be yelling out. You had to be hard.'

Graduation felt like an anticlimax. There was no celebration. The minister of health, Arnold Nordmeyer, turned up and pinned on the medals, 'then it was back up to the surgery'.

Margaret McLean was posted to Masterton. 'We had to pay our own fares to wherever we were posted and find our own accommodation.' She struggled to cope on her own because the supervisor was in hospital. One day the principal dental officer turned up unexpectedly and she was told she had to shift the next week to Westland. 'I had just set up a flat in Masterton but you had no say — you had to go where you were put.'

There was no one to meet her when she arrived in Hokitika. The clinic was a mess, with half the equipment lost, and there was a huge backlog of children who had gone untreated. The isolation and loneliness of the place had driven the previous nurse to drink. Margaret worked 'from 7.30am to dark. Children had to be treated in one day [transport was curtailed as a result of the wartime petrol shortage] . . . The children used to eat onions because they thought nurse wouldn't treat them but nurse ate onions too.' Evenings were spent writing up dental history charts.

She soon learned that knowing the people in the district and their histories was vital. 'There were feuding families so you could not bring in children from different families at the same time.' The mass killing of seven people by local farmer Stanley Graham in 1941, which had been prompted by a feud between neighbours, was still fresh in people's minds.

Though she'd trained on the new electric drill, it was back to working on the treadle. 'They gave a lot of trouble. You had to be mechanical to keep your equipment in top condition. You had to improvise — a lot of the parts were German-made, like the Kava handpieces. With the war on you couldn't get parts.'

Surprise clinic inspections by head office had long been routine, but they were infrequent as there was only one inspector for each island and nurses traditionally warned colleagues up the line that the inspector was on the way by sending a telegram with the cryptic message 'A case of apples is arriving'. However, as the service expanded so too did the inspections. A number of dental nurses, seemingly chosen for their fault-finding skills, were promoted to dental nurse inspectors. Like most nurses, Margaret grew to loathe visits from the inspector. 'They came to catch you out rather than constructively help you. They would turn up at a clinic early to see if people arrived in time. You were docked a half day's pay. We just hated her, absolutely negative. Her pettiness made me cringe.'

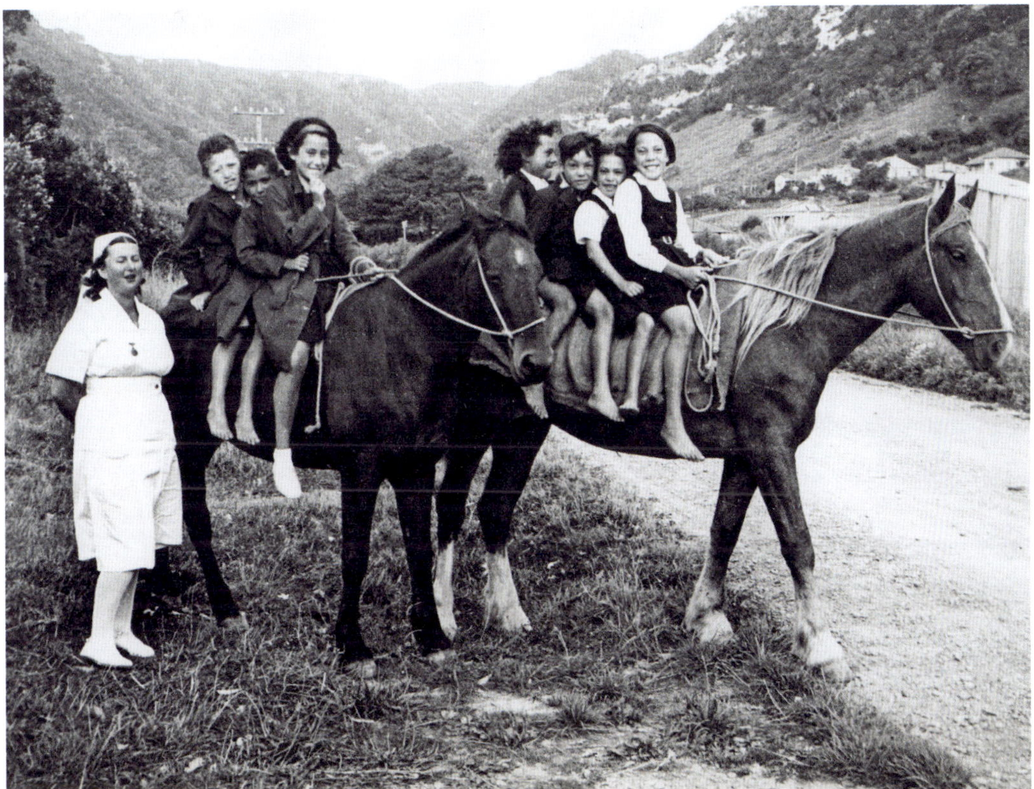

School dental nurse Urquhart with some of her patients, Te Araroa, north of Gisborne, circa 1940s. Dental nurses often had to travel by horseback, too.

Any minor irregularity in dress would be denounced as unprofessional, yet, as Margaret found, the starched uniform and veil became a problem after a while. 'Starched veils caused dandruff and hair loss. A lot of people lost their hair and got a bald patch on top. The starch and perspiration could cause skin complaints.' A more serious hazard, as some nurses discovered, was veils catching fire while heating the amalgam for fillings. At the Hokitika clinic the headmaster liked to see Margaret without her uniform. 'He would always wait until I was changing into my uniform in the morning. He was a dirty old man.'

Though it was strictly forbidden, she treated some adults, as the nearest dentist was over 150 kilometres away. 'I did fillings for quite a few adults, they couldn't afford it otherwise. You had hermits coming out of the bush.'

Like her predecessor at Hokitika, she had periods of despair. 'There was nobody to turn to. You couldn't ask for help because you were expected to know.' At weekends there was little to do: 'On wet Saturdays I played poker with the policeman, priest, baker and commercial traveller.' She jumped at the chance of some entertainment: 'It was nothing to go 50 miles to a dance.'

For some, though, isolation provided the best experiences of their careers. In 1940, newly graduated nurse Margaret Austen was stationed in Addington, Christchurch, when she received a buff-coloured OHMS (On His Majesty's Service) envelope. She opened it with trepidation — what had she done wrong? Had she been spotted when she sneaked a day off to go to the races? The enclosed letter, she read with some relief, was simply a transfer, telling her to report to Oaro. But where in the world was Oaro? She discovered it was a small coastal settlement north of Christchurch near Kaikōura. At the time it was mainly a camp for the unemployed, who were drilling tunnels to extend the main railway line north. On arrival she was given the key to her lodgings, a small army hut, the timber walls extending only a metre in height, with the remainder canvas that reached up to the roof. 'I can still vividly remember in stormy wet weather the creaking of the walls, the flapping and whining canvas, the beating of the rain on the iron roof. Shivering, I often wondered if I would be swept out to sea.'[5] Next day she picked her way over the stony road to find the clinic, aware she was being scrutinised by the women in the huts; the men were all away at work.

The clinic turned out to be similar to her bleak hut. 'As I opened the door the bare essentials seemed to magnify themselves before me, a dental chair, foot drill, sink and cupboard and stove.' Her heart sank when she saw the Primus stove — how would she ever get it to work? She turned on the tap but no water flowed. A visit from a plumber 'with a disarming toothless grin' fixed the problem, but her initial excitement at being sole charge and treating her own patients had dissipated. It was going to be a hard slog.

> For many in the camp times were hard, these people had emerged from the years of the depression, only to be thrust into World War II. Life consisted of having the bare essentials — a toothbrush was sheer luxury, as I was soon to discover. However my stomach always revolted at my having to work in a filthy mouth and so a tooth cleaning programme was the first on my agenda before examination. News soon got around that the new nurse made the poor kids clean their teeth with a rag before she got going. One morning when Johnny was due in along came his big sister with a note, torn off the corner of the newspaper. All it said was 'When you have 13 kids you won't worry about dirty teeth nither'.
>
> Another poor urchin hadn't been in the bath for weeks, his face was black and grimy, with sticky jam around his mouth, so out came my rags, soap and water and he was given a long overdue wash before I could venture to say, 'open wide'. The following day he brought me a sooty piece of brown paper and scribbled across it was 'My boy ain't no rose, drill him, don't smell 'im.'
>
> After a day of many extractions and large compound fillings, toothache and fiery looking abscesses, it was a happy relief to lock the door at night. I enjoyed the solitude of my own palace before starting out for an evening meal at the camp cookhouse.[6]

In the cookhouse Margaret was confronted by a sea of rugged men's faces. Seeing her anxiety, the cook took pity on her and set a table in the kitchen — 'a hot smoky place where big black dixies sat on enormous coal stoves, their contents bubbling as they sent off delicious aromatic odours too subtle to guess what they contained'. To her surprise, cookhouse meals proved to be a sumptuous feast night after night. 'Never before have I tasted venison or fresh fish caught a few hours before and crayfish that had been wriggling in crayfish pots at day break.'

Despite the isolation, she came to love the place. 'Often the nights would be dark, wintry and wet as I made my way home, across the Oaro Bridge and past the rows of army huts to my own little four walls, but I always felt secure and safe with these people. The men would call out "Goodnight, nursie", as they passed by, never once scaring or molesting me.'

In Europe, Hitler's forces were on the offensive and the Allies in retreat. The New Zealand government introduced conscription. Men aged between 18 and 45 were once more liable to be called up by ballot. 'Conscription came in not long after I had been at the Oaro Clinic and this really upset my register,' remembered Margaret. 'It was impossible to attach the correct surname to many children. When their respective father was called up in the single men's ballot, the child, or in many cases children, would revert back to the mother's maiden name or better still adopt the name of another new father.'

Social activities were non-existent, but she found life was full of fun and adventure. 'The beauty of the snow tipped mountainous ranges which ran down to meet the golden sand of the rugged beaches, the clean azure blue skies, and seas, sometimes gentle, other times angry, grey and treacherous made this place a part of New Zealand untouched by modern civilisation.'

In 1940, despite the grim press reports, the war seemed a long way off. Then on 7 December 1941 Japan bombed Pearl Harbor and, as the *Evening Post* observed, 'The war in a single night advance[d] menacingly towards us.'[7] Within months, Japanese troops had swept through the Philippines, Burma, Malaya and the Dutch East Indies. When Singapore fell, the bastion of the British Empire in the Far East, New Zealand suddenly felt vulnerable. With its military might, such as it was, bolstering the British in Europe, only God was left to defend New Zealand and He wasn't making much headway against the forces of the god emperor Hirohito.

In cinemas women were urged to do their bit for the war effort. *Women at War*, a short film by the state-run National Film Unit, reached new heights of bombast:

> War needs women's skills as well as men's strong arms, women's endurance as well as courage from New Zealand men, women's speed in execution of small motions as well as man's ability to plan the great campaigns and spell the words of war. Death! Destruction! Fire! Famine! No longer dainty hands and pretty dress, steel now for the guns. No longer lily-fingered loveliness, steel fingers now, dirty fingers now, working fingers now, bombs now, metal now . . . Women at work, working for war, women counting minutes, clocking in and clocking out and the endless stream that feeds the machines and makes the machines of war. Women in overalls, women in uniform,

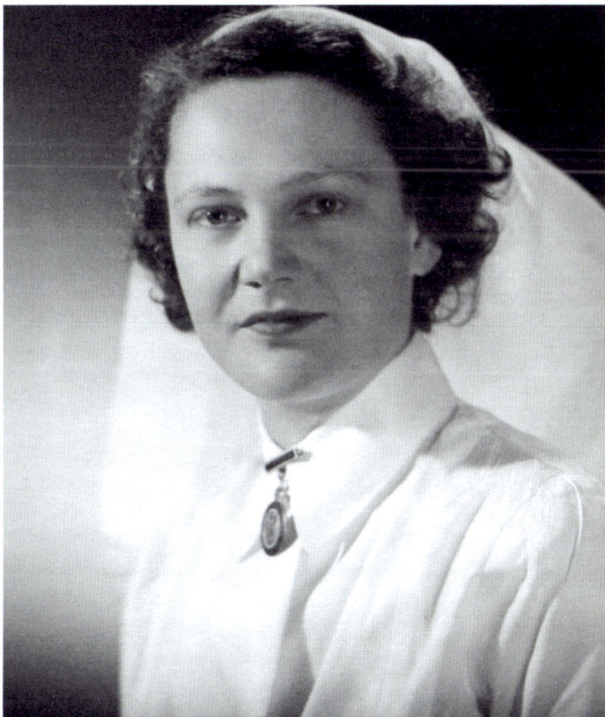

'The first thing we dental nurses noticed about the Americans above everything else was their wonderful teeth. We were besotted by the beautiful teeth.'

— Marjorie Orchiston

> marching, women in the ranks, women in the factories, women taking part in the twentieth century's biggest parade, women with heads held high. Women who work for war!'[8]

In the end women had no choice. The government introduced manpower regulations to force civilians to work in designated essential industries that included everything from munition factories to freezing works and mental hospitals. It proved more controversial than military conscription: parents were reluctant to let their daughters shift to the cities and work in factories, and women did not want to work long hours in repetitive jobs that paid half the wages of men doing the same work.

Despite propaganda about civilians getting behind the war effort, defaulting and absenteeism became so prevalent that manpower officers, along with police, were given authority to question people they suspected of skiving in their homes and in public places such as cinemas, hotels and billiard halls. Manpower began to visit hotels, hoping to catch those playing truant.

Dental nursing suddenly became attractive to the daughters of the wealthy, some of whom who had never done even domestic chores and did not wish to risk their 'lily-fingered loveliness' making bullets and grenades. They were resented by the other trainees. 'They hated the work but it was better than working in a factory, and they left as soon as restrictions were lifted,' Margaret McLean recalled. In the hostels they kept to themselves, 'never did their own washing, never boiled an egg. Some sent washing home to be done by the maid.'

Though dental nursing was not her first choice either, Marjorie Orchiston was not one of the wealthy. A farmer's daughter from Pahiatua, she says she was not very popular when she was born. The family had just bought a farm when the depression came and the last thing they wanted was a girl. She had her heart set on being a teacher but was turned down by Teachers' College because her birthday was outside the admissions period that year. 'I just floated around and didn't know what to do. Then my mother saw an advertisement for dental nurses.'[9] Greatly taken with the idea of wearing a veil, Marjorie applied.

She began training at the Tomato House in 1940, but the Willis Street clinic opened soon after. 'Patients were cancelled for a fortnight and we junior nurses were sent to the new building to scrape paint off the banisters and get it ready for opening.' Like many, she was not a fan of the building. 'It was so wrong for a place for children . . . It should never have been built.'

But there was one good thing about the new premises: Marjorie got to practise her musical skills, playing the popular songs of the day on the piano at lunchtime while staff tucked into wiener schnitzel or Hungarian goulash prepared by an Austrian refugee chef for whom Dr Bibby had secured a work permit. That winter Marjorie whisked diners back to the Old Country, even if they'd never been there, playing wartime favourites such as 'A Nightingale Sang in Berkeley Square'.

Though the piano playing assured she had no problems with manual dexterity, Marjorie was not mechanical, an essential trait when operating in the field where you had to maintain equipment. Only dogged persistence got her through. 'The lecturer came along and unscrewed a piece of equipment and dropped it on the floor and you had to put it together again. Any normal person would have put the screws in a row. I tried so hard and was so hopeless and I spent all my lunch hours practising.'

In June 1942, American troops began arriving in New Zealand to strengthen the Allies' hand in the Pacific war. Thousands were disgorged from troopships in

Auckland and Wellington. Their arrival went unreported in the media because of strict censorship laws that meant even weather forecasts were banned. Only recipes appearing in the press for lemon and pumpkin pies, waffles and doughnuts gave any clue to the encampment of the new troops. It was not the best-kept secret — short-wave radio listeners were well aware of the American arrivals from the broadcasts of Tokyo Rose, the English-language propaganda disseminated by the Japanese to demoralise troops.

Marjorie found out when she spotted the ships in Wellington Harbour. From the roof of the clinic you could see down into the city. 'The word went around and we couldn't wait until half past four to rush into town.' Wellington was packed with 'tickle and giggle girls', a snide term for office girls, originally typists from T&G Insurance. The Marines, dapper in their tailored uniforms, looked like Hollywood soldiers, provoking guilty comparisons with baggy-arsed Kiwi troops in their rough khaki smelling of mothballs, heavy boots and lemon-squeezer hats. Only the finest physical specimens were accepted in the Marine Corps — a missing tooth was enough to warrant rejection. It was an attribute that did not get overlooked. 'The first thing we dental nurses noticed about the Americans above everything else was their wonderful teeth. We were besotted by the beautiful teeth.'

The Americans injected new life into the drab, blacked-out capital. They literally threw their money about, flinging coins from trams for kids to scramble after. Enterprising schoolboys set up shoeshine stalls on the pavements. Black Americans had the surreal experience of having their shoes shined by a white boy. Though the six o'clock closing of pubs was a serious obstacle to a good night out, the Marines smuggled alcohol into dance clubs, where management turned a blind eye and police did not visit.

Coffee places and milkbars with names like Hot Dog and California sprang up. In the Hotel Cecil, near the railway station, the American Red Cross served ham and eggs, doughnuts and real coffee, from 7 a.m. to 11 p.m. The Green Parrot Cafe in Taranaki Street became a late-night hangout after the movies, where Marines wolfed down steak, raw tomatoes and glasses of milk.

Wellington would never earn the epithet of 'the city that never sleeps', but most nights it was still awake after midnight. In the Majestic Cabaret, the favourite venue for a big night out (Artie Shaw and the US Navy Band had famously played there), the staid foxtrot gave way to the uninhibited jitterbug (not to be attempted with full skirts, some clubs warned). Society and T&G girls flocked to the Majestic, but you could always tell the dental nurses because of the black silver nitrate stain on their hands, recalled Marjorie: 'There was no way you could get it off.'

Though they made fun of the T&G girls, dental nurses were no more immune to the charms of the Americans. As official war historian Nancy Taylor wrote:

> These charms were augmented by money. American pay rates were higher than New Zealanders', and many coming from the islands and due to return there had substantial amounts of back pay and every intention of spending it. For a 'date', a posy of flowers might be sent, the young man might bring sweets or chocolates, he would certainly be lavish with cigarettes; a sheaf of roses or other flowers might arrive a day or so after a pleasant evening or as a 'thank-you' to a hostess. There were meals at hotels, and rooms for private entertainment; liquor was somehow acquired, there were taxis, one went places. It was fun to dress up and be admired, fun to talk with the girls at work about one's American and his buddies, fun to flourish cigarettes and gum, perhaps parade a slight accent. It was exciting to be squired by men from far away, whose place back home would lose nothing and possibly gain much in the telling. With such largesse suddenly replacing Saturday nights at the pictures with the girl-friends, it was small wonder that some young women were swept off their feet.[10]

However, in the oral history *Women in Wartime*, Ali, then a young married woman, recalled her less romantic view of the Americans:

> My first impression was either how young or thin they seemed to be or how middle-aged and fat. Cheeky they certainly were . . . In those days girls didn't, but believe me there were plenty of naughty girls who did, and that included their mothers. The hotels were fully booked . . .
>
> Most of the servicemen had tablets of sulphanilamide (sulfa drugs which preceded penicillin) in their pockets. These they doled out to their girlfriends, who believed they were a form of contraception, and of course they became pregnant. The birth rate soared. The servicemen were really cheeky. They would approach you, saying, 'Hello babe, hello honey — going my way?' They would try to take your arm or put their arm around your waist. You became quite callous and adept at thumping them or kicking them in the shins.[11]

But dental nurses had limited opportunities to find out whether the Yanks were Romeos or sex pests. At The Mansions, under the gimlet eye of Miss Pengelly, enjoying a social life was a risky business, necessitating use of the fire escape — and suspension or dismissal if caught. Marjorie Orchiston made regular use of the fire escape, 'with the help of a very nice policeman who helped you up. The Mansions was about four stories high and once I got in on the wrong floor, two instead of three, got my leg stuck in the window, and the poor nurse [inside] nearly died on the spot. She shouldn't have left the window open.'

Like everything in a dental nurse's life, social life was conducted according to a strict pecking order. 'The seniors went to the Officers' Club, the intermediates went to Webby's [a popular night spot], which had some officers, and the juniors went to the Blue Triangle, the YMCA.' The division had nothing to do with age or worldliness — some of the juniors were older than the seniors. As a junior Marjorie became a regular at the YMCA. 'I used to play lots of hymns like "Onward, Christian Soldiers" and

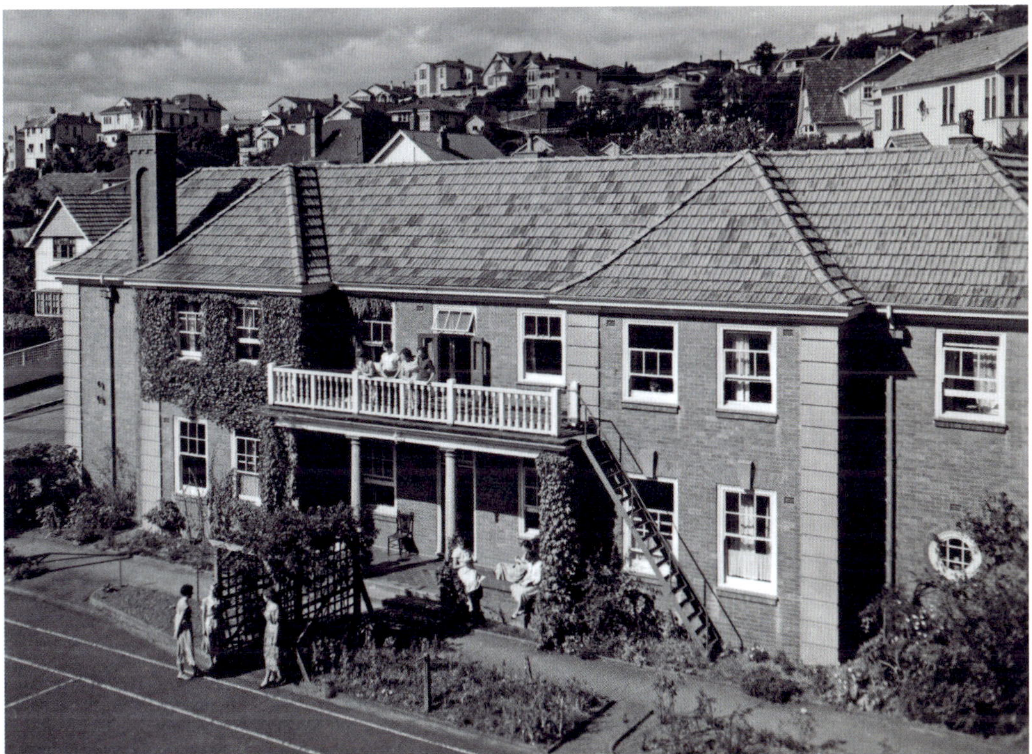

Student dental nurses catch some sun at The Glen Hostel in Kelburn, Wellington.

dance around with soldiers in their big army boots.' She felt sorry for the New Zealand soldiers who had no money and couldn't compete with the Yanks, who'd turn up on a date with a bunch of flowers. 'I remember we were visiting friends at the Kelburn hostel and some New Zealand soldiers turned up. One of them had a whole bush he'd pinched from the Botanical Gardens.'

The scarcity of silk stockings put a dampener on social life. Silk was reserved for parachutes. 'Attractive as they may be silk stockings are not essential and life will go on without them. Substitutes will be found but aeroplanes and parachutes are essential to modern war,' women were told. 'Those who believe that in the midst of the most frightful war in the world's history civilian life can remain untroubled and unchanged are living in a fool's paradise.'[12] However, no self-respecting woman wanted to go bare-legged and many employers took exception to it. As Australia's Dame Enid Lyons observed at the time, 'There exists in the mind of every woman the belief that the most undistinguished ankle becomes a thing of beauty in silken hose, and that even the most graceful without it deteriorates into a mere joint.'[13]

Marjorie remembers women experimenting with stockingless creams. The camouflage cream coloured their legs and was supplied with an eyebrow pencil to draw a line down the back of each leg to mimic a seam. The advertisements claimed it brought the 'comfort of bare-legged freedom with the elegance of the sheerest hose'. As the cream was too expensive for regular use, some women resorted to Bisto gravy mix, a cause for regret when it rained.

In 1940 the American chemical company DuPont began marketing nylon stockings. Nylon, a new synthetic silk 'as strong as steel, as fine as the spider's web', was derived from coal. American women bought them in the millions but none were sold in New Zealand due to wartime import restrictions. US Marines, however, seemed to have a ready supply, and their largesse with nylons was yet another wooing advantage they had over local soldiers.

In light of all of these inequalities, New Zealand soldiers bore a simmering resentment towards the Americans, which came to the boil one Saturday night in 1943. The Battle of Manners Street, as it became known, was triggered by a group of redneck Marines drinking in the Allied Services Club.[14] Seeing some Māori servicemen enter they blocked them from buying a drink. They goaded them as 'black curs', and the inevitable scuffle broke out. The Marines removed their brass-buckled belts and started swinging. The mêlée spilled into the street and turned into a riot embroiling more than a thousand servicemen and civilians. The violence, which spread up Cuba Street and towards Courtenay Place, took eight hours to quell and left two Marines

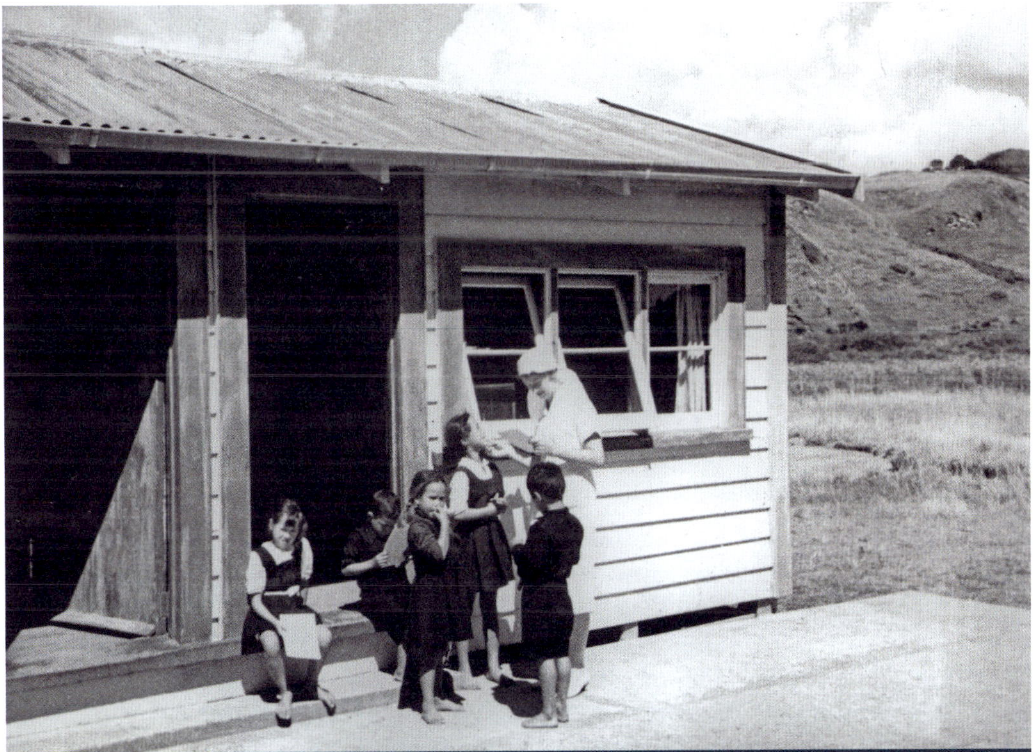

A dental nurse chats with school children at the Cape Runaway dental clinic in the early 1940s.

dead and many injured. Marjorie and her friends nearly ended up in the middle of it. 'We got out pretty smartly so we didn't see much of it. American military police came and started bundling soldiers into vans.'

At graduation, Marjorie was asked where she would like to be posted and expressed a preference for a Māori community on the East Cape, anywhere but her home town. She was furious when she was posted to the comatose little town of Eketahuna, just 100 kilometres or so from Pahiatua. 'When I arrived in Eketahuna, all the young blokes who weren't old enough for overseas service came to meet the bus. And as the

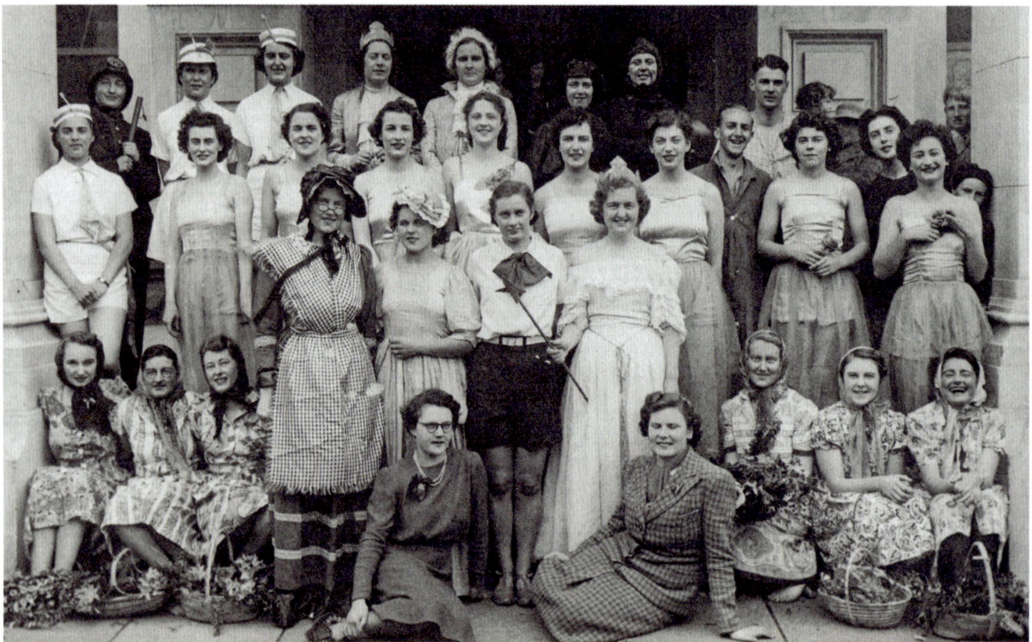

Marjorie Orchiston (seated, centre right) with the cast of her pantomime, an extravaganza of dental education that featured Little Bo-Peep, the Old Woman Who Lived in a Shoe, Bertie Germ and the Fairy Queen, among others.

big shearing shed was within walking distance at lunchtime, they all came and had lunch with me which was very flattering.'

She boarded at the Eketahuna Hotel. 'The proprietor's father had nothing to do but bore everybody and make a nuisance of himself. He said, "Now Marge, would you like to come into my office" and when we got in the office, he said, "What about a little square gin — did you ever have Dutch gin? Very good for your kidneys." I didn't stop to find out. You learned very quickly.'

A 7.2 earthquake provided some relief from the monotony. The other inhabitants of the hotel — a couple of commercial travellers, a barber, and two women schoolteachers — were unfazed. 'It was like something had really happened at last in the small town. They set up kerosene tins in the backyard to cook with. The earthquake was an exciting event.'

Every week Marjorie had to visit her sub-base at Woodville, 40 kilometres away.

The two-hour train ride was a journey she never looked forward to, given that 'it stopped at every tiny station picking up stock all the way to Woodville'. One afternoon, she boarded a carriage to find it full of American troops, for whom she became an object of close scrutiny. 'In those days I smoked and I got a cigarette out and they all rushed at me to light it. I had no means of escape whatsoever.'

> They didn't know where they were going and had no idea what to do for the weekend. They got out of me that I was on a committee that ran dances and there was a dance that Saturday night. I thought, 'Oh I shouldn't have said that' . . . When we got to the railway station and my father — I could have killed him — he'd come straight off the farm and he had his trouser legs tied up with string and a couple of dogs and the old farm truck. He said, 'What are you doing with all those Americans?' The Americans piled into the town's two taxis and went off to town. 'See you tomorrow night!' they shouted.
>
> Next night at the dance, the young men in the town would have nothing to do with me — I was a traitor to the human race, I think. All the girls had come and older women who'd heard about nylons and things. In those country dances everybody went. They tucked the babies down in the cloakroom and the kids slid around the hall on sacks and cushions between dances. At the end of the dance the girls had all learned to jitterbug and so forth, and were having the time of their lives. The old farmers had learned about American farming. My father even invited one for a cup of coffee next morning to learn more about farming in Texas. It was the most successful dance evening the small town had had for a while.
>
> I'll never forget that train ride with the Americans. They were only kids about 18 or so. They knew they were just going to slaughter up in the islands. They were so yellow with that awful drug for malaria.

The drug was Atabrine, a substitute for the anti-malarial quinine, supplies of which were cut off when the Japanese occupied Java. Atabrine had many unpleasant side effects, including yellow skin. Soldiers did everything to avoid taking it, with the result that four out of ten soldiers serving in the Pacific were hospitalised with malaria.

Though she stuck at it and later became a tutor sister at the clinic, Marjorie never felt fulfilled in her dental nursing career. A musician and short story writer, she was drawn to dental education where she could use her creative talents. With children in the chair, she would often make up stories to distract them, somewhat to the annoyance of the other clinic nurse, who liked to listen to the radio. It was the heyday of Bertie Germ, the lurking enemy ever ready to lay waste to children's teeth. Germ, only a syllable short of 'German', inspired the patriotism of health department educators. A popular poster of the time, 'Bombs for Bertie', shows a bomber raining down fruit and vegetables to nobble any unwitting germs.

Marjorie was determined to do her bit to annihilate Bertie. She devised a pantomime that was performed by dental nurses in the Concert Chamber of the Wellington Town Hall. It was an extravaganza of dental education like no other and drew school audiences from all over the city. The newspaper reviews were enthusiastic.

> It is some time since Wellington children have been treated to a real pantomime and certainly a long time since they saw such an entertaining one . . . The story is told in simple language and mime how a small boy Tony allowed the Germ Army to invade his teeth because he did not keep them clean and how he added to his naughtiness by sucking his thumb. The Toothbrush Army, spick and span, in blue and white defeated the evil Decay Spirits in their black and scarlet suits. When Tony reformed and promised to use his tooth brush, he was crowned Knight of the Ivory Kingdom by the King and taken to fairyland and the magic woods. The cast included Bo-Peep, the Old Woman in the Shoe and her children, Golliwog, Spider, Bertie Germ, and Fairy Queen among others. Attractive ballets were plentiful and many songs were sung with enthusiasm . . . Every scene and action in the pantomime was created for the purpose of bringing vividly to childish minds the urgent need there is for all boys and girls to give their teeth constant care and attention.[15]

It was a triumph for Marjorie, who'd written and produced the show, but, as it turned out, a bittersweet one. The National Film Unit decided to film a dress rehearsal for its *Weekly Review*. To fit the segment, she had to cut and rewrite on the spot, a feat that impressed the film-makers. 'They offered me a job. It was what I really wanted and I was over the moon. But Head Office refused to let me go because the dental service was an essential service, as was the Film Unit.'

The war found Kath Salter in Huntly with a pile of work to do.[16] Huntly had 17 schools and 800 children, half of whom had never had any treatment. 'Well, dear, they always

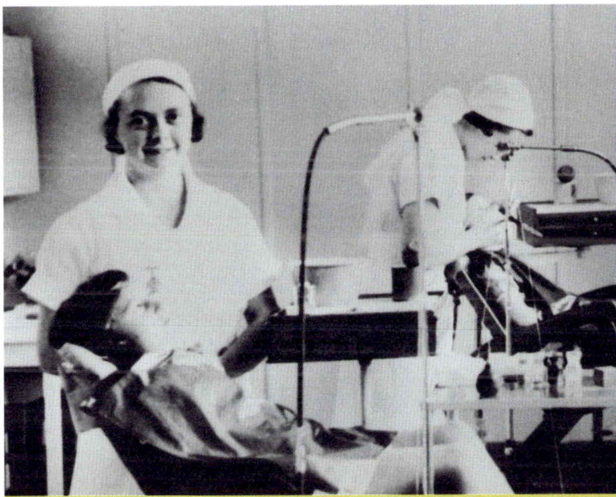

Kath Salter in her clinic. During the war she was stationed in Huntly, where there were 17 schools and 800 children to treat. 'I never worked so hard as I did in Huntly, where I ran to work at 8.15, never had a proper lunch and crawled home at 5.30 each night and rested before going out to Red Cross meetings at night.'

choose the best girls for the worst jobs,' said her friend Madge Grocott.[17] Kath soon found out what she meant. The clinic was a walled-off corridor facing south, so the light was poor. There was a cupboard and steriliser, and an old couch where mothers would come and watch her work. 'The anaesthetic supplied was only one per cent strength. The department was too scared to issue anything that might cause reactions. It was made up in Wellington and sent out to us.' The heavy, leaky syringes didn't help — 'you hoped the anaesthetic was going down the gum and not your wrist'.

In Huntly, she found that children's teeth were completely broken down. 'They were dental cripples. It was nothing to see children with dentures in high school. If they did get a denture it acted as a splint and the jaw didn't develop at that age. I could recognise young women with a deep cleft and collapsed bite and sharp chin because they'd lost all their teeth and the bite had been lost. The molars would be extracted and the bite would collapse and lower teeth would be hitting the upper roof. They probably had terrible trouble even taking a denture.'

She knew she was often inflicting pain, but there was no other way to fix up the children's teeth. 'I remember having to struggle for an hour to get a lower six [molar] out of a 12 year old boy in the back blocks.' She travelled to remote schools in the surrounding Māori communities, working in a dirty classroom with a clapped-out stove. 'You froze to death and had to jam a duster in the door to keep out the wind because it had no lock. The fog was so bad that you couldn't operate after 3pm and everybody had nits or scabies or impetigo. I had to carry water in buckets and use an outside latrine and put white paper on a packing case for a table.' There was no lavatory — 'I had to hold an umbrella over the mother while children went to the toilet under a hedge in the pouring rain.'

It was not the efficient dental service the department was boasting about in its new Wellington clinic. When the dental inspector called he could only laugh weakly and back out. 'One thing, Nurse Salter, you'll always be good at camping.'

Kath was not a happy camper, but she made the best of it. She learned te reo Māori, though children were scolded for speaking it in school. 'Sir Apirana Ngata said, "If they don't know the English language they'll always be second class citizens, they'll never compete with the Pakeha. Let them be proficient in English and then they can learn their own language."' Kath developed a glossary of essential phrases, which was published in the *Gazette* to help other nurses in Māori communities. Be brave, be strong — Kia toa, kia kaha. Open your mouth — Hamama to waha. Enough, be quiet! — Kati te turituri. And spit — E tuwha. However, another nurse who was serving in the Far North wished the glossary had been more precise. 'We suggest Nurse Salter supply us with the Māori version of "Spit in the basin" not just for "Spit".'

Kath was fascinated by the Māori customs she observed. 'Never boil handkerchiefs on the cooking fire and always wash male and female clothing separately and hang male clothing on one side of the whare and female on the other. When baby teeth "came off" they were buried with the umbilical cord under the family's special tree.'

To get around the more remote areas, Kath went by launch or on horseback or a combination of both. In wartime it was often hard to get petrol for the launch. 'You had to travel according to the moon and the tides.' And being small, she hated having to ride a big horse. 'I'd be riding across bogs on a horse with one eye. They always used to race home so they would take off on me.' On one occasion she was thrown off when the horse smashed through a fence. 'I thought I was going to be kicked. I put my back out and I was in agony for three weeks.'

In the Pacific, Japanese forces were closing in. Kath had a kit prepared to go bush in the event of an invasion. Troops were stationed in the area 'in leaky World War 1 tents, and not enough changes of clothes amid the fog in the Waikato. It was miserable in winter.'

To help keep up their morale, she performed in concert parties. In the clinic she'd have sheet music for songs like 'Over the Rainbow' and 'Wish Me Luck as You Wave Me Goodbye' propped up so she could learn the words as she did the fillings. 'We'd climb up on the forces' stage and sing to thousands and my knees would be knocking. Then we'd take food and feed all those poor guys.'

It was a busy life. 'If I hadn't been as strong and physically fit I could never have worked as hard as I did in Huntly where I ran to work at 8.15, never had a proper lunch break and crawled home at 5.30 each night and rested before going out to Red Cross meetings.'

The war brought extra work for everyone — dental nurses were expected to do voluntary aid work in the evenings and at weekends — and chronic shortages made life more difficult. Radio star Aunt Daisy came to the rescue with her butterless and eggless recipes when basic foods became luxuries because meat and dairy exports had been stepped up to help the war effort in Britain; it didn't help that the resident American troops, like teenagers (which many were), were eating New Zealand out of house and home. Petrol rationing, which did not end until 1950, made travel more difficult. After the fall of Malaya and the Dutch East Indies to the Japanese, rubber became scarce. To obtain a pair of gumboots you had to prove you owned at least 12 cows, and a hot-water bottle required a doctor's certificate, as these were reserved for the sick and injured. In hospitals night staff had to make their rounds with candles and storm lanterns because torch batteries were so scarce. Even simple things like combs became unprocurable, a problem for women with the high-maintenance hairstyles of the 1940s.

With so many colleagues serving overseas, dentists were overworked. To make an appointment, you had to book three months ahead and put up with minor pain until it was urgent. The shortage, though, proved a boon for children whose parents could not afford dental treatment. In 1941 dental nurses were finally given permission to work on children's front teeth, something dentists had strongly opposed for financial reasons.

In the *Gazette*, dental nurses were urged to help the war effort by conserving their supplies.

> Take a packet of burs in your hand and you hold a microcosm of our whole economic system. What are burs made of? FINEST STEEL . . . Steel is a vital factor in this great struggle for victory.
>
> Let us consider the other stores in our cupboards. Mercury — precious and hard to procure . . . save every drop of that precious mercury to be redistilled.

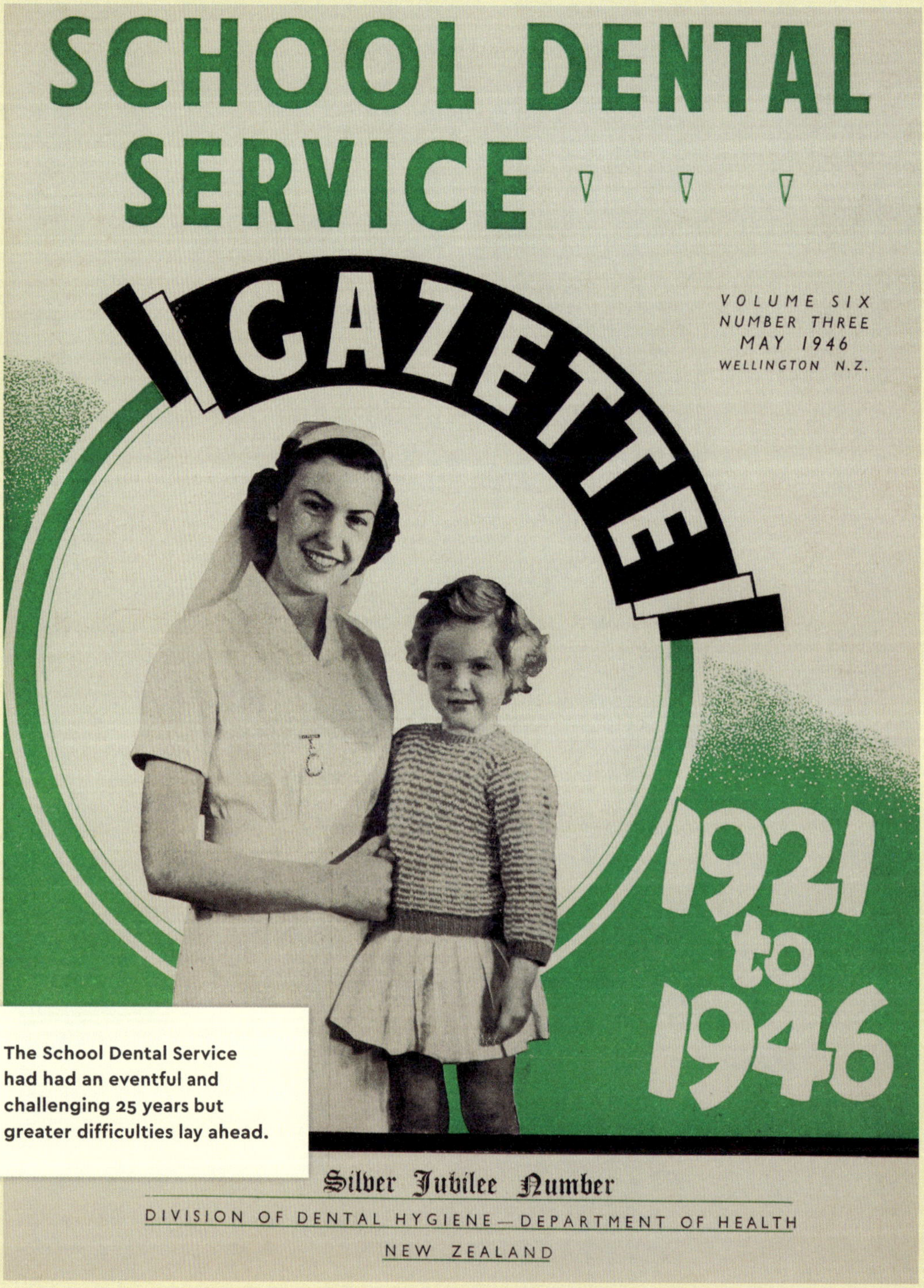

The School Dental Service had had an eventful and challenging 25 years but greater difficulties lay ahead.

> Cotton — we have cotton wool, cotton wool rolls and gauze among our stores, and the chief source of cotton-supply these days is from Egypt, thence to England to be made up into the materials we know. Think of our boys fighting to keep those vital places free.
>
> We use silver amalgam, copper amalgam cement and zinc oxide — every one of them imported . . . Go canny with the drugs, keep them well corked, save our bottles when empty and corks too. Cork comes from Spain and Morocco: there won't be any more.[18]

At 11 a.m. on 15 August 1945, news reached New Zealand that the Japanese had unconditionally surrendered. The *Evening Post* quoted British prime minister Clement Attlee, who affirmed that 'the last of our enemies is laid low'.[19] The newspaper reported that 'Wellington got away to a split-second start with its VJ Day celebrations. Hardly had the first four dramatic words of the British Prime Minister's announcement died away than ships' sirens, locomotive whistles, motor horns, and minor noises broke forth in a lusty chorus of jubilation. By one minute after 11 o'clock showers of paper and streamers started to pour forth from tall windows, and quickly settled on the damp streets. Five minutes after the historic hour the main streets, particularly Willis Street, were jammed with people. It seemed as if everyone had spontaneously downed tools, and obeyed the natural impulse to gang up and celebrate.'[20] In the Willis Street clinic it was graduation day — a double celebration for graduating nurse Lesley Kerr. 'I remember all of us throwing our dental instruments into the air and really going berserk.'[21]

After the celebrations, however, the wartime shortages continued for most of the decade. For the School Dental Service the years ahead would bring the most serious and intractable shortfall — people.

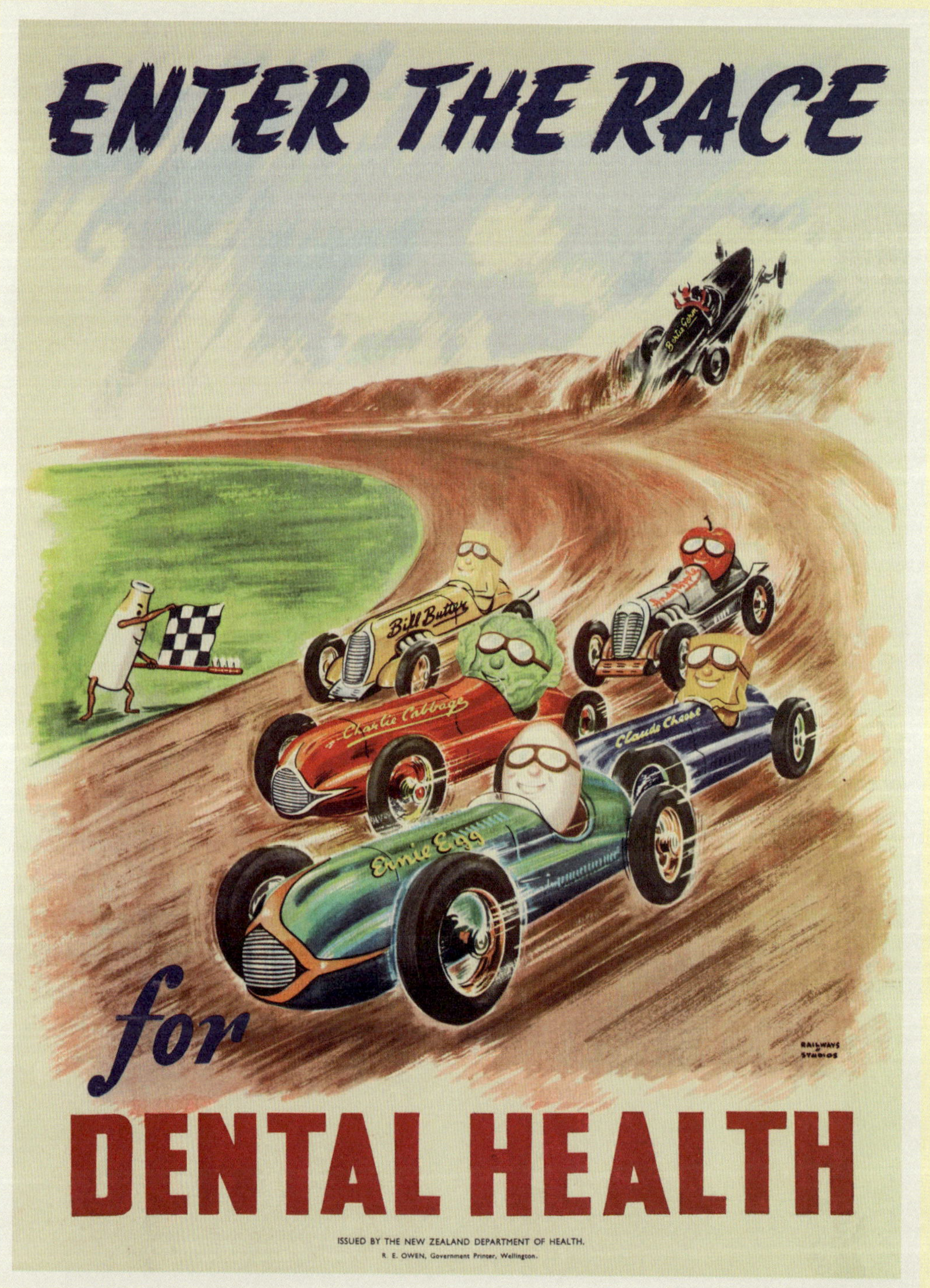
ENTER THE RACE
Bill Butter
Charlie Cabbage
Claude Cheese
Ernie Egg
for
DENTAL HEALTH
RAILWAYS STUDIOS
ISSUED BY THE NEW ZEALAND DEPARTMENT OF HEALTH.
R. E. OWEN, Government Printer, Wellington.

5

THE BABY BOOM YEARS

One evening in 1950 Pauline White, just turned 17, boarded the MV *Maori* at Lyttelton to travel to Wellington.[1] Like her parents, who were South Canterbury farmers, she'd never been to the North Island, let alone the capital. As she bunked down on the overnight ferry there was much to think about.

She was about to embark on a career as a school dental nurse. Had she made the right choice? At secondary school in Timaru, the head teacher had encouraged her to go to university. But she knew that was out of the question; she didn't even raise the possibility with her parents. With five other children in the family, money was scarce. As a dental nurse trainee, she would have an income. Small as it was, she reckoned she could be self-supporting. With such thoughts swirling through her head and the steady chug of the engines as the ferry ploughed through the dark waves towards Wellington, it's probable she slept fitfully. Before dawn, white-jacketed stewards were waking passengers with steaming tea in thick cups bearing the green Union Steam Ship Company crest and a water biscuit to nibble on.

Later, in the early morning light, passengers gathered on deck as the ferry entered Wellington Harbour, past Barrett Reef, where three years earlier the *Wanganella* had run aground and been stuck for 18 days and where 18 years later the *Wahine* would founder with the loss of 51 lives. The ferry slipped into the busy port, through the freighters and passenger ships, all with their distinctive coloured funnels, berthing at the inter-island wharf at 7 a.m. sharp. Had Pauline been familiar with the city, she might have caught a glimpse of the Willis Street clinic where she would spend the next two years. If she was a little apprehensive about the prospect, the health department booklet *The School Dental Nurse* had been reassuring: 'The career of a School Dental Nurse offers many attractions: good prospects, good holidays, and good pay . . . Life is varied and happy . . . with plenty of opportunities for recreational activities such as swimming, basketball, hockey and other sports.'[2] There were many pictures of nurses happily engaged in work and study or relaxing in the nurses' lounge and hostel. The booklet was in sharp contrast with the more prescriptive one issued 10 years earlier that spelled out the rigorous curriculum trainees would have to master, emphasised personal responsibility and warned of the need for 'full cooperation with those in authority'.

Times had changed. In postwar New Zealand, employers could no longer afford to be so dictatorial; workers, especially women workers, were in short supply. American writer James A. Michener pinpointed the issue in his 1951 book *Return to Paradise*.[3] Michener, who'd spent time in New Zealand as a naval intelligence officer during the war, returned in 1950 to write a sequel to his bestseller *Tales of the South Pacific*. He was flabbergasted at the 'ridiculous' competition for workers in postwar New Zealand:

> Employers must bribe help to work and are lucky if beginners stay long enough to learn a trade. Consider one advertisement of thirty-nine lines, begging girls to come to work. Twenty-five relate to the bonus system, the newly decorated tea room, provisions for time off, assurance of constant radio music during working hours plus the plea, 'Bring your parents with you if you would like their opinion of the working conditions.' The ad ends: 'What Girl Could Ask For More?'
>
> Apparently many do, because another shop offers, in addition to the above: free permanent waves, daily carfare, taxis home on late nights, tickets to the movies twice a week, and — illegally — an extra two weeks' pay above vacation pay if the girls will consent to report to work on Monday after the annual holiday!

It wasn't just shops that struggled to attract female staff. Upper-class families found it difficult to get decent hard-working servants, unlike during the Great Depression. Workers had other aspirations. In this 'socialistic paradise' that was closed for business on weekends, Michener wondered who would do the work as the country was loath to take any immigrants but British. 'Tragically, of every hundred Englishmen who do arrive as immigrants, as many as forty go right back home. Their reasons: no houses to live in; the beer is too weak; we can't stand those dreadful New Zealand weekends.'

Since the war New Zealanders had been breeding like Central Otago rabbits. However, the baby boom, 'one of the the most spectacular in the western world',[4] boosting the population from 1.7 million to more than three million in the space of three decades, came too late to relieve the chronic labour shortages of the 1950s, though it did create an oversupply of customers for the School Dental Service.

To add to the problem, many women resigned from the service when their

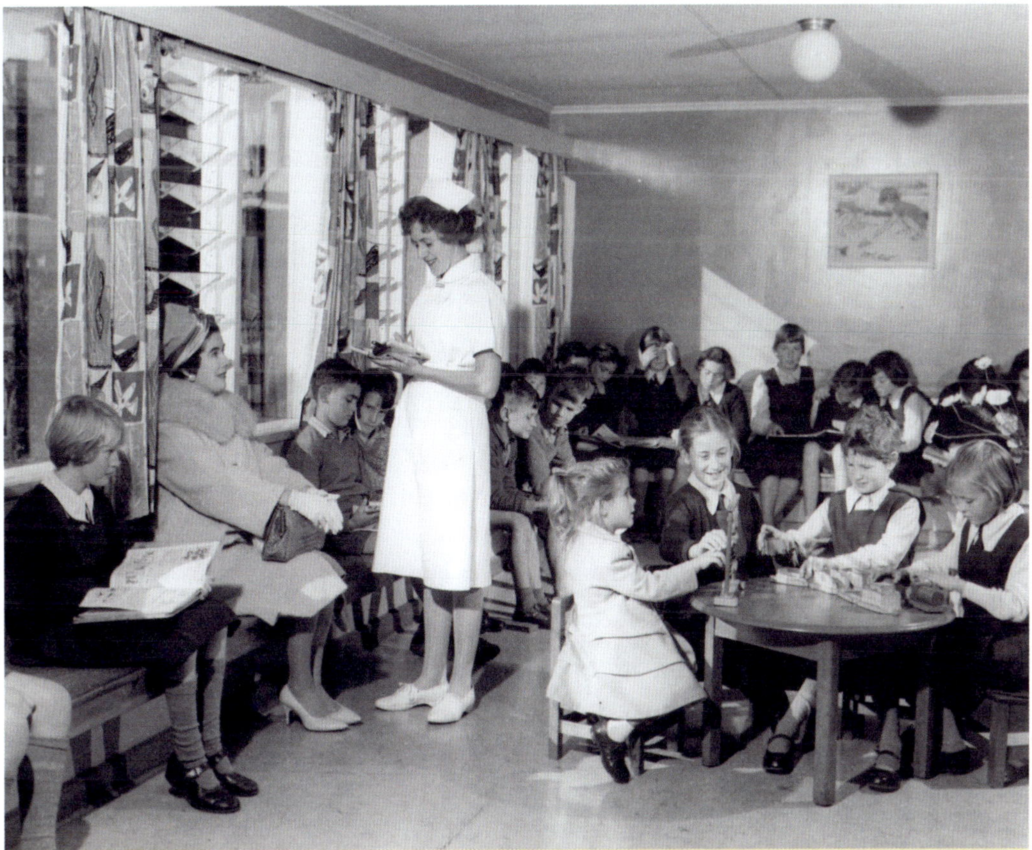

The baby boom years put a strain on the services — too many mouths to drill and not enough dental nurses.

husbands returned from the war. Men regarded it as a slight to their manhood to have their wives go out to work, and women may have felt they had enough to do keeping house and caring for children. Certainly they weren't sitting around drinking endless cups of Bushell's Coffee Essence, 'the fragrant answer to a housewife's dream'. Housework was hard slog without labour-saving devices. The family washing took a whole day: first chopping wood to heat the water in the copper, then scrubbing clothes on a washboard, rinsing in cold water and laboriously wringing out each item by hand before hanging it out. Ironing took another day since there were no easy-care synthetic fabrics. In 1956, over 40 per cent of households still did not have an electric washing machine. Then there was the shopping: with no refrigerator, no supermarkets and no weekend shopping, women made the rounds of grocer, greengrocer and butcher three times a week. It was time-consuming putting food on the table, though radio advertisements promised women could 'see less of the kitchen and more of the family with Gregg's Instant Puddings'.

Women who had to work to supplement the family income found workplaces were far from female-friendly. Though the government was forced to change its position and allow married women to be permanently employed in the public service, it continued to discriminate against them. Until 1971 women were taxed at the higher secondary rate and were ineligible for the concessions available to married men. Often overlooked for promotion, they were also paid less than their male colleagues. (This gender pay gap remained legal in the public sector until it was abolished by the Equal Pay Act of 1960; pay equity — under law, at least — extended to the private sector in 1972.)

With only a small pool of women workers, the School Dental Service faced stiff competition from teaching and regular nursing. In 1953 the National Film Unit produced a lavish colour recruitment film entitled *A Friendly Career*.[5] 'Schools throughout the Dominion are preparing girls for adult life . . . few girls will wish to remain at home until the wedding march ushers them into a home of their own, so upon leaving school they'll be faced with a choice . . . For careers being made available to girls today there is none more congenial, more satisfying than that of a school dental nurse.'

Pauline White found it congenial. Certainly, the discipline was strict, but she'd been used to that after her years at Sacred Heart Girls' College in Timaru. One incident stood out in her training years. One morning she arrived at the clinic not feeling well and was told to spend the rest of the day getting some sun on the roof. 'I came out in a rash and they took me down to the doctor. They knew straight away it was measles and I was taken by ambulance to the Fever Hospital.' The isolation hospital set among trees on the top of Mt Victoria had first been used to house ill returned servicemen from the First World War. In those days, before vaccination and immunisation, it quarantined patients suffering from scarlet fever, measles, influenza, chickenpox and later epidemics, including polio. In the early 1950s, though, it was practically empty.

'I was put in a ward of eight beds and I was the only one in it,' Pauline remembers. 'The place rattled and banged in the Wellington wind all night. It was really the most scary place to be in on your own. The nurse didn't want contact with me, she'd just bring the meals and run.' The hospital was later said to be haunted by Sister Slippers, the ghost of a nurse who shuffled through the wards in her slippers after dark. Pauline

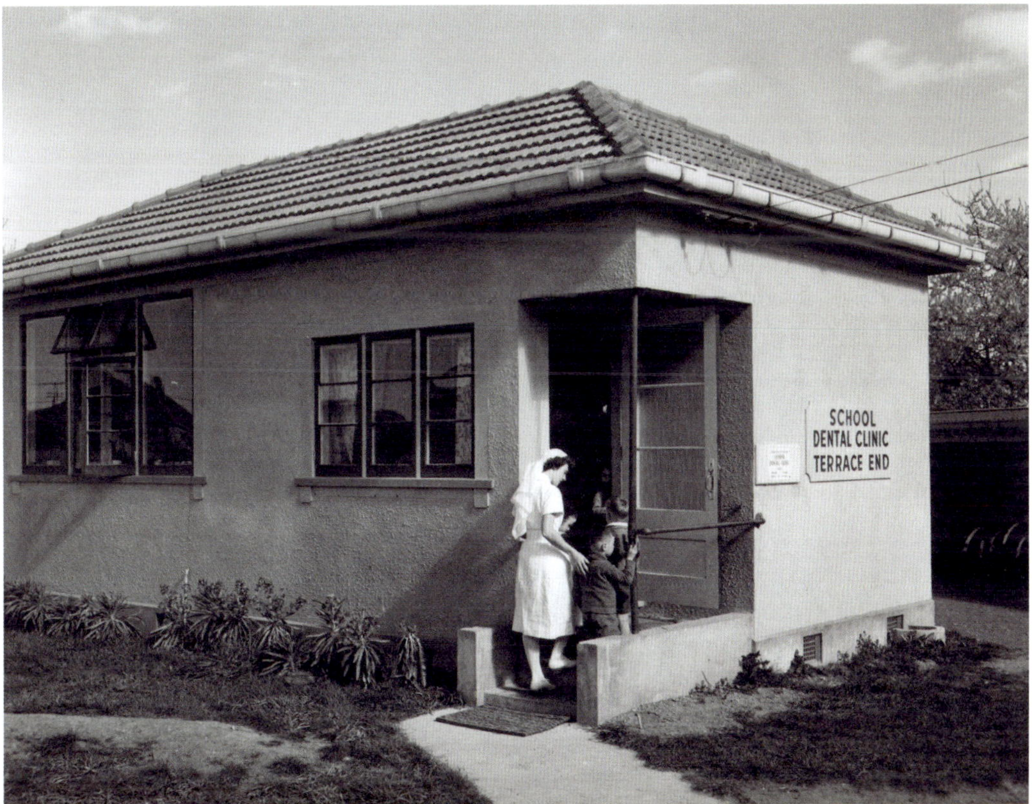

Terrace End dental clinic in Palmerston North. Dental clinics were on school grounds but often far from the main buildings.

did not see any ghosts, but was relieved when she was able to return to the hostel. A week later she contracted chickenpox and was quarantined in the hostel for a week. It was an occupational hazard. 'When you're a nurse you're exposed to everything, poking in people's mouths you have a greater chance of picking up things.'

Just 19 when she graduated, Pauline was dismayed to be posted to a sole charge clinic in Dunedin. 'They were so desperate in my day for nurses that you were sent to wherever was the greatest need.' Six months later, she was posted to the small settlement of Tokanui, some 60 kilometres from Invercargill. It was a lonely life. She boarded with an elderly woman and her brother. Social life was non-existent.

'The [community] hall had burned down so there was nowhere to meet. It was a dry [alcohol-free] area, too. I could go into Invercargill after work on Friday night but I had to come home again on the nine-o-clock bus as there was no bus out there until the afternoon of the following Monday.'

The work was relentless. 'I had about six contributing schools and the children had the worst teeth I've ever struck anywhere. I was getting children who needed massive extractions.' She'd trained on an electric drill, but all the work now had to be done on the treadle drill. 'If you can imagine standing on one leg and treadling with the other all day it was not very good for the spinal column. It ruined my back, and I've had that ever since.' She also contracted glandular fever, possibly from a patient, and was off for six weeks.

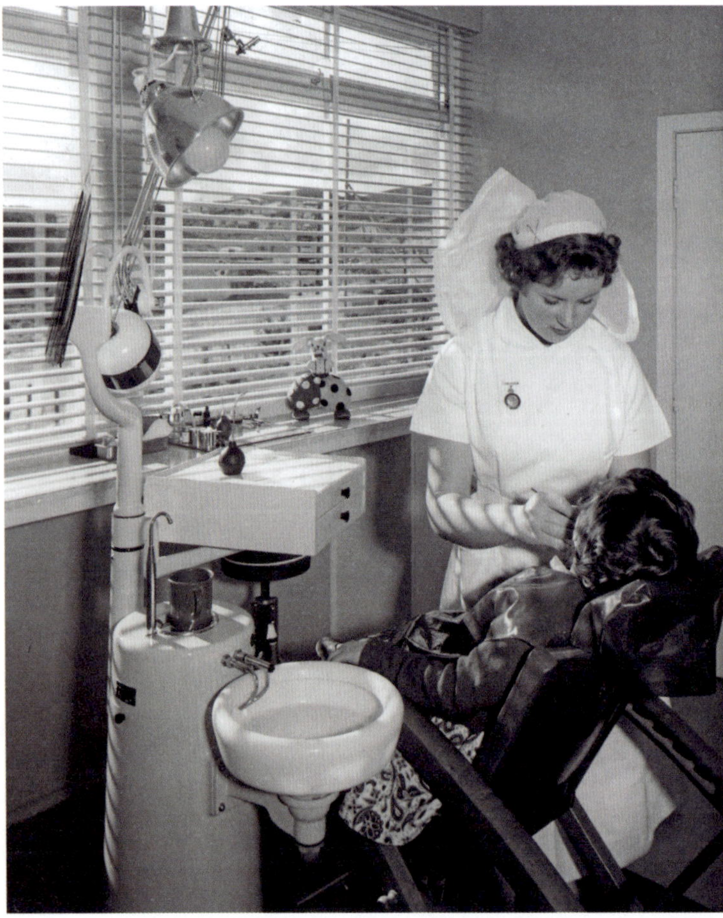

By the 1950s, clinics were starting to become better equipped with electric drills, but many dental nurses still had to rely on the pedal-powered drill, especially in rural areas.

Like most dental nurses she deplored the clinic nickname 'murder house', but admits that dentistry in those days was far from gentle. 'We knew it was painful for them and that made the job emotionally difficult too. You didn't want to but you knew you were hurting them to a degree to make things better for them.'

In *The Dreaming Land*, a memoir of growing up in the 1950s, Martin Edmond relived the experience of visiting the dental clinic.

> Another fear, far more justifiable, is of dental nurses and, by extension, of dentistry itself, which is incubated under the terrifying ministrations of one Nurse Cattell. She is a large, freckled, gingery, cheerful woman who expresses her gratitude to my parents for letting her board with us (where did she sleep?) by summoning me on a regular basis to the Murder House, there to drill and fill the gaps between every one of my twenty-odd baby teeth. I have the metallic taste of fillings always in my mouth and when I smile it is a metal smile. Certain constants enter my days at school: the dread of anticipation: that sinking feeling when a child returns from his or her spell of torture and my name is called; hours spent reclining in the chair with my mouth open, watching the woven steel cables whirr fast and then slow above me while Nurse Cattell pumps the pedal-powered drill with her feet. In my desperation I set myself to memorising the coloured poster on the wall called *Enter the Race for Dental Health* in which Bertie Germ, in a black racing car, crashes out while Arnold Apple, Bill Banana, Claude Cheese, Charlie Cabbage and Ernie Egg zoom past the winning post where a bottle of milk waves the chequered flag. I don't know when or even if my parents become aware of this unfolding atrocity; nor when Nurse Cattell (I always think 'cattle') leaves us.[6]

Pauline White spent the early 1950s moving from clinic to clinic in the lower South Island. 'If you got through the work before the next six months review you'd be transferred to another clinic, which happened to me.' It was a busy time with pockets of excitement. Pauline remembers how the whole country felt elated when Edmund Hillary planted the Union Jack on the summit of Everest in 1953. With his donkey smile, the Auckland beekeeper was no advertisement for New Zealand dentistry, but to his credit his teeth were all his own. Americans were later to marvel that a celebrity could have such bad teeth.

The excitement over Hillary's triumph was soon eclipsed by the imminent visit of the newly crowned Queen Elizabeth and her handsome Greek husband Prince Philip, who arrived two days before Christmas 1953 and stayed for five weeks.[7] It was the first visit to New Zealand by a reigning British monarch, and the spruced-up country was a riot of Union Jacks and red, white and blue bunting. Sheep were dyed red, white and blue. Householders were advised when and how to plant blue lobelias, red salvias and white begonias. The queen got a taste of the boring, dutiful life that lay ahead of her when she visited 46 towns or cities and attended 110 separate civic functions. Everywhere, thousands who had stood for hours along the route frantically beat the air with paper flags as the queen's cavalcade passed. Pauline was in Invercargill, the last stop on the royal tour, and there she was, waving from the balcony of the Grand Hotel. Pauline remembers it as one big happy Southland party. The *Southland Times* reported: 'Invercargill was thronged by one of the biggest crowds in its history, an eager and excited crowd which today will gather to welcome the Queen to the southernmost corner of her wide Empire.' And then she was gone. Thirty-eight days of visits to dairy farms, hydroelectric stations, irrigation projects, woollen mills, canneries, car assembly plants, race tracks and hospitals. But alas, not to the School Dental Service. Colonel Saunders was despondent: 'It was a matter of great disappointment, at least to all in the service that Her Majesty was not afforded the opportunity of seeing a type of dental health service unique in the British Commonwealth, and essentially of New Zealand origin.'[8]

Disappointment aside, the unique service did attract lots of praise from overseas delegations of dental experts, although one expert, Dr Allen O. Gruebbel, visiting on behalf of the American Dental Association, was less complimentary. It may not have come as a surprise: American dentists were opposed to state dentistry. In his report published in the association's journal in 1950 Gruebbel was blunt about the evils of the New Zealand system: 'Political, cultural and economic consequences of socialism are strikingly evident in New Zealand. Excessive social legislation has greatly increased the power of central government and has lessened individual freedoms; it has encouraged mediocrity and has stifled the urge to excel; it has discouraged personal initiative and has caused heavy dependency on the State for individual needs; it has immensely increased the tax burden and, thereby, has reduced opportunities for capital investment in individual enterprise and commercial expansion.'[9]

Such statements made it easy for Saunders and the health department to dismiss Gruebbel's discourteous report as an extremist view, but they also ignored valid criticisms. Gruebbel had described dental clinic material and equipment as inadequate and old-fashioned. He also identified the big weakness in applying a military 'theirs not to reason why' approach to training people entrusted with the dental health of the country's children.

> The deliberate effort to create a subprofessional outlook and attitude among school dental nurses is paradoxical and illogical. Although the school dental nurse is expected to provide a scientific health service, a considerable portion of which is of a surgical nature, she is given no scientific training, she is not encouraged to read scientific books or publications and she is not given an opportunity for continuing her dental education. School dental nurses are expected to diagnose Vincent's disease, gingivitis and anomalies, but they are given very little scientific training for making such diagnoses.
>
> School dental nurses are trained to perform the mechanical operations involved in cleaning, filling and extracting teeth. The scientific aspects of these operations are deliberately excluded from the course of instruction in order that school dental nurses will not develop an attitude that they are members of a profession . . .
>
> Parents in New Zealand have a false sense of security regarding the dental health of their children because of the belief that their dental health needs are being met. The public cannot be expected to know dentistry's role in a complete health service so long as dental treatment for children is limited largely to filling, extracting and cleaning teeth.[10]

New Zealand parents were, however, more than happy to send their children to the school dental nurse. Since most demand was coming from Auckland, a dental school was hastily established in Mount Eden Road in 1952. Auckland dentists soon had student nurses turning up to collect their patients' discarded teeth. One beautiful day Nurse Dale Morton set out for Queen Street with her brown paper bag and preserving jar with screw-top lid.

> It gave me an opportunity to wear my newly acquired two piece grey suit. This had a pencil slim skirt with black wool fringes in layers down one side and a smart little weskit top. To brighten off my ensemble I topped it off with what must have been one of the world's most ridiculous hats. It would have been a knockout at the latest royal wedding. It was a boater covered with bright orange chook feathers. It was hideous but I thought it most chic at the time. Up and down flights of Queen Street dentists I wafted in my 'haute couture', adding to my foul Dettol-floating brew of brown stained decayed teeth at every practice stop. Unfortunately I must have not screwed the lid on tightly enough. As I passed the main doors of the prestigious Smith and

> Caughey's department store the soggy brown paper bag let go of its odorous contents. They spilled out with a hideous crash all over the pavement, floating in the stinky pink Dettol.
>
> Quelle horreur! What was a girl to do? I hurriedly retrieved the remains of the glass and paper and took off. Teeth were scattered for yards and I was not going to scramble around on hands and knees picking them up. My red face would have clashed horribly with my hat and I must move on and compose myself elsewhere. After gazing vacantly into shop windows further down the street I felt sufficiently recovered to return and watch what the elegant customers of Smith and Caughey were making of the unusual street decoration. I remember having to stifle my laughter as I pretended I was waiting for someone. Bewildered business men in tailored suits, chic young things on their lunch break, all gave puzzled glances at the pavement! I will never know how they rationalised the dozens of horrible little blobs crunching under their shiny shoes. In those days Queen Street was quite elegant.[11]

Along with more training places, dental nurse recruitment was stepped up, with advertisements in the press, stalls and shop window displays. Dental nurses were constantly urged to '[d]ouble your contribution to New Zealand Dental Health by recruiting another suitable Dental Nurse'. A recruitment drive started in schools on a principle similar to the Jesuit tactic of catching them young: 'It is often at a very early age that career decisions are made, and impressions of a well-conducted and happy clinic will imprint themselves firmly on the young mind,' nurses were told. It would be their job to encourage girls in primary and intermediate schools to become dental clinic monitors. The monitors were given a badge and sometimes a written-off uniform and veil, and helped out with chores such as sterilising and tidying the clinic.

Though the military discipline and regulations did not change, some concessions were made to make the service more attractive. Nurses no longer had to forfeit 100 pounds if they left before their three-year bond period was up. Uniforms, cardigans, shoes and stockings were provided at the cost of the department instead of being issued on payment. Nurses working in remote locations and in areas where living conditions were substandard received special allowances.

Just as dental nurses were struggling to keep up with the demand for their services, a magic bullet appeared that would stop tooth decay in its tracks — or so it seemed. In the early 1900s an American dentist, Frederick McKay, had discovered that sodium fluoride occurring naturally in some water supplies was staining children's teeth.[12] However, it also had a positive effect: it prevented tooth decay. Scientists hypothesised that adding fluoride to water supplies at lower concentrations would eliminate the staining effect while still preventing decay. In 1945, the city of Grand Rapids in Michigan decided to test the hypothesis by adding fluoride to its water supply at one part per million. Scientists reported an amazing result: tooth decay in children born after fluoride was added to the water was reduced by 60 per cent.

The School Dental Service took notice, and in 1949 instructed nurses to topically apply sodium fluoride to teeth as a routine procedure. In 1953 New Zealand became only the second country to experiment with adding fluoride to the water supply. To test the results, Hastings, which had its water fluoridated that year, agreed to be the guinea pig while nearby non-fluoridated Napier, with its identical water supply, would be the control. The experiment was to run for 10 years, and after just 27 months the health department was reporting 'spectacular results' of 50–60 per cent reductions in tooth decay among Hastings children.

One person who needed no convincing about the benefits of fluoridation was Auckland dentist John Colquhoun, who had closely followed American scientific studies on the topic. A softly spoken man with a strong social conscience, he saw fluoridation as a way to reduce disadvantage in dental health for those living in low-income areas. As an Auckland city councillor, he was able to persuade the council to fluoridate the city's water supply despite fierce opposition from some fellow councillors and the newly formed New Zealand Anti-Fluoridation Society.

In 1971 Colquhoun was appointed principal dental officer for the Auckland Health District. With access to the treatment records and dental decay rates of 98 per cent of the city's children, he was able to report a decline in children's tooth decay in the city following fluoridation. He found it gratifying that the biggest benefit appeared to be in low-income areas. Colquhoun quickly became the country's leading advocate of fluoridation. His health department bosses were so impressed that in 1980 they sent him on a world study tour so he could become their expert in the field and lead a campaign to promote fluoridation in those parts of New Zealand that had thus far resisted it.

Before he set out on his travels, health officials confided to him some unexpected data: school dental clinic records were showing that children's tooth decay was now declining at the same rate in both fluoridated and non-fluoridated areas. Nevertheless, they felt sure that when they'd collected complete data for the country it would still show the benefits of fluoridation, albeit not the 50–60 per cent previously claimed. The tooth decay decline in non-fluoridated areas they attributed to the use of fluoride toothpastes and fluoride supplements, and from fluoride applications to the children's teeth in dental clinics. As a keen fluoridationist, Colquhoun readily accepted their explanation, but on his world tour he discovered that health officials in the US, Britain and Europe had been puzzled by the same phenomenon: tooth decay was declining across the board without water fluoridation. Like their New Zealand counterparts, they were convinced that larger-scale surveys would still show the benefits of fluoridation.

Colquhoun returned to New Zealand, still an ardent fluoride advocate, and was appointed chairman of a new national Fluoridation Promotion Committee. Before throwing himself into the role of chief fluoridation promoter, he decided on some further research. As he later explained, he was shocked by what he found:

> I looked at the new dental statistics that had been collected while I was away for my own health district, Auckland. These were for all children attending school dental clinics — virtually the entire child population of Auckland. To my surprise, they showed that fewer fillings had been required in the non-fluoridated part of my district than in the fluoridated part. When I obtained the same statistics from the districts to the north and south of mine — that is, from 'Greater Auckland', which contains a quarter of New Zealand's population — the picture was the same: tooth decay had declined, but there was virtually no difference in tooth decay rates between the fluoridated and non-fluoridated places. In fact, teeth were slightly better in the non-fluoridated areas. I wondered why I had not been sent the statistics for the rest of New Zealand. When I requested them, they were sent to me with a warning that they were not to be made public. Those for 1981 showed that in most health districts the percentage of 12- and 13-year-old children who were free of tooth decay — that is, had perfect teeth — was greater in the non-fluoridated part of the district.[13]

Colquhoun was in a quandary. His professional reputation had been built on fluoridation, but he could not ignore this new evidence. The argument that children in non-fluoridated areas were benefiting from fluoride in other ways no longer

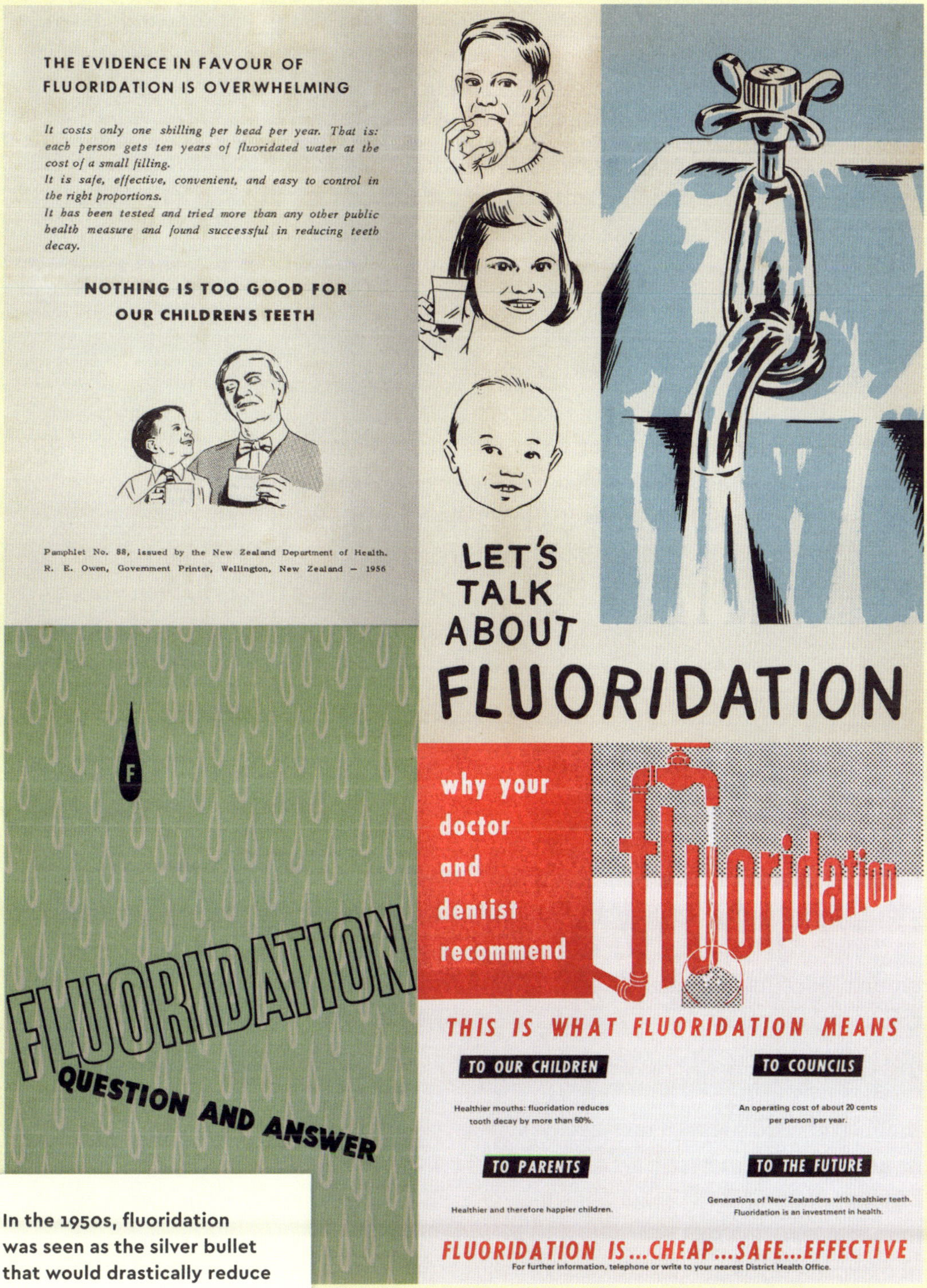

In the 1950s, fluoridation was seen as the silver bullet that would drastically reduce tooth decay in children.

seemed convincing to him. He knew that in Auckland very few children used fluoride toothpaste, many had not received fluoride applications to their teeth, and hardly any had been given fluoride tablets. Examining the records of the large numbers of children who had been treated in school dental clinics from the 1930s on, he found that tooth decay had begun to decline well before fluoridation had been introduced, and that the decline continued after all the children had received fluoride all their lives, so the continuing decline could not be because of fluoride.

Colquhoun also discovered that a quarter of the children in fluoridated Auckland had mottled teeth, or dental fluorosis, caused by excess intake of fluoride. It seemed to him that if fluoride toxicity could affect tooth-forming cells it might also affect other parts of the body. 'I could not persuade my superiors to do anything about the situation and finally I appeared on national television . . . We had the children there, the television cameras went into the clinics and showed the nation what fluoride is doing to the children's teeth. Of course that caused an uproar.'

Colquhoun felt he had no alternative. 'When you work in a health service and are promoting the health of children, in my case the oral health of children, and you suddenly discover that what you've been doing is poisoning those children — that was the crucial point in my career when I became publicly opposed to water fluoridation. When there is some possibility of harm as well as the mottling of the teeth how can you justify giving a dose to everyone in the community, infants, young people, old people in the water supply?'

He took early retirement from the Department of Health. After a lifetime of advocating for fluoridation, he became the poster boy for the anti-fluoridationists on whom he had previously poured scorn.

After retirement Colquhoun continued his anti-fluoridation crusade, acquiring a PhD in the history of fluoridation along the way and reviewing published studies on the subject. He argued that many studies had been poorly designed, with non-random selection of subjects and communities and inherent bias because they were conducted by ardent fluoridationists. His contribution was as welcome as a blowfly at a barbecue.

His investigations led him back to the 1953 experiment with school dental nurses that had excited so much interest in fluoride. Using the Official Information Act, he gained access to health department files related to the Hastings study.[14] He was astonished by what he found: 'In effect, it was a rigged experiment.' School dental nurses in Hastings had been given strict instructions to change their usual method of diagnosis on what constituted tooth decay. Before the experiment they had filled

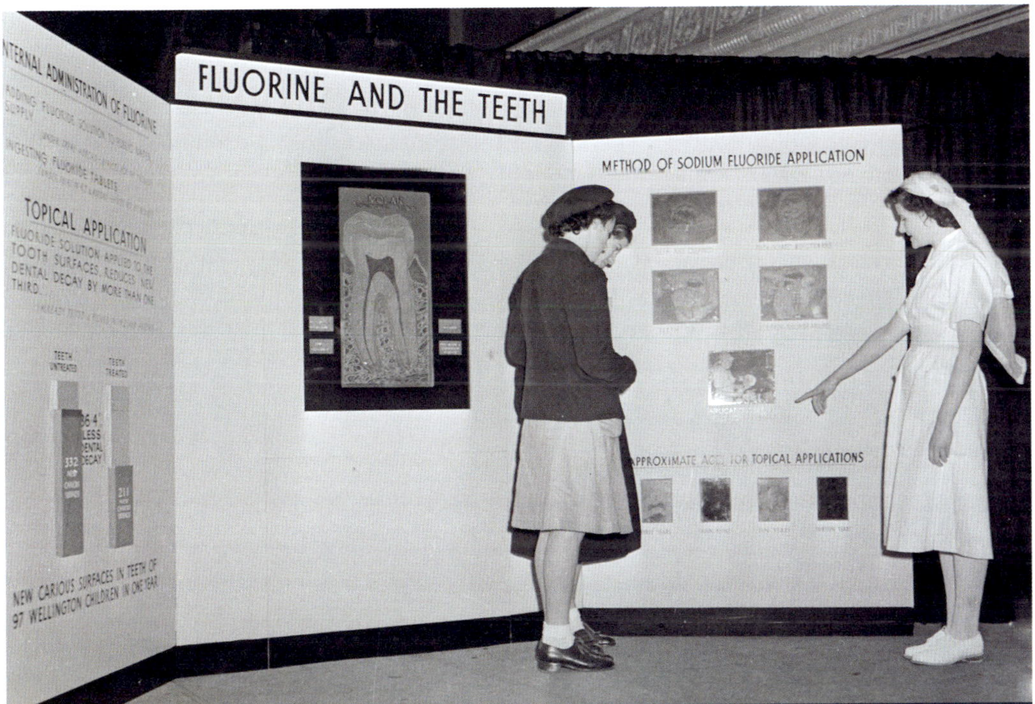

In the 1960s dental nurses were drafted as propagandists for fluoride at a time when water fluoridation attracted vociferous opposition.

(and classified as 'decayed') teeth with any small catch on the surface, before it had penetrated the outer enamel layer. After the experiment began, they filled (and classified as 'decayed') only teeth with cavities that penetrated the outer enamel layer. This moving of the goal posts brought about an apparent sudden drop in 'decayed and filled' teeth among Hastings children. However, when early results were compared with the control city, it was found tooth decay had actually declined more in Napier, despite the fact that dental nurses there were using the old, more stringent method of diagnosis.

How could this be? 'The claimed excuse,' Colquhoun said later, 'was that a previously unknown trace element, molybdenum, had been discovered in some of the soil of the control city, making tooth decay levels there unusually low, but this excuse is not supported by available information, from the files or elsewhere, on decay levels throughout New Zealand.'[15] Napier was dropped and the experiment continued without a control.

It is clear from Colquhoun's investigation that in 1953 school dental nurses were used to participate unwittingly in a rigged study by being ordered to abandon their meticulous method of diagnosis to make tooth decay appear less prevalent in fluoridated Hastings. Later they were drafted as propagandists for water fluoridation. An editorial in the *Gazette* in 1963 advised dental nurses to indoctrinate children with the aid of a new filmstrip called 'Fluoride Fairy':

> [D]esigned for our younger age groups, [it] introduces the subject in its true perspective as another important method of controlling dental decay. This is the starting point from which the next generation can learn to appraise its benefits through scientific facts. If all the suitable water supplies have not already been fluoridated, by the time these children have a voice in community affairs it will be too late for those who have not lived within its influence to gain very much improvement in their own dental health. With the greater appreciation of this modern approach, however, they will accept it in the same way as previous generations have come to accept the school dental nurse herself not for themselves but for their children and their neighbour's children.[16]

Water fluoridation attracted vociferous opposition from a wide spectrum of disparate individuals: scientists who worried that it could cause skeletal deformation, cranks who feared it would encourage left-handedness and effeminacy, personal rights advocates who thought it an affront to individual liberty. If parents believed fluoridation would protect their children's teeth, they argued, they could buy fluoride tablets.[17]

The Hastings experiment took place at the height of the Cold War. New Zealand troops had helped repel communist forces in the Korean War and later fought against communist insurgents in Malaya. The United States subscribed to the domino theory: that is, that communism, if uncontained, would spread across Asia. China was the first domino, toppling Korea, Vietnam, Laos and Cambodia. Next predicted to fall were Thailand, Malaysia, Indonesia, Burma and India.

In 1951, worried Commonwealth countries set up the Colombo Plan Co-operative Economic Development in South and Southeast Asia to counter the spread of communism. School dental nurses were co-opted to join the fight. Once the poor Asian masses saw how well their children's teeth were looked after, they would surely think twice about throwing their lot in with the communists. Students from Asian countries came to train in Wellington and New Zealand dental nurses were sent overseas to set up clinics and train local girls in school dentistry.

In 1953 Kath Salter, now a dental education tutor sister, agreed to go to Ceylon (present-day Sri Lanka) for six months to organise the treatment and running of dental clinics. Kath had toughed it out running clinics in remote parts of New Zealand, but nothing had prepared her for the chaos, squalor and politics of 1950s Ceylon.

On arrival, she was taken to a district health office:

> Dark dirty rooms with a clerk screwing up vitamin C and Aspro tablets in bits of newspaper, and decanting rancid shark liver oil into beer bottles and pushing them through the window bars to patients. Two senior medical officers (SMOs) were examining queues of children – swollen spleen, malaria, rough skin on legs – lack of vitamin B, whitish tongue and under eyelids – anaemia, or hookworm, swollen belly – pellagra or worms. The SMO took me to the Secretariat where I met two Directors of Health. The Government had changed and the previous man wouldn't leave for 6 weeks, till he had sorted every file in case anything could be held against him. The new man welcomed me but didn't know a thing about the proposed scheme. The SMO begged me to 'throw my weight about as much as possible, as when I left everything would fizzle' because the influential head of the dental hospital was very much against school dental nursing. As were all the dentists. There was no finance available and all the plans and specifications sent from N.Z. had disappeared.[18]

Some of the equipment was broken, but Kath had long had a No. 8 wire attitude and that wasn't going to stop her. To repair the handpiece of a drill she 'actually bought a piece of black-market telephone wire [cross-country lines were often denuded and the copper sold], filed it down with a nail file then tapped out the old rivet with the shaft of a straight bur. Replaced the new cog, tapped in the copper wire and smoothed it off.' She found that some equipment parts had been flogged to the Amalgamated Dental Company, so she went to buy them back.

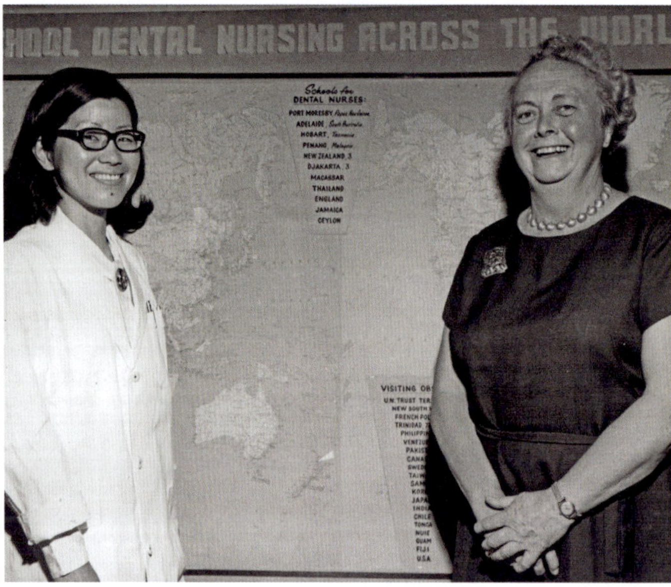

After setting up a school dental service in Ceylon (now Sri Lanka), dental health education tutor Kath Salter became the go-to person for overseas projects. She is pictured here in 1972 with Fumiko Toma, a dental officer visiting from Japan, before setting off for a five-year assignment in Jamaica.

> [It] was a tiny shop down in the slums where I threaded through the piles of rotting rubbish, sick cows, importuning beggars and stinking corners, which were obviously used as urinals! The nice Chinese gentleman took me to his wife's restaurant and kept topping up a huge glass of whisky and plying me with exotic dishes. He had heard I was trying to battle in a huge dental order and nothing I could say would persuade him it was a government order and nothing to do with me. He also smiled and waggled his head until I could see two heads!! An inexperienced drinker, I still think I did well not to pass out!

Once she had got six clinics functioning — 'begging material for uniforms, finding a little man in the slums who would make dental chair cushions' — she worked on setting up a training school and hostel, battling bureaucracy and scouting for suitable premises. Eventually Saunders, keen to learn how she was getting on, paid a visit.

> I was greatly relieved that Mr Saunders had visited, as I was in despair and felt no one in N.Z. would ever understand the horrendous problems. We were shown an empty building with the floors thick in bat and pigeon dung and cockroaches. One clinic had no windows and the only equipment was a dental chair without a head rest, the itinerant dental officers travelled from country

hospital to country hospital. The idea was to fix these shabby rooms up as a hostel. I could see Mr Saunders' eyes getting bigger and bigger.

Sick and dispirited, and feeling I might go home and everyone would say, 'Poor Salter, I guess she did her best,' when at the last minute I had to report with the lady SMO to an old building with 12 feet high walls, broken glass on top. This place backed on to the slums but was near the eye hospital. Could we plan it for NZ staff and order all the equipment for a classroom and dormitories for 15 students? and NZ would be asked to supply staff and technical equipment. My heart sank at the thought of teaching and living-in as virtually a house mother. However, I felt it was at least a start.

After her five years in Ceylon, Kath returned to New Zealand with amoebic dysentery and a reputation for getting things done. She went on to work in Jamaica and Guyana, lecturing in dental education.

Jackie Humm was 16 in 1957 when she left her home town of Blenheim to begin her training as a dental nurse. She flew to Wellington on an NAC Heron. After living in a small town all her life she was not prepared for the hustle and bustle of the city. 'It was a real culture shock. There were trams and buses going up and down and masses of people. I was really freaked out.'[19] Her mother stayed with her overnight at the Salvation Army People's Palace. 'When my mother left I cried all the way down Willis Street. I was petrified. It lasted all afternoon. It was so claustrophobic. I felt like a little girl lost in the woods.'

The dental clinic looked huge and very imposing. 'I hadn't seen anything like it before. Inside everybody was milling around, waiting, looking a bit lost. There was another girl from Blenheim and I stood by her.'

She was directed to live at the Hunter House, a hostel in Hobson Street in Thorndon. In the hostel there were four or five girls to a room. It was the perfect antidote to loneliness and fear of being adrift in a big city. She soon became knowing in the ways of hostel life and the necessary subterfuges. 'One matron came in and ripped the sheets off someone suspected of fire escaping. People went out quite often and they would stuff the pillow in their bed.'

That year Marty Robbins' 'A White Sport Coat and a Pink Carnation' topped the Lever Hit Parade. After the drab war years, colour was in. Being paid to train, 'thirteen pounds in our hands to spend a fortnight and nothing to pay back', Jackie was able to

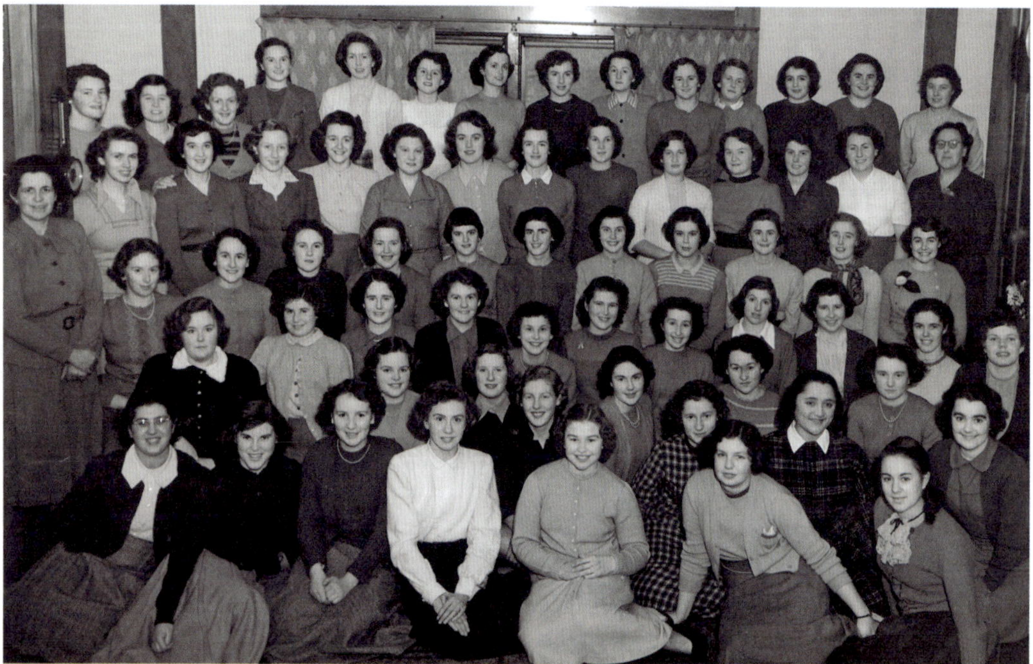

The intake of dental nurse students at the Hobson Street hostel, Wellington, in February 1950. Student numbers were 203 that year, but had doubled by the late 1950s as demand increased.

splash out on fashionable clothes: 'a very bright pink overcoat and a bright yellow one'.

Sex was being talked about more candidly than before thanks to the work of American psychologist Albert Ellis, who in 1958 published the influential *Sex Without Guilt*. 'The first book on sex education came out and we'd go up to the top floor of the training school and someone would read out parts of the book while we listened boggle-eyed. Sex didn't enter our world.'

Elvis Presley was scandalising respectable folk with a twist of his pelvis and his suggestive pout. The 'menace to young girls' was starring in a new movie. 'You had to be 18 to see *Jailhouse Rock* so we all dressed up and went down by tram to Courtenay Place in our very best. "Are you 18?" "Of course," we said and they let us in.'

Six months later Jackie was transferred to the public service hostel in Woburn, Lower Hutt. Commuting each day on the railcar unit to the Wellington Clinic didn't

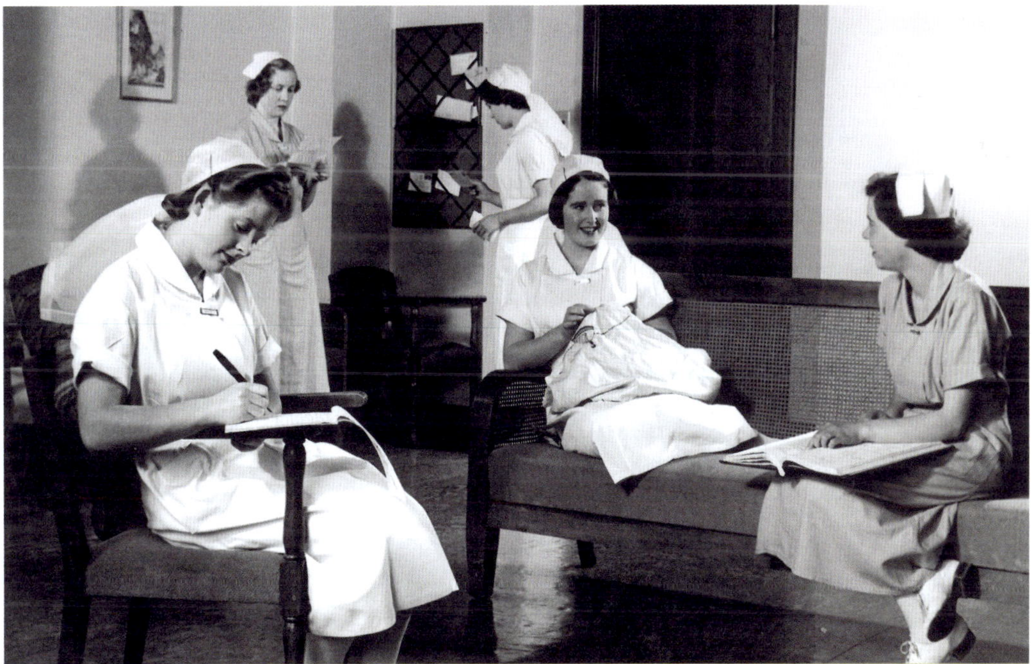

Student dental nurses in the lunchtime lounge at the Willis Street clinic, 1950s.

leave much time for a social life — not that much was on offer in suburban Lower Hutt. 'During the week we would go for a walk after dinner and buy an ice cream.' And curfews of 9.30 on Friday night and 10.30 on Saturday curtailed any social life in Wellington. Jackie spent her Saturdays lying in bed smoking. Sometimes she went out with boys who came over the hill from Featherston and Masterton, but any romantic trysts had little chance to blossom under the vigilant eye of the matron. 'It was hilarious watching the farewells at the door with the matron watching.'

The Woburn hostel became the setting for Maurice Gee's young adult novel *Hostel Girl*, a 'chilling story of obsessive love set in Lower Hutt' according to the blurb.[20] It features 14-year-old nurse Ailsa, the matron's daughter, who shares a room with beautiful and aloof room-mate Gloria, a trainee dental nurse. Gee based it on the experience of his wife Margareta, who lived in the hostel when her mother was matron there. Gee describes 'the dining room at half past five with the roar of 300 voices all around, the clatter of 300 knives and forks, and mutton, mashed potatoes, grey cabbage on the plate, with jam sponge and custard to follow'.

Ailsa dreams of a little house in Wellington, halfway up a hill, with the city down below, and a job, maybe in a government ministry; and 'no grinny nurses, shrieking nurses, crying nurses, or ones who thought they were too good for the hostel, no rules, no curfew, no peeping toms and no sharing a room at the start of each half year with someone you'd never seen before'.

At the clinic Jackie was getting intimately acquainted with teeth in a way she'd never dreamed of before. 'Teeth set in plaster so you could look at it from the side, the front, the top and get to know the shape of the tooth, the planes of the tooth.' Then it was time to recreate it. 'Soap carving used to take place in the lower depths of the training school and we used to sit and sing all sorts of songs while we did the carving. Songs from *The Student Prince*, which was popular at the time.'[21]

When Jackie finally got to work on actual teeth in real patients, she found the laborious process of inspection of her work at every stage frustrating and she felt sorry for her patients. 'You'd hold up your number until the tutor came, stand to attention, state our problem and then we were allowed to stand at ease. We were not encouraged to ask questions because we were young girls and didn't have a brain really. We were handmaidens.'

Her first patient was a boy with the unforgettable name of Ramsbottom-Isherwood. 'He had a three six — a six year molar — and I had to use the treadle engine to do the tooth. There was little in the way of anaesthetic and that poor boy made four visits of one hour's duration each until the tooth was completed. I'd do the prep work then I'd put zinc oxide into it and cover it up. Next week he'd get on the bus and come back. It was barbaric. No wonder there was a negative response [to dental nurses].'

Though electric drills were commonplace before the Second World War and were used in the Willis Street clinic, treadle engines continued to be used in the dental annexe in Tinakori Road. 'You put your foot on the foot control and you'd pedal like mad, try to go as fast as you could. The poor child sitting in the chair with their mouth open, everything going well and then you missed your beat and it would jump and go backwards.' The nurses wondered whether it provided exercise — 'we'd always stop and look at the right leg to see if the insole had grown'. It was 1962 before Jackie got to use an electric drill.

The training focused entirely on teeth and little on their possessors. 'We weren't given a great deal of information about how children grow, how they think, what fears

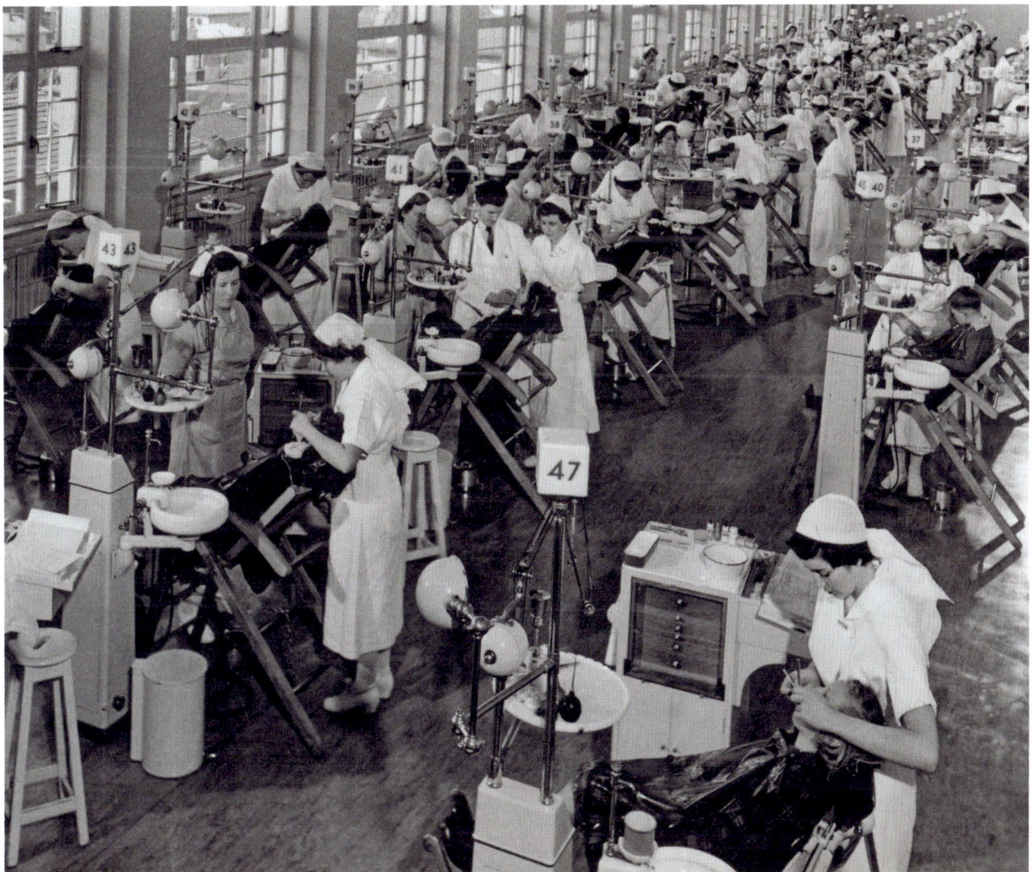

A busy day in the Willis Street clinic. Note the young dentist inspecting the nurse's work while she stands to attention, hands behind her back.

they had. We couldn't apply anything like that. We were there as dental nurses and we were dealing with teeth. Everything else was secondary. Some nurses would not have been familiar with children at all.'

Pain relief seems not to have been a priority. Posted to a South Canterbury clinic, Jackie quickly found that anaesthetics had been a serious omission in her training. Faced with a child with an infected molar that had to be extracted, she knew she would have to attempt a nerve block, something she'd never been trained to do. When infected teeth in the lower jaw need to be extracted, she explained, 'you cannot place a needle in the area of the infection. You have to give a nerve block and the whole area will go to sleep and you can remove the tooth. The infection is not touched and the cavity clears up and the child is over the problem.'

She knew the theory: 'the lower jaw is divided into two. You place the needle at the very back of the mouth, the soft tissue where a lot of nerves supply cheeks, tongue and teeth. It's a matter of being taught where to place the needle and the technique of moving it so that anaesthetic is dispensed at the back of the mouth and channelled so it affects the nerves that supply the mandible. There is a tunnel in the jaw and from that little tunnels run to each root below the canine and nerve. The mouth will go to sleep from front to back. It lasts a long time.' It took her an hour to administer the nerve block. Fortunately for the patient, her attempt was successful and she was able to extract the tooth without unnecessary pain.

Jackie got into dental nursing because her aunt was one and 'it just clicked'. Ngaire Mune drifted into dental nursing despite her first visit to the dental nurse turning out to be a big disappointment. It began when her mother's two sisters came to stay. 'Both of them had had their teeth out. It was quite a common thing that women would get their teeth out in preparation for marriage. A rite of passage, I suppose.' (At the time, even young women with a perfect set of teeth would have them replaced with dentures to spare their husband future expense. Getting a full set of dentures was also a popular twenty-first birthday present. And up until the 1950s, the standard treatment for periodontal disease was to extract all teeth and replace them with dentures.)

The young Ngaire was fascinated by her aunts' gummy mouths. 'You had to wait three months for the gums to harden before getting fitted with dentures. I just loved feeling their mouths because they dribbled a bit and they had black sockets and little pink bubbles. They said gum disease had caused decay so all their teeth had been removed.'[22]

In the summer of 1944 it was five-year-old Ngaire's turn to go to the dental clinic and her aunt took her. 'I said to my auntie, "It's a good job I've got my red twinset on" and she asked why. "So the blood won't show." I thought I was going to get all my teeth out. But the dental nurse said, "You've got a perfect set of teeth, there's nothing to do so you can hop down." I was not best pleased. I thought she didn't know what she was talking about, that I'd been short changed.'

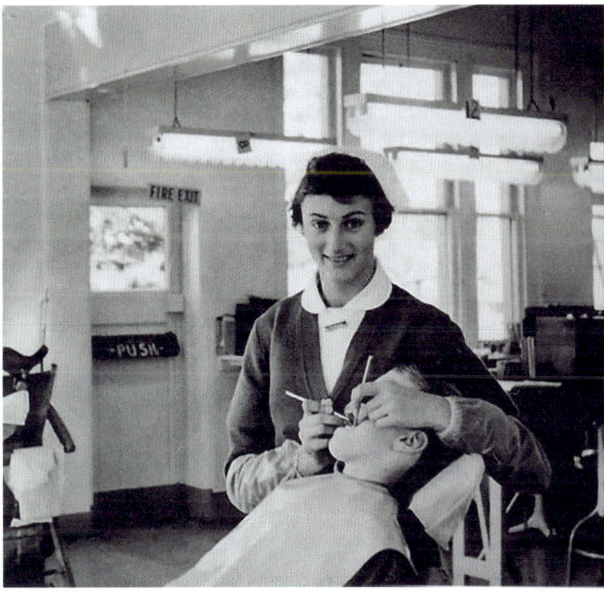

'I said to my auntie "it's a good job I've got my red twinset on" and she asked why. "So the blood won't show." I thought I was going to get all my teeth out.'

— Ngaire Mune

After this initial disappointment, Ngaire had no desire to emulate the dental nurse in her choice of career. 'A lot of the people [I went to school with] who became dental nurses were what I call dental nurse groupies, they always used to run errands for the dental nurse or they cleaned the clinic. I wasn't like that at all.' At 15 she was in the sixth form when her mother pulled her out of school. She'd enjoyed school and had her heart set on becoming a teacher. Instead, she went to work for the health department pricing doctors' prescriptions. By this time her parents were embroiled in a messy and public divorce. The court had ordered her to live with her mother, while her brother went to their father. A pharmacist friend in the department showed Ngaire an ad for dental nurses in the *Public Service Gazette*. 'He'd met my mother when she came into the office. She was a very troubled woman and he didn't like her. He thought that I'd be better if I got away.'

Ngaire applied and was accepted for training. However, the new Auckland training school had too many applicants. Was she prepared to study in Wellington? Ngaire was delighted to get away from home in Auckland. 'It was a bit of a gamble. In some ways it was a fortunate accident.'

Though conformity was a touchstone of the 1950s she found the School Dental Service had made a fetish of it. As a new junior student she was presented with a typed screed of rules. They ranged from the length of time they were permitted to take a bath, to conversation ('to be restricted to what is necessary in connection to the work'), to knitting, and to books other than textbooks ('must not be carried around in satchels'). Then there was the all-important method of address, which 'when speaking to a senior nurse or other student nurse is "Nurse —". Christian names are not permitted. Dental officers will be addressed as "Miss" or "Mr" using the surname. Dental Tutor Sisters will be addressed as "Sister" using the surname.' And:

> Students are expected to rise and stand to attention when spoken to on duty, or when addressing a member of the staff, another nurse, or a member of the public.
> The position of attention is defined as follows:
> Standing erect, feet together, hands clasped behind back.[23]

As she wrote later, 'Right from the start, the ABCDE of dental nursing was drummed into us regularly and emphatically — Attention to detail, Best behaviour, Conformity, Discipline and Excellence . . . I had great difficulty with the C word — conformity — a euphemism for total obedience . . . Why did I lose the right to use my Christian name? Why must I place instruments in the drawer in a prescribed manner if this does not suit my work process?'[24]

In a *Gazette* editorial titled 'Accent on Conformity' nurses were warned of the dangers of original ideas, which,

> however stimulating they may be, should not entirely exclude the orthodox, nor should the urge for change at any cost be given unlimited rein . . . insistence on conformity can be thought irksome by self-reliant and independent natures, yet, when applied in a logical sense, no more is expected than the voluntary submission to higher authority in the interests of a common cause; an attitude of mind which, it is hoped, officers at all levels in the Service will continue to adopt . . . [I]n the final analysis, however, there is no more valuable asset to the Service than individual loyalty and an earnest endeavour by all officers to conform to official practice. To regard unquestioning obedience, in these circumstances, as a surrender of personal liberty is to misconstrue the meaning of the term. Liberty, to quote an appropriate truism, is not freedom to do as one pleases, but the right to do as one should.[25]

Conformity, however, meant invisibility. 'As long as we conformed we were nameless and faceless,' says Ngaire. 'To prove this I bet several of my fellow students that if I turned up for duty with green eyebrows, but otherwise impeccably turned out, nobody would notice. Well, of course the children noticed and thought it was a huge joke, but otherwise my bright green eyebrows went unnoticed and unremarked. That was until the new principal [dental officer], an earnest young dentist, paid an unscheduled visit to the surgery where I was working. I was out of his view loading the steriliser when a fellow student dashed past and hissed that I'd better wash my eyebrows off — quick! And I did. Apparently the principal was overheard remarking to the tutor sister that my eyebrows were green. She vehemently denied that any of her girls would "be so silly". I lost the bet, but we all had a good laugh.'

It took a while for Ngaire to get used to hostel life. 'A lot of the girls liked the hostels because they came from boarding schools and it was what they were used to.' Hostels full of young women were a magnet for peeping Toms. She remembers how they set a trap for one:

> At 32 Hobson Street there was a big room at the top of the house we called the barn. It had eight or 10 girls in it, and one night somebody woke up and saw somebody peering in. I think he might have come two or three times. So the nurses rigged up a bucket with a mixture we used to put on ulcers. It was called acra violet, a purple and yellow colour. It was set to trip should he come up the fire escape. I don't know whether he had inside knowledge but the bucket tripped without catching anybody. Instead it trickled down the white paint of the building, which didn't make us popular.
>
> I was in a lean-to below. My roommate had one end and we were feet to feet, heads against the wall and all this excitement going on upstairs. We hung a sign outside our window, 'Peeping Tom, we're in here'. But he never appeared after that.

The acra violet may have been a useful peeping Tom deterrent, but another off-label use proved less successful. 'A friend of mind had black hair and of course we all dyed our hair because it was fashionable then. But her hair was so dark she couldn't get a colour that showed up. So she rinsed in acra violet to see if that would work. It worked so well that her scalp turned purple too. It wouldn't come off and she had to use rubbing alcohol to get it off, which burned her scalp. It also stained the porcelain wash-hand basin.'

Clockwise from top: An electric portable drill used when dental nurses had to travel to outlying schools; real teeth were collected and set in plaster of Paris, both in blocks and in dummy jaws, for students to practise drilling and filling.

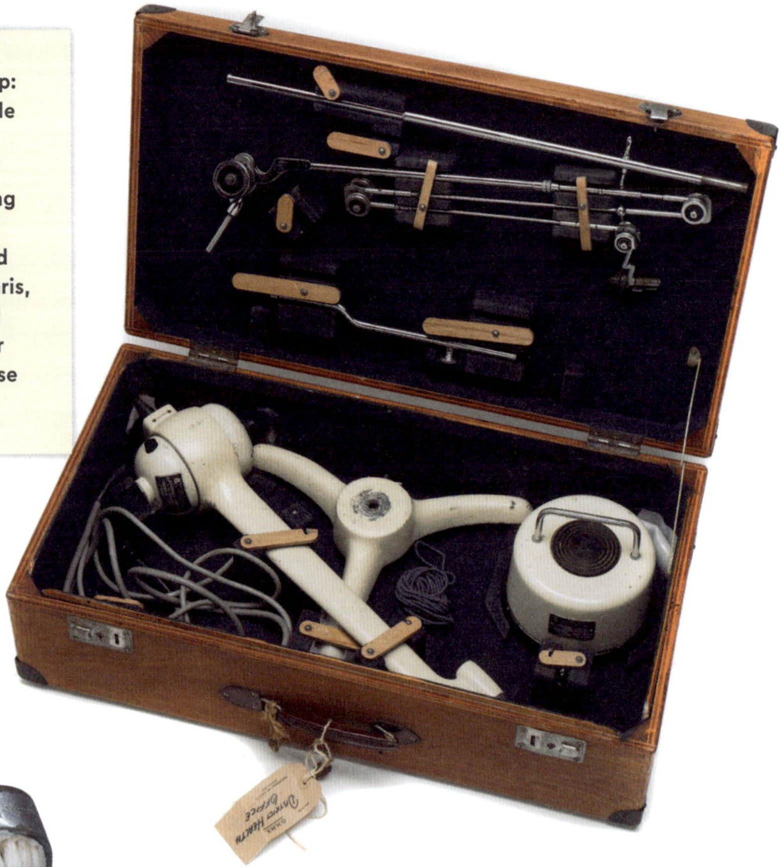

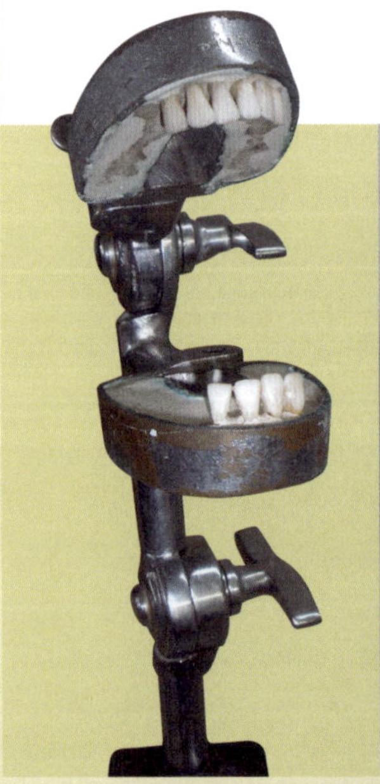

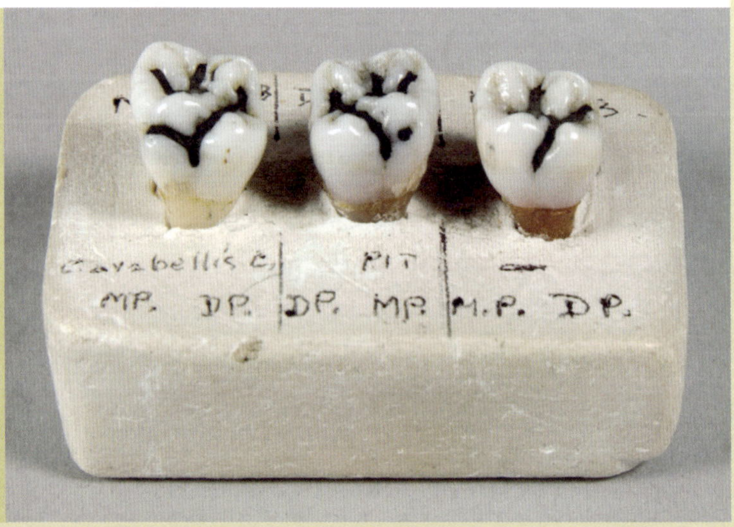

Within their curfew hours, the nurses did their best to live it up. There were plentiful party invitations from university student hostels. 'Once we got invited to a new restaurant opening, got drunk, danced on tables and never got invited back. My favourite tipple was Horse's Neck, a mix of brandy and ginger or Pimm's. The men swilled flagon beer.'

She was the only Aucklander and once a month there was the chance of weekend leave if you got a note from your parents. 'But no way was I going to go back home. Other girls covered me in their note and I went to a lot of different homes. The people were so nice to me.' In the Christmas holidays she hitchhiked round the South Island.

During her training, she struggled with the tooth-carving ritual.

> One of our first student assignments was to carve a set of deciduous and permanent teeth out of laundry soap. We were given a set of real permanent teeth on a wire ring, and a set of outlines for the deciduous teeth and our task was to reproduce realistic teeth exactly to scale. The only tools we had were three small carving instruments and a pair of callipers. Michelangelo may have said that every block of stone has a statue inside it, but believe me, not every block of soap has a tooth inside it. The trick was using a set of basic cuts, patience, and perseverance — delicate roots often snapped off so it meant starting over. In an era where no decent young lady went without a petticoat, rubbing the tooth with our nylon petticoats gave the perfect final polish.

From soap carving of teeth she progressed to drilling and filling real teeth set into plaster of Paris gums, in a dummy jaw that was 'a capricious animal with a tendency to snap closed on fingers, or swivel, and crash teeth first onto the bench'. After collecting teeth from local dentists — 'Some had huge, grossly decayed cavities, some had chunks of bone attached to the roots and some had shreds of torn gum floating around them like pale pink, diaphanous skirts' — she had the task of sorting and cleaning them, boiling and scraping off any residual soft tissue. 'We were responsible for setting up our own jaws, and we needed several sets. The teeth had to be put in the correct anatomical sequence, and correctly spaced and aligned. When the jaws were closed the occlusion (bite) was expected to be reasonably normal. This could be a frustrating task as the plaster of Paris gums needed to be the exact consistency. Too stiff and it set before all the teeth were in place; too soft and the teeth wouldn't stand upright.'

Operating on actual patients had its unpleasant side, too, when it was your week to clean out the slop buckets.

> Between each patient, individual spit bowls were emptied into a lidded, white enamel slop bucket that contained a coarse sieve. The sieve separated the liquid, made up of water, saliva, and blood, from the solids that were mostly pieces of gauze, cotton wool rolls, small bits of amalgam and extracted teeth. At the end of each day we would put the solids in the rubbish bin and then empty the viscous, gloopy liquid down the drain. The bucket, the lid and the sieve were scrubbed with soap and water and rinsed with Chenol, a thick, brown disinfectant made from coal tar, which had an intense smell, much like a powerful version of Jeyes Fluid, and clung to everything it touched. We affectionately called it Chenol Number 5. Chenol was harsh on the skin too, and we were provided with heavy-duty protective gloves to use. But we were more scared of the evil lurking inside those gloves than of anything we might find in the slop bucket, so most of us chose to tackle cleaning the slop buckets with bare hands.

Ngaire saw it as good training 'because when I graduated, I was required to travel into rural areas carrying with me my treadle drill, wooden chair, slop bucket and everything else I might need'.

It was 1959 and dental nurses were still having to use treadle drills invented a century before. In 1949 John Patrick Walsh, a New Zealand dentist who hated going to the dentist because the drills were uncomfortable and painful, invented the air-turbine high-speed drill. Lack of research funding, however, led to the drill being developed in America. As Tom Brooking writes, 'If the New Zealand Government had been more awake to the invention's possibilities, we could have claimed the dental drill for our own, even if the Wright brothers really did fly before Pearse!'

A 1959 *Gazette* editorial lauded the invention

> that dentists everywhere were turning to . . . when used correctly the rate at which enamel can be cut and the ease with which it is done has to be seen to be believed. The efficiency of the instrument is almost incredible but like all instruments that are manually operated it has its dangers. There is always the human element to contend with. The tooth cuts so quickly and so effortlessly that it is imperative to see precisely what one is doing at all times;

> to work by feel alone is barely possible . . . As far as the School Dental Service is concerned an early changeover to high speed equipment is unlikely. There are many good reasons why we cannot afford to be unduly hasty, and they are not all related to cost (although a simple multiplication of 800 times £240 would give some idea of what it would cost to equip every clinic at the present time).[26]

No mention of the unnecessary discomfort and pain that another generation of children would have to endure.

The School Dental Service management remained as stiff and immovable as the starched uniforms dental nurses struggled into on cold mornings. But a tornado of social change was gathering strength elsewhere, and sooner rather than later it would make landfall in New Zealand.

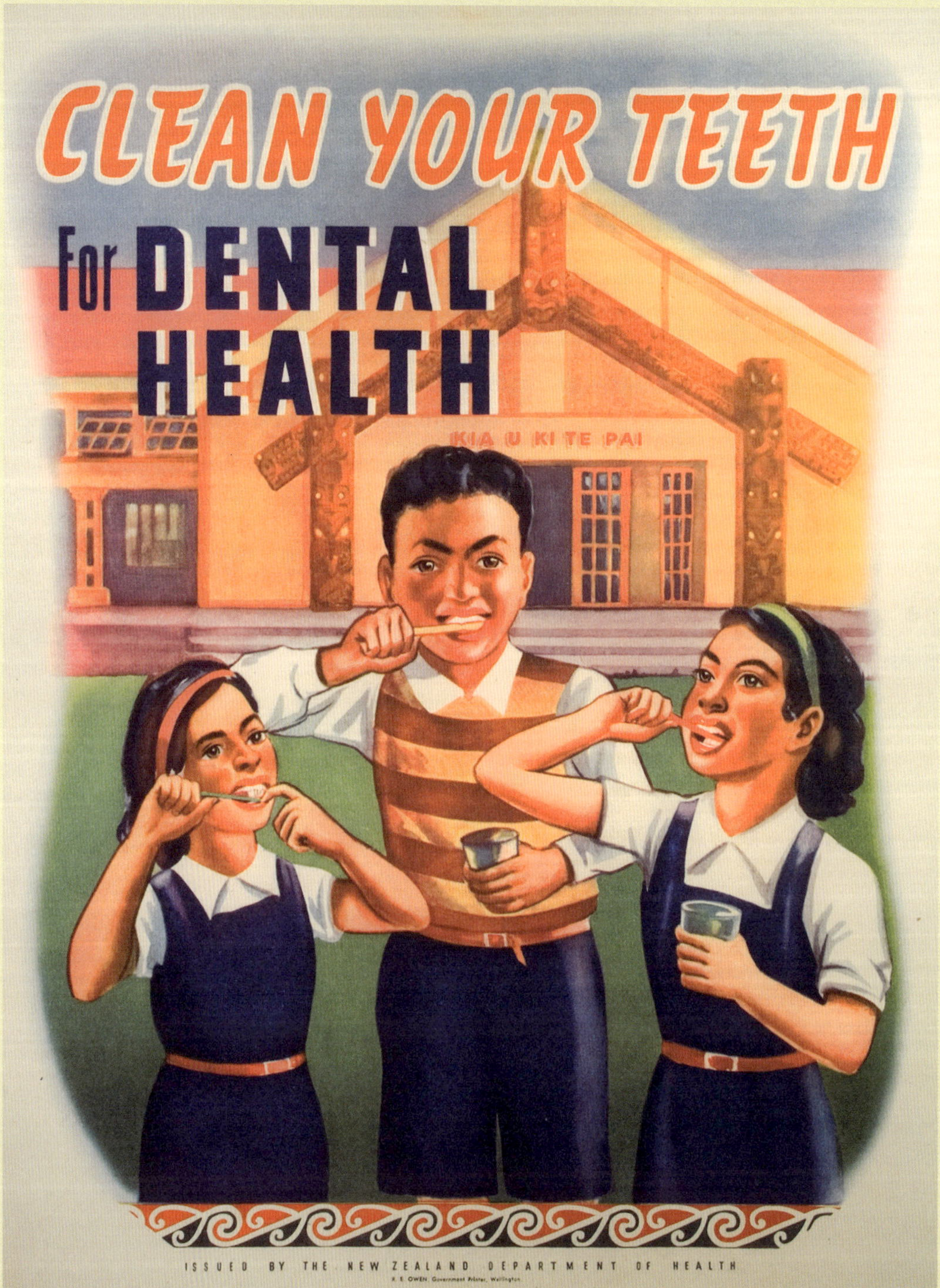
CLEAN YOUR TEETH
For DENTAL
HEALTH
KIA U KI TE PAI
ISSUED BY THE NEW ZEALAND DEPARTMENT OF HEALTH
R. E. OWEN, Government Printer, Wellington

6

'WE WERE COOKIE-CUTTER PEOPLE, REALLY'

Comedian Robin Williams once famously remarked that if you could remember the sixties you weren't there. For most people, though, who didn't 'tune in, turn on, drop out', the decade was unforgettable: a heady explosion of catchy music, liberating ideas, political turmoil, cultural upheaval and wild optimism.

Rebellion was in the air. Dental nurse trainees wandering through Auckland's Albert Park on a Sunday afternoon may have stopped to listen to the entertaining rhetoric of anarchist Tim Shadbolt, the bombast behind Ausapocpah (Auckland University Society for the Active Prevention of Cruelty to Politically Apathetic Humans). In Wellington, bohemian types frequented folk and coffee clubs such as Chez Paree, where local troubadours strummed and sang standards by Bob Dylan and Joan Baez. Later, on their way to the Willis Street clinic, the dental nurses passed Resistance Bookshop, a hangout for serious, bearded young men and young women in Indian peasant dresses, the smell of incense wafting from the doorway. In the window, titles that you wouldn't come across in Whitcombe & Tomb were displayed: *Karl Marx: Theories of surplus value*; *Baba Ram Dass: Be Here Now*; *Women's Rights: A practical guide.*

For dental nurses, there was only one book that mattered: *Department of Health School Dental Service Standing Instructions.* The big blue book of cyclostyled pages, published in 1966, was their bible. Like the holy book of fundamental Christians, it was to be observed as literal truth, not open to interpretation. Unlike the Bible, it was subject to regular amendments, all of which had to be recorded as inserted with 'Full Signature' and date. The index contained 422 different instructions, from 'Absence from place of employment, penalty for unauthorised' to 'X-Ray, Annual chest, for School Dental Nurses'. All these were to be 'strictly observed in all aspects'.[1]

Although school dental nurses were employed by the Department of Health and were under control of the district's principal dental officer, the lack of day-to-day male

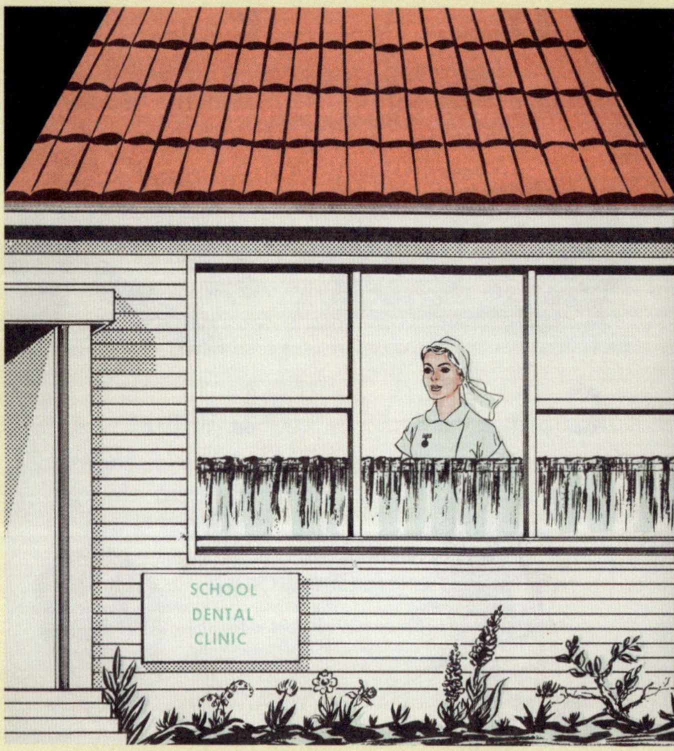

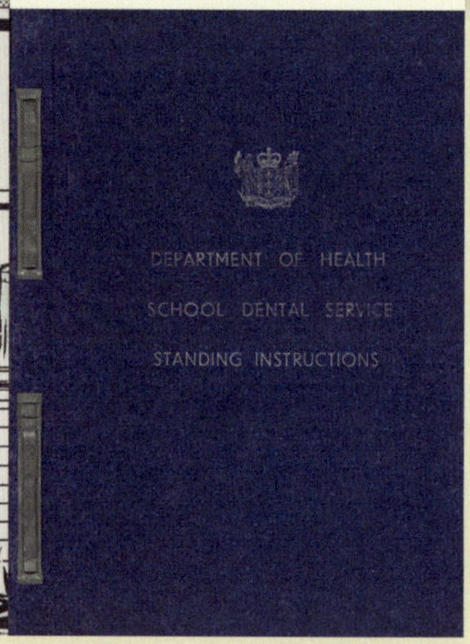

Left: A panel from a Health Department leaflet advertising the School Dental Service. Below: The dental nurses' bible, *Standing Instructions.*

supervision was considered an unacceptable risk, so the (usually male) head teachers of the schools they were attached to were enlisted to spy on them. 'Head teachers are authorised to exercise supervision over the dental staff attached to their schools to ensure correct observance of punctuality and hours of work and they are to bring to the notice of the Principal Dental Officer any shortcomings in these or other aspects.' Nurses were required to advise head teachers of their movements when visiting outlying schools. A nurse acting on her own initiative was not to be encouraged.

The dress code remained as formal as ever. 'The wearing of uniform in the street is not permitted except in the course of duty.' Nurses should note that 'wristlet watches, bangles, rings, including earrings etc. will not be worn whilst on duty. The white organdie veil will be worn forward and fastened in such a manner that it will not slip back while operating . . . Individual hair styles will not be acceptable as reasons for the incorrect wearing of the veil.'

And on it went. 'The medallion will be worn 3 inches down from the base of the neck and 2 and half inches to the right of the midline.' 'Tarnished medals should be regilded,' and 'the small cost must be met by the nurse'. 'Service uniform cardigans, if worn, must be buttoned over the uniform. Half sleeves are to be worn with the cardigan while operating. Half sleeves will not be worn without the cardigan nor are cardigans to be worn with the sleeves rolled up.' 'Service buttons are to be worn for fastening the belt.'

In a concession to the times, perhaps, nurses were allowed to buy their own white shoes — within reason. And what type of white shoe had you in mind, a shop assistant might innocently ask. 'Low or Cuban heel (not wedgies), straight, inner sole, lace-up canvas or leather uppers, these to be plain with rounded toe and without elaborate decoration or excessive openwork. Soles to be of leather or hard rubber (not sponge rubber).'

The department provided 'a personal issue of two pairs of white duty stockings' each term. Unlike other requisitioned store items, however, the department generously conceded that they should be regarded as personal items and need not 'be written off or otherwise accounted for at a later date . . . It is to be noted, also, that under normal circumstances articles of uniform are not to be requisitioned until those to be replaced are certified as unserviceable, i.e., "written off" by the Principal Dental Officer or the Dental Nurse Inspector.'

The department was less generous when it came to minor breaches of discipline. It warned nurses that under the State Services Act 1962 it could impose a penalty of up to £10 ($400 in today's money). As *Standing Instructions* advised, minor offences that could be penalised in this way included: overstaying leave, being absent without leave for short periods, being late on duty, failing to observe correct hours, having a clinic that was dirty or untidy, and being incorrectly dressed for duty.

In case they needed reminding, nurses were advised that 'slapping of unruly children is forbidden irrespective of the provocation. Officers who fail to carry out this instruction will render themselves liable to instant suspension from duty.' Dirty children, however, could be sent home. 'In cases where children exhibit lack of bodily cleanliness the attention of the head teacher may be drawn to the fact, with a recommendation that the child be sent home for necessary treatment before dental treatment is attempted.'

Every minute of the day's activities had to be logged. 'The whole of each working day from 8.30am to 4.15pm is to be accounted for in the Daily Record.' As well as keeping meticulous patient records, the nurse was expected to maintain an inventory of dental equipment 'kept ready for inspection' showing the correct quantity of each item on charge to the clinic. Drills, instruments and other equipment had to be oiled, cleaned daily or weekly. 'The cost of an engine arm, handpiece or any other item of equipment which has become defective through neglect may be a surcharge to the officer concerned.' Little wonder, then, that dental nurses dreaded the frequent inspections. There was wide scope for fault finding if that was the aim, and more often than not it was exactly that.

Throughout the 1960s, school dental nurses continued to model the subservience and blind obedience expected of them, and to accept the low pay and the inadequate resources that made their work harder and sometimes unpleasant for their patients. But a new generation of school dental nurses, less inclined to acquiescence, was pouring out of the training schools. It would take only a few individuals to light the fuse of their discontent.

When she began her dental nursing training in 1964 Pam Horncy knew nothing about the antiquated rules and regulations dental nurses were still expected to observe, though she was later to become a leading figure in the campaign to change them.[2] A lonely girl growing up on a farm outside Kaukapakapa, 80 kilometres north of Auckland, she was more interested in pop music than politics. From the farm 'up a skinny old metal road' the cataclysmic events of the decade were the faintest tremors. 'I was ironing a dress Mum had made to go to a cabaret with my brother's friend when the news came over the radio about Kennedy's assassination.' However, the sounds of sixties Britain and America — 'Love me Do', 'Big Girls Don't Cry', 'Summer Holiday', et al. — resonated, albeit tinnily, when her parents presented her with a transistor radio for passing School Certificate.

She'd latched on to dental nursing as a career when two dental nurses had come on a recruiting visit to the local high school. At 16, though, she was told she was too young. Not wanting to stay on at school, she found a job as nurse aide at the local maternity hospital. 'They used to lay the women on the side and my job was to hold a leg up. It was a dead weight. The women weren't concerned; they just wanted to get the thing out.' She felt privileged to witness the births, but had to leave because the irregular shifts played havoc with her body clock and she developed chronic insomnia. Until she was accepted for dental nurse training a year later, she worked in a shop. Enrolling in training school meant moving to a hostel in Auckland, but she'd already lived away from home while working as a nurse aide.

'It was a life ruled by bells, a bell to wake up, a bell for breakfast, at the training school a bell for lessons to start, a bell at lunch time, a bell to mark the end of lunch time, and so on.'

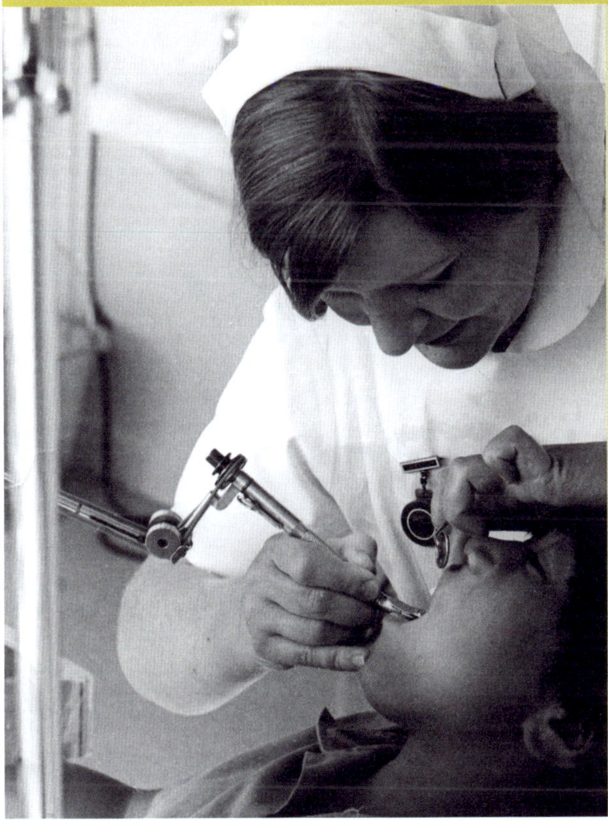

'We didn't use anaesthetic [for fillings]. When I think back I cringe. We never talked about the pain we were inflicting. It sits very uncomfortably. I guess we told ourselves it was for the greater good.'

— Pam Horncy

Pam adapted quickly to her new regimented life, but she found it hard to warm to many of the tutor sisters; she described them as 'hard old tarts. They were from a different era. They would have been confronted with working conditions and a worse state of dentition than we ever had to, so they had to be hard to deal with it all. They were particularly hard on people who were struggling with the actual practice. They didn't have any involvement in the theoretical side of it. It was all dental officers who taught and set the exams.'

She gained an insight into the problems earlier school dental nurses had had to face when, on graduation, she was posted to Northland, where she made regular visits to Te Hapua, a tiny settlement up the Cape. 'Te Hapua didn't have electricity but they had a little school so we had to get the milk truck to take up a lot of the equipment. We used Rockgas for sterilising and a treadle drill.

'We didn't use anaesthetic. When I think back I cringe. We never talked about the pain we were inflicting. It sits very uncomfortably. I guess we told ourselves it was for the greater good.' Still, the alternative was the prolonged pain of toothache, abscesses and extractions. Pam was proud of her work, of the profession. However, the wider world beckoned. Friends were leaving and returning on what cartoonist and columnist Tom Scott would later popularise as 'the big OE'. She boarded a ship to London, returning three years later via the hippie trail, and resumed work in a clinic in Henderson at the start of the next school year.

Maggie Morgan began her school dental training the year Pam Horncy graduated.[3] The two never met while training, but they would soon become comrades in arms and lifelong friends. The Auckland intake that year — 87 students — was huge and had to be split in two because the lecture space was inadequate. (The postwar baby boom was still putting pressure on the School Dental Service.) But even among that big intake, Maggie stood out: the blue-collar girl from the wrong side of the tracks. In Auckland, Newton Gully, where she'd grown up, was notorious — a working-class area full of sly-grog shops and frequented by criminals and communists.

Adman and author Bob Harvey had also grown up there in the 1950s. In his biography *Wild Westie*, Harvey talks about 'the filth of Newton Gully. The houses faced the wrong way so the sun only came in the back porches. Sanitation was limited to just an outhouse for each dwelling. Refrigeration was unheard of so food was always warm and went off quickly in the heat. Long periods of sickness were common.'[4]

Maggie recalls the big rats in the streets. 'I can remember my mother running out in the street with a spade and killing rats. She'd see a rat in the gutter and she'd be out like a shot with a spade and give it a whack on the head.'

Like many in the area, the family was anti-establishment and anti-police. They moved to nearby Grey Lynn, where her father was building a house that he never would finish. The quarter-acre section was filled with gorse. 'Mum beat it down and planted a vegetable garden that kept us going because Dad was only sporadically working for himself. He couldn't obtain employment with anybody because he was an alcoholic.'

When Maggie decided to try dental nursing, it was having the school holidays off that attracted her. Her experience with the School Dental Service up till then had been all bad. 'When I went to the dental nurse, the pain was terrible, [so] I worked out ways of not going. When I was called, I'd go to the cloakroom and hang around there and try to work out how much time had passed.' If she had any other aim in becoming a dental nurse it was to treat children better than she had been treated.

The school careers adviser had helped her gloss over the fact that her father was mostly out of work and in the pub by describing him on the form as a drainage contractor.

One afternoon she was called for an interview and ushered into a room where three people were seated by a window. 'I was facing the window and I couldn't see them very well, they were just dark silhouettes. The careers adviser had advised me not to wear my glasses but they quickly worked out that I had a cast in my eye and asked if I wore glasses. They also inspected my hands and asked if I did crafts.' Manual dexterity was considered an essential attribute.

From the start, she stood out from the other girls taking up dental nursing that year. 'They'd make fun of the clothes I was wearing, clothes my mother had made for me in form 2 because we had no money.' As a day girl, she remained excluded as most students lived in hostels, but it also meant she had another life beyond the training school. 'My brother and I were very active in the Progressive Youth Movement.' The Auckland PYM was the unofficial youth wing of the Maoist Communist Party of New Zealand and was notorious for scuffles with police at demonstrations. It adapted its manifesto from a prose poem by Tim Shadbolt, which began, 'Fuck your war / Fuck your petty morality . . . Fuck your politicians — representing big egos and small minds.' The PYM toned it down by replacing 'fuck' with 'damn'.[5] The manifesto ended, 'Damn your monied class politics, your churches, your system, your filth / You offer us your world / It stinks and you aren't making it any better so / Fuck off and let us try. We are the young and it's our world.'[6]

When the United States ramped up its involvement in the Vietnam War in 1964, sparking worldwide protests and demonstrations, the Auckland PYM and Maggie and her brother were in the thick of it. 'Mum supported our stand and helped us paint placards.' When President Lyndon Johnson arrived for a 24-hour visit to New Zealand in 1966 to shore up support for the war, he was rapturously received. More than 200,000 New Zealanders lined the route of the motorcade to Parliament. In Auckland Maggie Morgan was one of a much smaller number protesting and chanting, 'Hey, hey, LBJ, how many kids have you killed today?'

Her political activism was tolerated at the training school but left her feeling isolated. Like inmates in a prison, trainees had access to only one phone for personal calls and Maggie was often taunted with snide comments, such as 'talking to your commie friends again?', by other trainees waiting their turn. She did, however, find moral support in an unlikely quarter. 'I got on the bus one day and John Colquhoun [the training school dental officer] was on the bus as well and we both ended up at the

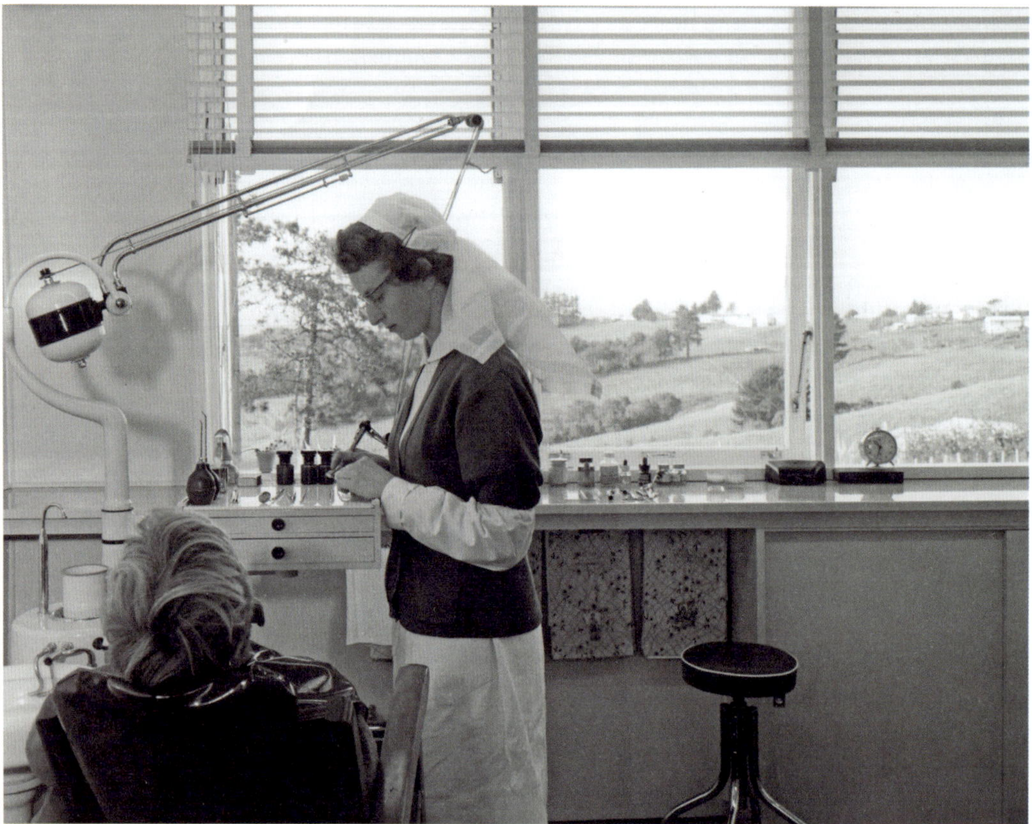

Dental nurses had to wear their uniforms correctly at all times; they never knew when an inspector would turn up.

same demonstration against Johnson's visit. He was very good to me after that.'

She had no time for the others. 'The dental officers and their sycophantic tutor sisters were absolutely horrid to the students. They were bullies so if you were not the right class, or hadn't the right look or you were struggling to complete the practical work they were just hideous.'

Maggie struggled with the work. Unlike the hostel girls who had a set period of study each evening, she found it hard to study amid the chaos at home, and the practical work was demanding. 'Working with live patients was fairly scary stuff. You knew what to do in theory but you've got this real patient, the pain, the wriggling, the cotton rolls, the whole nine yards. I really struggled with the practical and only just made it through the final exam.

'When I graduated my mother was embarrassed about our house so she took a photo of me across the road at our neighbour's verandah.' Though she was prepared to go anywhere, Maggie was surprised to be posted to the clinic at New Lynn Primary School, not far from her home.

An editorial in the *Gazette* at the time reminded nurses what was expected of them at the school:

> With workers in every field of employment, it is established custom that staff are permitted to have a tea break, usually confined to about 10 minutes. It is therefore quite acceptable that a school dental nurse will observe a similar custom. In fact, if she is wise, she will usually have a cup of tea in the mornings with the school staff, thereby getting to know them as individuals and improving her public relations.
>
> Where the dental nurse is to draw the line, however, is concerning eating at this time. It would be very imprudent, indeed, for her to take something to eat just as a matter of course. On special occasions such as staff farewells or end-of-year functions and the like, nurses should join in the festivities, but they should be restricted for those occasions only. Every nurse should know perfectly well that her tea habits are observed by the pupils and it is undermining her own teaching to the children if she does not observe the principles she is trying to inculcate into the youngsters' minds. It is too difficult, if not impossible, to reason with large groups of patients that the nurse could possibly do one thing herself and forbid the children to do likewise. It is therefore safer and indeed more effective for the dental nurse to refrain from daily eating between meals within the sight of children.[7]

'The Morning Tea Break' editorial continued: 'When it comes to a cup of tea during the afternoon the position is somewhat different.' Nurses, it implied, should be getting on with the job, not wasting time in the staffroom. 'It is . . . timely to remind officers that they are working in a privileged Service which has shorter working hours and much more leave than all other branches of the Public Service, outside the teaching profession itself. Any seeming restriction on the behaviour patterns of the tea breaks are not so arduous as they might appear to be on the surface.'

Maggie found the heavily starched uniform took a bit of getting used to. It had a double layer in front to fit any size bust, 'and when they were starched the top layer stuck out so you appeared to have a giant bosom'. A male teacher at morning tea used to position himself so he could sneak a look between the layers. 'He couldn't see much but he thought he was going to.'

Maggie graduated in 1968. 'Miniskirts were coming in, so we started to decrease the length of the skirt and got into trouble with the dental nurse inspector. You could get away with a little bit of shortness because you had white stockings but when witches' britches came in you couldn't get away with it because they came down to your knees. I had red ones with black lace on them. I put them on one day and of course my uniform was too short. It wasn't too bad when I was standing still but I had to take a dental health lesson that day and the kids all fell about laughing because they could see my knickers.'

In her 2004 novel *Music from a Distant Room* Stephanie Johnson describes the life of a school dental nurse in the 1960s. The protagonist Nola Lane, dental nurse and winner of beauty contests, loves her job despite the fear she instilled in children.

> The children were afraid of her. She knew this and it broke her heart a little: it chipped a corner of it, though not enough to overwhelm the pride she felt in her white uniform, the red cardigan, the crisp gauze veil that stood away from her shoulders; not enough to temper her quick, professional strides in her street shoes each morning across the asphalt and up the concrete path to the wooden clinic; not enough to stop her pausing by the step to admire the garden of cineraria tall behind a pattern of pansies that she had made herself, coming into school on the weekends to do it; not enough to dim the pleasure she felt in laying out fresh picture books for her patients to enjoy in the tiny, shiny brown waiting-room, or in renewing the exhorting posters on the walls; not enough to permit any slackening in her clinical standards: her hygiene, the maintenance of her equipment.
>
> Neither was she haunted by the fear of the children, by their tears and stricken faces, though she felt for them. Eyes and noses were tenderly wiped with the white chin cloth at the end of appointments, crude dolls were fashioned out of cottonwool rolls with pen marks for eyes, arms and legs cut away from the body with her sharp scissors, and balls of glistening mercury were tweezered out of the Drop Bottle to slip about in tiny, empty pink bur boxes. Sad and difficult kids would leave clutching one or other of these trophies in one hand, in the other a piece of paper inscribed with a name that was not their own, and a number.[8]

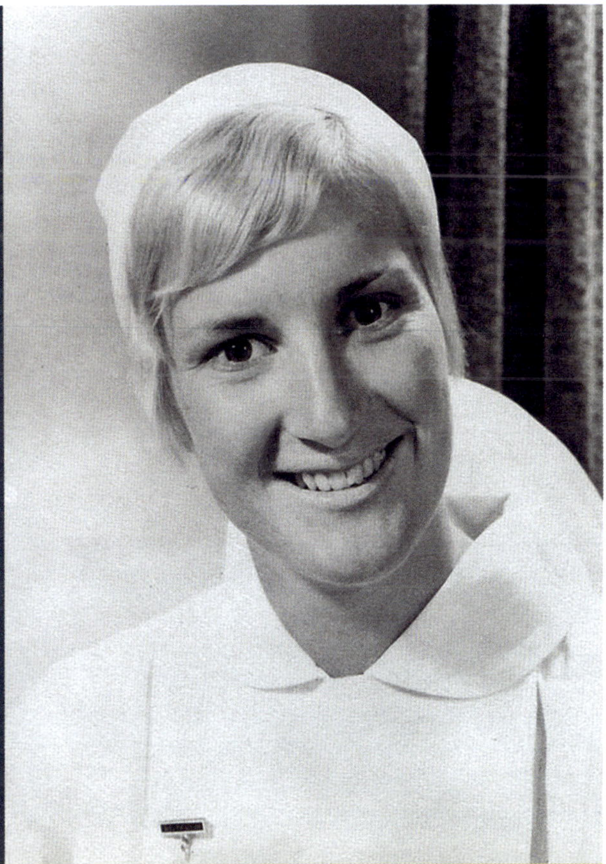

As a teenager, Annette King was fascinated with dental nurses and got a job cleaning the dental clinic. Alone in the clinic Annette would dress up in the nurse's uniform and drill holes in stones and plug them with whatever she thought was dental filling. Then she'd relax with one of the nurse's Du Maurier cigarettes.

Annette King could identify with the children's suffering. 'I had bad baby teeth and the experience was terrible.'[9] And yet the idea of becoming a school dental nurse was irresistible. 'My grandparents lived next door to us and they used to have the dental nurses as boarders when they came to service the local schools. I admired them so much because they'd go off to work in the starched uniforms [and] seamed stockings with their veils on.'

At 14, she recalls, 'I got the job of cleaning the dental clinic each night and on the weekends.' Alone in the clinic she'd dress up in the nurse's uniform and drill holes in stones and plug them with whatever she thought was dental filling. Then she'd relax with one of the nurse's Du Maurier cigarettes — 'but only one so she didn't notice'

— and soak up the atmosphere. 'I just loved the unique smell of the clinic, of eugenol [clove oil] and methylated spirits. It really got into my blood early on.'

Annette, though, wasn't the sort of young woman who would be a good fit in a service that prized compliance and unquestioning obedience in its employees. She might not, like Maggie Morgan, have come from the wrong side of the tracks, but the West Coast mining town of Murchison where she was born and grew up was not a place that produced the middle-class girls the service liked to recruit. She was, in her own words, 'always outspoken, opinionated and noisy', and got into 'terrible rows over politics' with her National-voting father, a linesman for the Post and Telegraph Department. In her final year at high school, in 1965, a teacher refused to teach her. 'My parents decided there was no point in my continuing to argue with the teacher so they sent me for my last year to college in Nelson.'

When she applied for school dental nursing that year she didn't think she'd be selected. 'I've never forgotten the woman who interviewed me, a Miss Everards, who was one of the original snaky dental nurse inspectors. She looked at my hands and she said, "Oh they're very big!" I thought that doesn't look very good. "What does your father do?" Oh, my father works in the P & T.' I got the impression I didn't come from a good enough family and I wasn't going to be accepted. It was a very awkward interview. In fact when I did start, out of an intake of 80, there were very few who came from ordinary working families.'

To do her training Annette didn't have to go to Wellington; a new training school had opened in Christchurch in 1959. The hostel was in an old turreted mansion called Holly Lea in Manchester Street. It had been the home of a wealthy Canterbury businessman, Allan McLean, who'd left it in his will to be run as a home for 'women of refinement and education in reduced or straitened circumstances'.

Whether teenage student dental nurses could pass as women of refinement and education was highly questionable, but they were often in straitened circumstances after a weekend of partying. And always hungry. There was a rota for sneaking down the fire escape and bringing back a big order of hamburgers from the local takeaway to scoff at one in the morning. Or 'there was a bin outside where the bread man delivered the bread and you could access it from the inside. We had one particularly skinny girl who could get through the hole into the kitchen . . . We'd be outside waiting while she would be getting tins of baked beans off the shelf, bread, butter, and so on. We'd have a midnight feast with stuff stolen from the kitchen. Then back up the fire escape to bed.'

Annette loved hostel life. 'We all shared clothes and the other thing we shared was hair dye — we had more bottle blondes in our hostel that you'd find naturally in life.

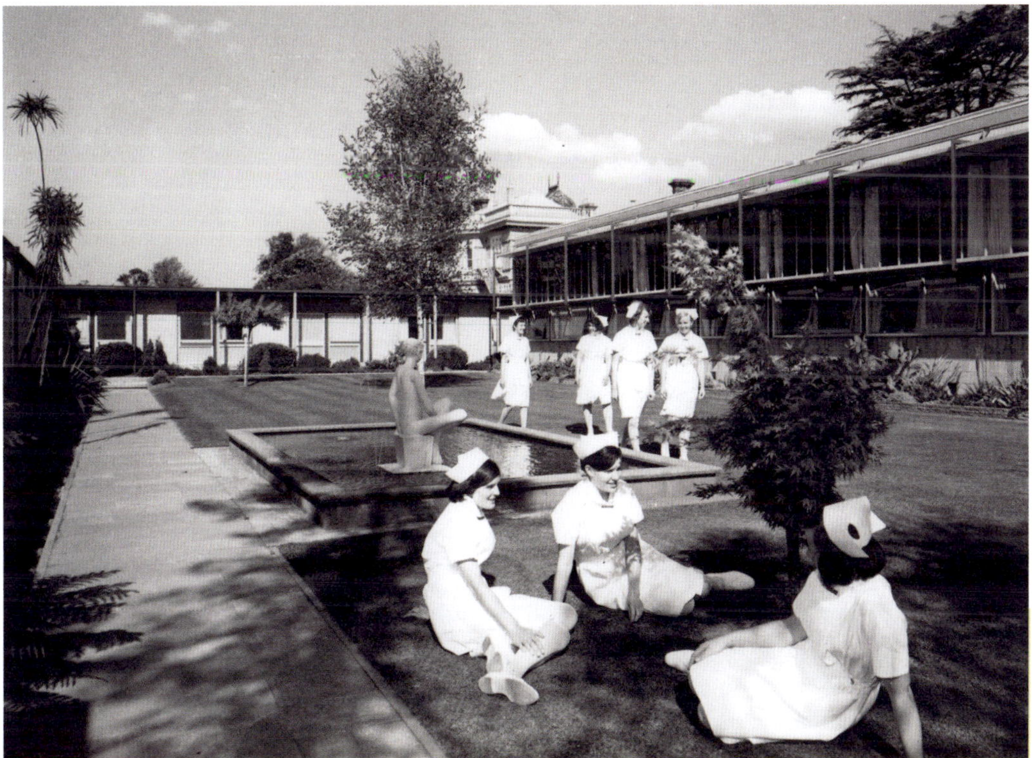

Student dental nurses relax in the grounds of the Christchurch training school during a break.

But on Saturday night most of us had purple hair. We'd put a drop of gentian violet in the water and dip your head in it and your bleached blonde hair came out slightly purple. And we'd head off to our latest party. By Monday the purple was usually gone.'

During the week a 9 p.m. curfew was strictly enforced by Miss Mannering, an Englishwoman who looked like a matron from central casting. 'She was a real tartar,' remembers Annette. Rosemary Kennedy, a fellow student who shared a turret room with three other girls, recalls some of the tricks they played on her. 'The matron was a big buxom woman who used to hang her underwear behind the shed in the hostel grounds. They were great bloomers and the girls sewed the legs up. Of course she couldn't go and complain to the principal dental officer because he would have asked to see the evidence so they got away with that.'[10] Another time they shut a dog in her toilet.

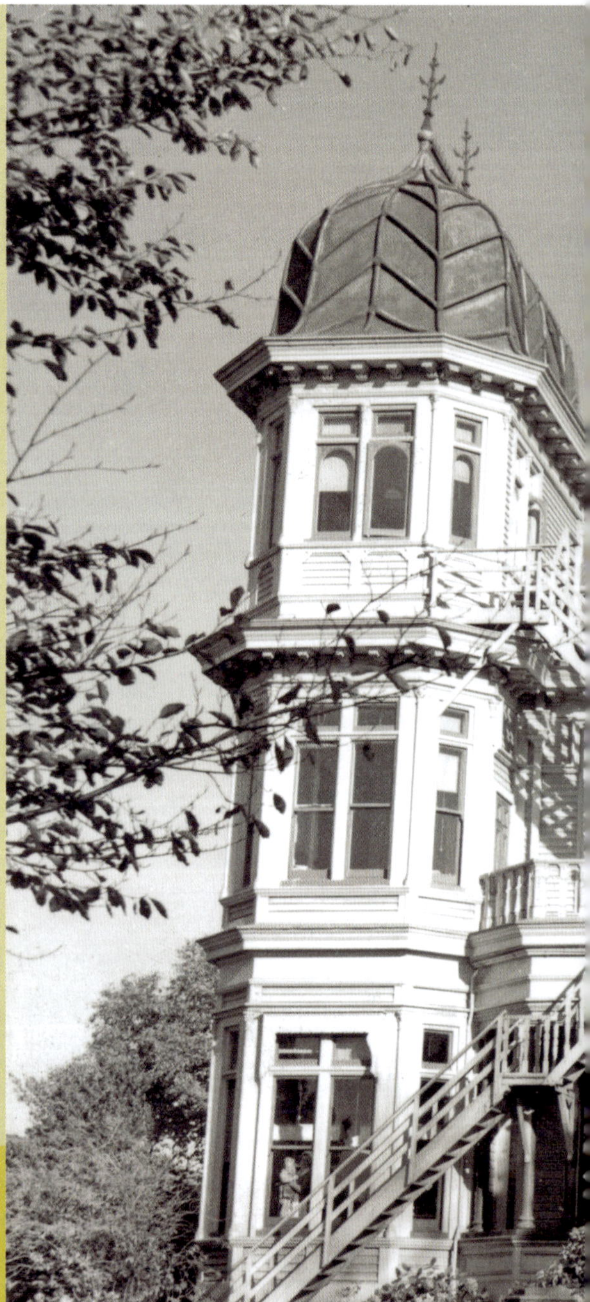

Holly Lea, the former mansion that became the hostel for student dental nurses in Christchurch. It was originally donated as a home 'for women of refinement and education in reduced or straitened circumstances'. Teenage student dental nurses were often in straitened circumstances after a weekend of partying. (The Category 1 heritage building was damaged in the 2011 Christchurch earthquake and has undergone significant restoration.)

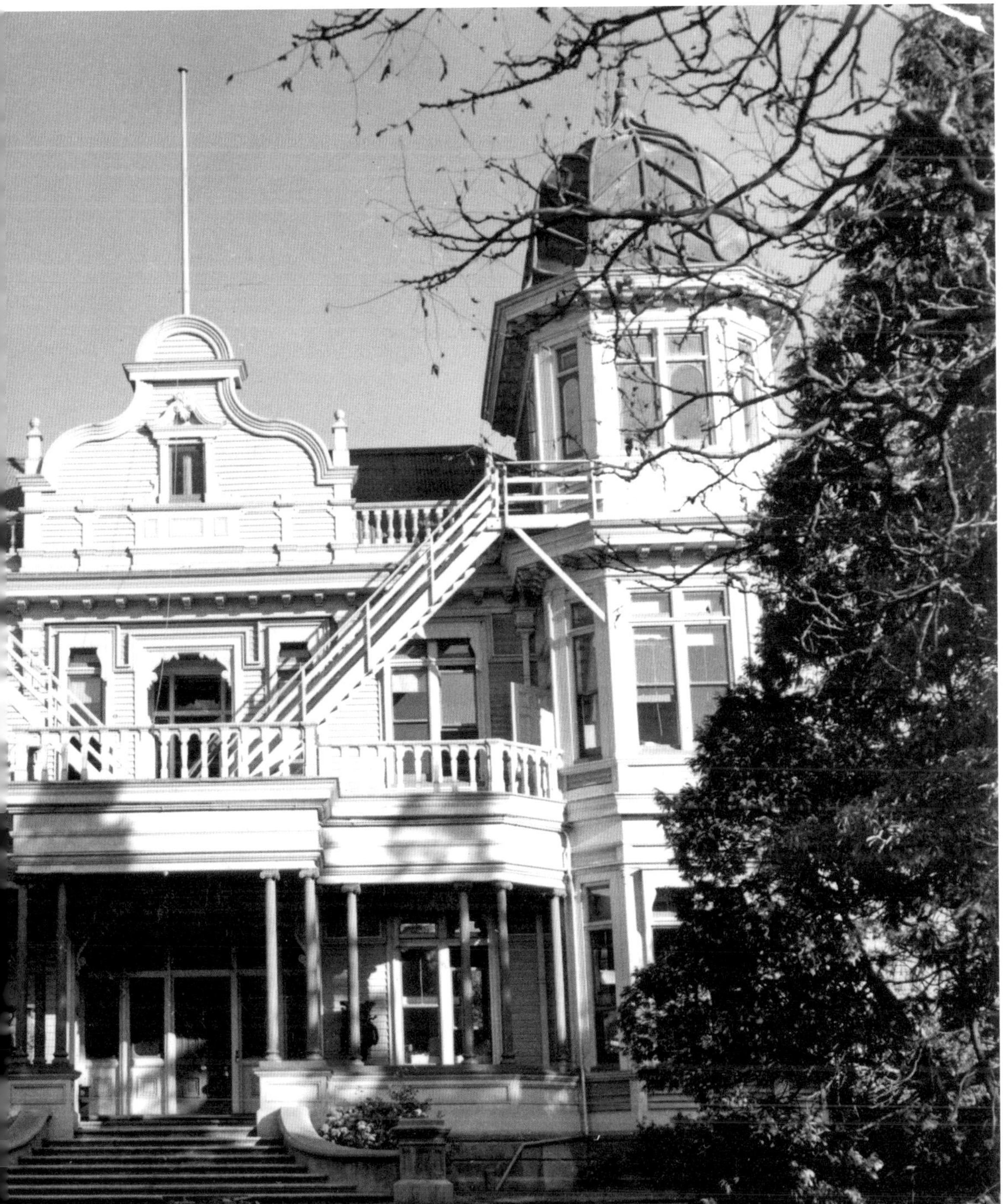

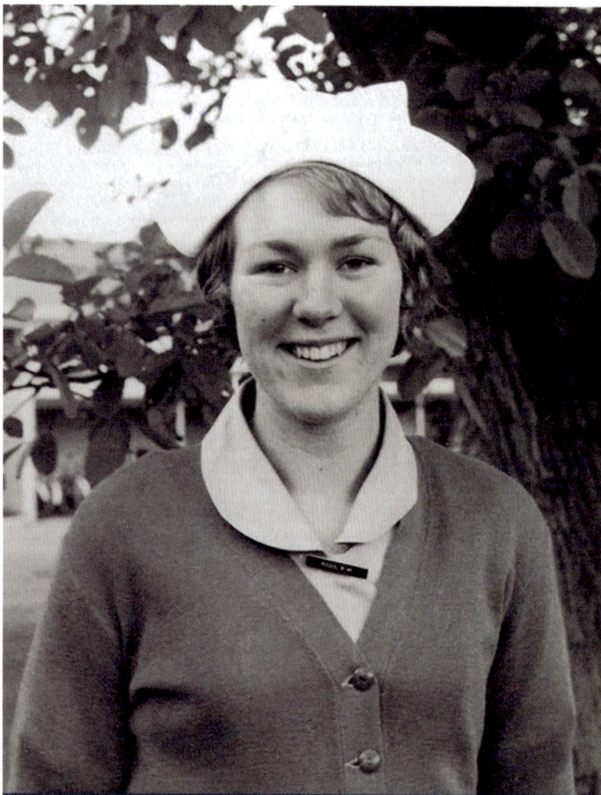

'The matron was a big buxom woman who used to hang her underwear behind the shed in the hostel grounds. They were great bloomers and the girls sewed the legs up. Another time they shut a dog in her toilet.'

— Rosemary Kennedy

When they got weekend leave, they would club together and stay at a motel, eight to one room. There was much fraternising with boys from Lincoln University. As Annette recalls, 'One of the challenges for Lincoln boys during orientation week was to steal the bath plugs from the dental nurses' hostel. Those baths could fit four of us and often four of us were in the bath . . . All of us smoked, it was just what we did, sitting in the big hostel lounge, ashtrays everywhere, puffing up. It was a great social life. I don't know how I ever passed.'[11]

Smoking, though, was confined to tobacco. Christchurch in the 1960s was a world away from the hippies of San Francisco and the Summer of Love. Twinsets and pearls, hats and gloves were the norm for most dental nurses. Rosemary remembers, 'There was always fish on Fridays and the Catholic girls would don black lace mantillas and go to church.' And there was old-fashioned bullying and sexual harassment. 'Billy Burgess, one of the tutors, would put his hand over yours pretending to guide you or he would nestle into you physically, forcing you into the wall to get away from him. Everybody knew that. They were underhand sexual techniques that today nobody would tolerate but we tolerated them because we didn't know that was unacceptable. One student got sick of Burgess and put a suspender belt on the end of the pointing stick for a lecture. And as the pointing stick was under the lectern he couldn't see the suspender on the end so when he picked up the stick everybody cracked up, laughing. He couldn't cope with it; bullies can never cope with a bit of something back.'

The memory of Burgess' dismissive arrogance, however, inspired Rosemary to further her education later and obtain a master's degree. 'We teach you what you need to know — you don't need to know any more,' he was fond of saying.

When she graduated, Annette King was posted to the last place she wanted to go: Pahiatua. The family had moved there after her father got a foreman's job in the P & T. At 19 she felt she was a real adult, and after two years of freedom she resented having to live at home again. 'They always wanted you to live with your family or nearby and you didn't get a say in the matter.' Annette had a boyfriend, a Lincoln graduate who was working in Nelson, so she applied for a transfer there. 'I wanted to get out of Pahiatua as fast I could.' A year after graduation she was married, with a daughter, and by the end of the 1960s she'd left dental nursing to look after the family. Though she would rejoin the profession early in the new decade, it was politics that she was increasingly drawn to, and the growing restlessness of dental nurses would provide plenty of scope for that.

Margaret Clarkson was another Christchurch graduate who would soon be drawn into the politics of the profession. Unlike King, she was counting on being sent to live close by her parents. 'My parents were living on the west coast of the South Island when I applied for dental nurse training. Then my father got ill and they had to go back to Wellington where we were from and so I wanted to be near my parents to help with my father.'[12] Instead, in 1964 she was posted to Waiheke Island, a place she'd never heard of. She'd never been north of Palmerston North and was horrified to find that Waiheke was nearly an hour's boat trip from Auckland. Waiheke had a scattered population of about 2000 people then. 'Quite a few of those people had a reputation for being pot smokers or criminals or people who had run out of credit and disappeared.'

On the plane to Auckland, she got chatting to a woman who took pity on the 19-year-old and took her to the ferry terminal. 'I had the address on a bit of paper and I asked for a one-way ticket. "Aren't you coming back, dear?" the ticket clerk asked. And my voice went all quivery and I said, "I don't know."'

She was met by Jill, the dental nurse she was replacing, who took her to a bach that had a dirt floor and two single beds. She was given a jug of water and told that the island only had tank water. 'Then we had a little bit of cold meat, a potato and some chopped-up lettuce. I remember going to bed and stuffing something in my mouth so Jill wouldn't hear me sobbing.'

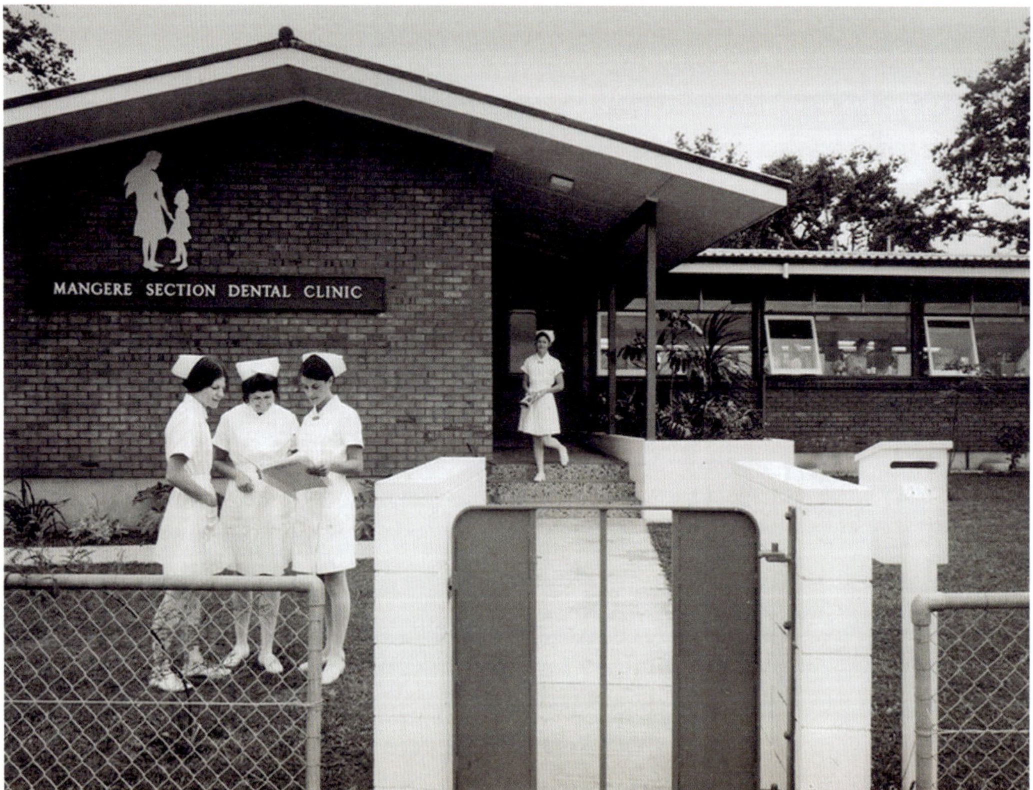

Section clinics were introduced in the 1960s. The Mangere clinic had 26 chairs, expanding the facilities of the Auckland training school.

The next day the bach owner told Margaret she wasn't taking boarders any more and she would have to find somewhere else to live. Jill took her to the three dental clinics for which she would be responsible — 'I was going to be the only dental person on the island for three schools' — and she found lodgings near the school. Then Jill left to return to Auckland. 'I was to start work with absolutely no support at all. There wasn't even a dentist on the island.' The clinic had been closed for months. The children's roll had to be organised, parents contacted for consent, stores and supplies ordered in quadruplicate. 'You were running a business completely on your own.'

'In the first week a great big man appeared at my door with toothache and wanted me to extract a molar. I would have had to stand on his chest to do it, and when I wouldn't do it, he was most upset because it meant he'd have to take a day off work and go across to Auckland.'

When the first school holidays came round Margaret was keen to get back to her family in Wellington and booked a flight, but the airline rang to say her cheque had bounced. 'The Health Department was paying my salary into the wrong bank and I had no money. The only money I'd been spending had been at the island's general store. Apparently all my cheques had been bouncing. I said to the owner, "Why didn't you say something?" He said, "I know where you live, you've got a job, you must have money somewhere."'

Margaret's feeling of isolation increased when the young teacher she shared a flat with got sick and returned to Auckland. Eighteen months later, she left Waiheke Island for a posting in Christchurch. After she married at 23, she became something of a matchmaker for dental nurses in the area. 'The young farmers would keep asking me when the next new graduates would be coming. I would arrange for the dental nurses to come with me to the upstairs bar of the Brighton Hotel to meet the young men.'

'We were cookie-cutter people, really,' she says. She was a conventional middle-class person in a conservative city, working in a profession that prized docility. Union activism, political awareness, militancy — all that was to come later, but not easily.

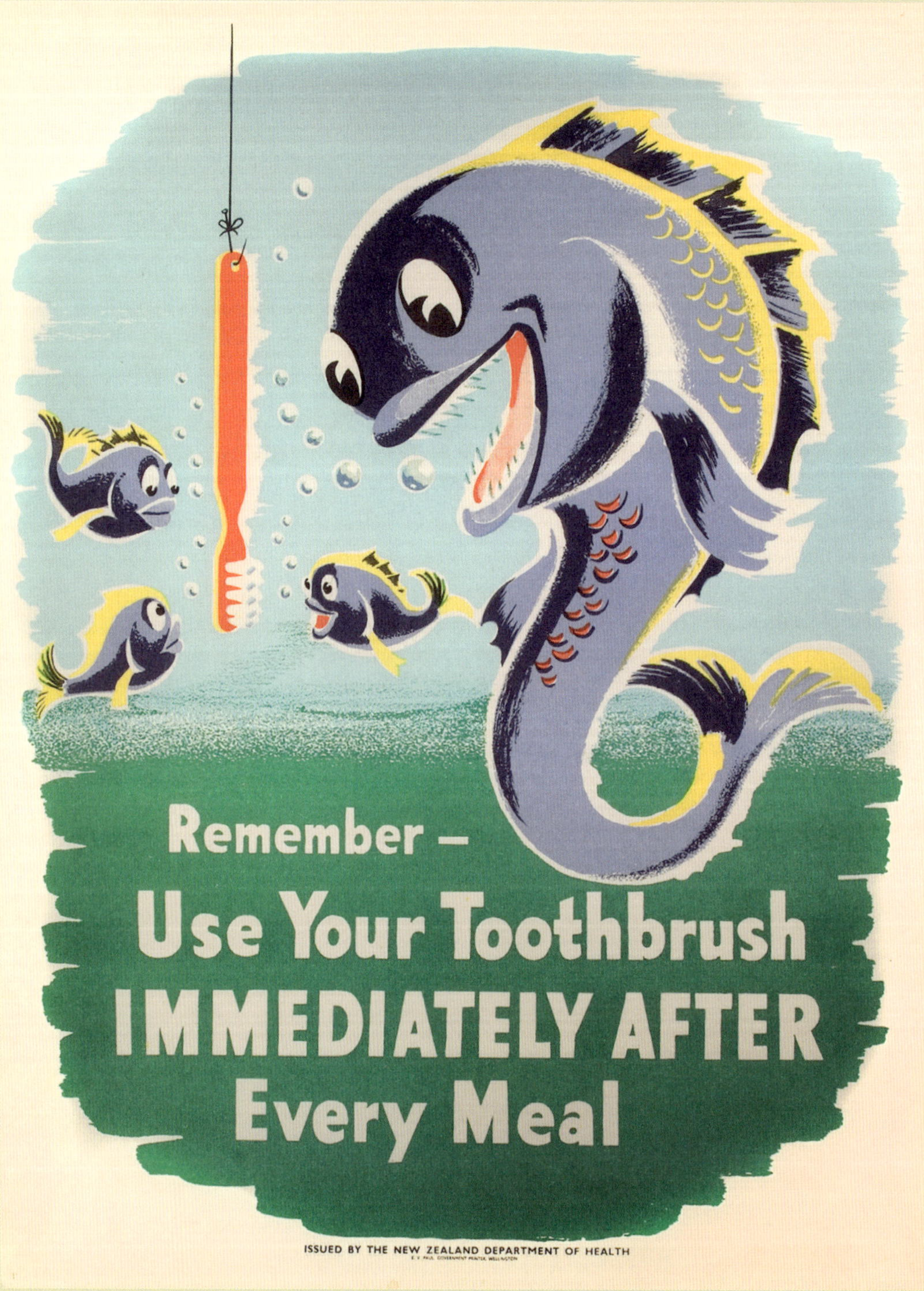
Remember –
Use Your Toothbrush
IMMEDIATELY AFTER
Every Meal
ISSUED BY THE NEW ZEALAND DEPARTMENT OF HEALTH

7

DISSENSION IN THE RANKS

Nineteen seventy-one was the year the School Dental Service marked its golden jubilee. The anniversary attracted little media coverage; the post office issued a special stamp and the health department published a cheap commemorative booklet written by G. H. Leslie, director of the Division of Dental Health.[1] He noted the contribution of the male dental officers who'd run the service over its 50 years, but few women got a mention unless they were matrons. The booklet, which included three pictures of Leslie himself, credited the New Zealand Dental Association for supporting the service despite the NZDA's initial bitter opposition and its determination to fight any expansion of the dental nurse's role or an extension of the service to treat secondary school students.

As Leslie was at pains to point out, school dental nurses were 'auxiliaries', foot soldiers in the war against tooth decay. There was, however, growing dissension in the ranks, a fact that was becoming apparent to him in his dealings with the Dental Nurses Institute. The institute, formed in 1935, had for decades been more of a social club than a professional body. A minute book from the 1950s is full of discussions about organising graduation balls and Christmas parties. Branches held one-hour monthly meetings, including supper and a talk. The September meeting of the Wellington branch in 1951, for example, was followed by a talk 'by Miss A. Leahy of her motor tour of Spain and the South of France'.[2]

By the 1970s, though, members attending institute meetings were venting their frustration at low salaries, obsolete equipment, intolerable conditions and lack of professional development. One remit asked: 'If high-speed drills are to go into intermediate schools in due course training would be necessary. Would it be possible to include the use of the nerve block in the same course?'[3] Another queried why they did not receive the reasons they'd been refused a transfer. 'We have to apply in writing. Couldn't we have a reply?'

If it all sounded like a genteel version of unionism, the institute president Mrs Mann was quick to disavow such a notion at the Dental Nurses Institute Delegates Conference in 1971. In the conference report, 'she stressed the Institute was not a "union" as such', but 'rather an organisation to promote fellowship among dental nurses, look after their welfare and represent them in an endeavour to iron out problems'.[4]

Leslie, the keynote speaker at that conference, was quick to endorse Mann's view. The institute, he said, was a place where nurses could voice their opinions, but 'I hope the rank and file of the service do not regard the Institute as a union. Militancy is all too common these days, there are signs of it even in the Public Service.'[5]

He supposed the world was changing, though. 'Those of us who were products of [the pre-war] era seldom question established practices, and when we did it was in a somewhat hesitant deferential manner.' Now was an era 'when young people have been encouraged to develop their own self wills and personalities, to analyse and think for themselves and to express their opinions'. He added that the 'outspoken forthright manner of young nurses' took a bit of getting used to. 'My first reaction was to bristle but I usually attribute this approach to youthful enthusiasm and overstatement rather than rudeness and disrespect.'[6]

Leslie seemed unaware that it wasn't just the new generation who was becoming disgruntled. Older nurses who'd worked overseas saw how New Zealand was being left behind, even though it had pioneered the school dental service model. Freda Patterson — she who had ingeniously rigged up an electric Singer sewing machine to a treadle drill — was now working in Canada.[7] No Canadian professional, she found, would dream of tackling the sort of dental work she'd been doing in New Zealand without a high-speed drill and adequate anaesthesia. When Freda returned to tutor in the training school in Wellington she found teaching methods and resources that were so outdated she resigned and returned to Canada to finish her career. Other nurses returning to the service after raising a family were staggered that so little had changed since they'd first practised.

Leslie, clearly unfazed by the rumblings of discontent, told the conference there was no likelihood that the New Zealand Dental School would stagnate: 'Senior officers are well qualified men and will not allow the service to become a back number. You will hear of improvements which are contemplated. The service cannot afford to rush into re-equipping over 1200 clinics, using vast expenditure of public funds without undertaking considerable investigation. What I always preach to visitors is that a service is not built on equipment alone, it is the staff that counts.'

In response to remits calling for advanced diploma studies for dental nurses and additional duties to increase their status, he channelled Henny Penny: 'This immediately raises issues which are in direct conflict with the original conception of a dental auxiliary whose sole purpose was to relieve a dentist of the day to day dental requirements of school children.' Allowing dental nurses to expand their role and gain further qualifications would 'blur the line of distinction between auxiliaries and dentists and would, eventually, have serious consequences for the New Zealand Dental Service and for the dental nurse and unfortunate repercussions throughout the world'.

The service, he went on, had succeeded because the rank and file were 'restricted to a clearly defined field of activity'. In other words, they did not encroach on dentists' business. He concluded: 'I hope the Institute will use its influence wisely to govern the attitudes of the school dental nurse in such a way that all assurances of their absolute dependency and loyalty are not just idle words.'

The institute, though, was not able to keep a lid on members' discontent, especially as the health department seemed indifferent to their concerns or to making improvements in the service. When Pam Horncy returned from her OE, she was struck by the low morale, the culture of complaint. A big gripe from nurses working in intermediate school clinics was pump chairs. 'The kids were way too big for the wooden chairs. New pump chairs [apparently acquired in a government contra-deal for butter or sheep meat] were sitting in boxes in the waiting rooms and cluttering up access to the clinics. They'd been sitting there for 18 months and still hadn't been installed.'[8]

Nurses were losing patience, too, with inspections. 'People started talking about the dental nurse inspectors and how trivial some of the issues were that they were picking them up on. If you had a dusty ledge right near the ceiling they would be saying that your hygiene wasn't up to standard. White shoes would invariably get black marks on them from kicking the foot-operated drill and the suggestion was: "Maybe you could put your feet in plastic bags." It also felt like an element of entrapment when you might be running five minutes late and there's the dental nurse inspector waiting for you at the door. There were a lot of women who had teenage children — they had been working mothers and they didn't like being still treated like they couldn't be completely trusted.' (The story goes that nurse Diane Holyoake, daughter of the then prime minister Keith Holyoake, got so irritated with a dental inspector that she bashed her over the head with her copy of *Standing Orders*.) Letters of complaint to the principal dental officer and the director of dental health achieved nothing. 'We felt we were getting nowhere and not being taken seriously,' says Pam.

To celebrate the School Dental Service golden jubilee in 1971, the uniforms for each decade were modelled, along with a description of the strict rules surrounding how they were to be worn. The high-fashion uniform proposed for the 1970s was purely wishful thinking.

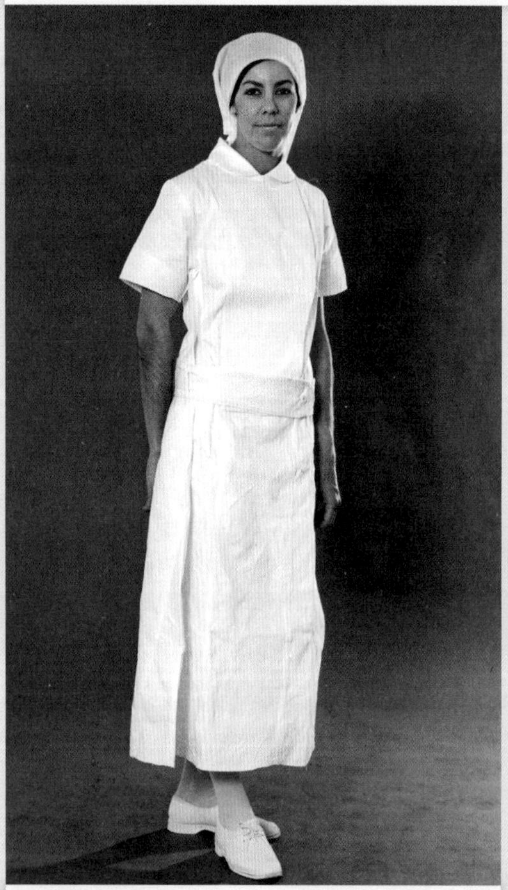

The 1920s

Uniform: Almost ankle-length.
No medallion.
Belt: Wide, low on hips. Plain white button, worn in centre.
Veil: Low on forehead, bunched into a pin, no hem, turned back at brow.
Stockings: Black or brown.
Shoes: Black or brown.
No lipstick.

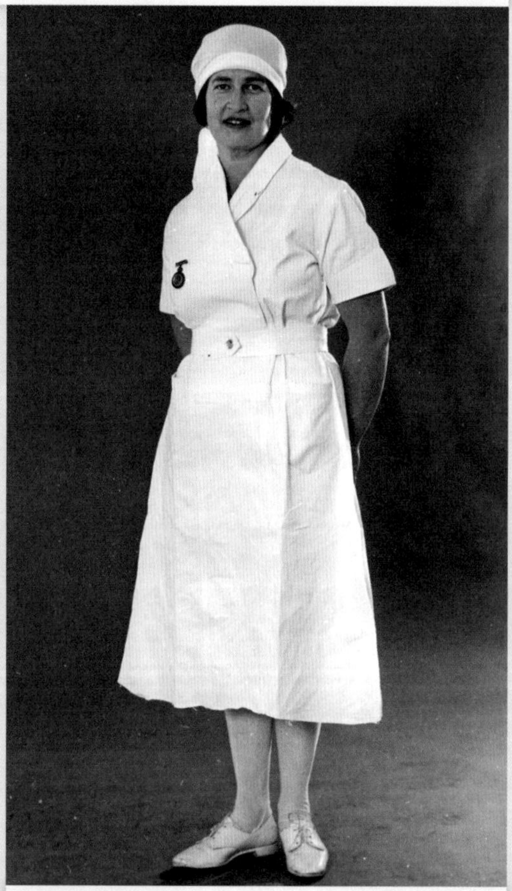

The 1930s

Uniform: Crossover shawl-collared neck-line. Medallion.
Belt: Wide, Service button worn centred.
Veil: Bunched into a pin. Mid-way down forehead.
Stockings: White lisle.
Shoes: White canvas, buttoned strap across instep.
A little lipstick, fairly dark shade.

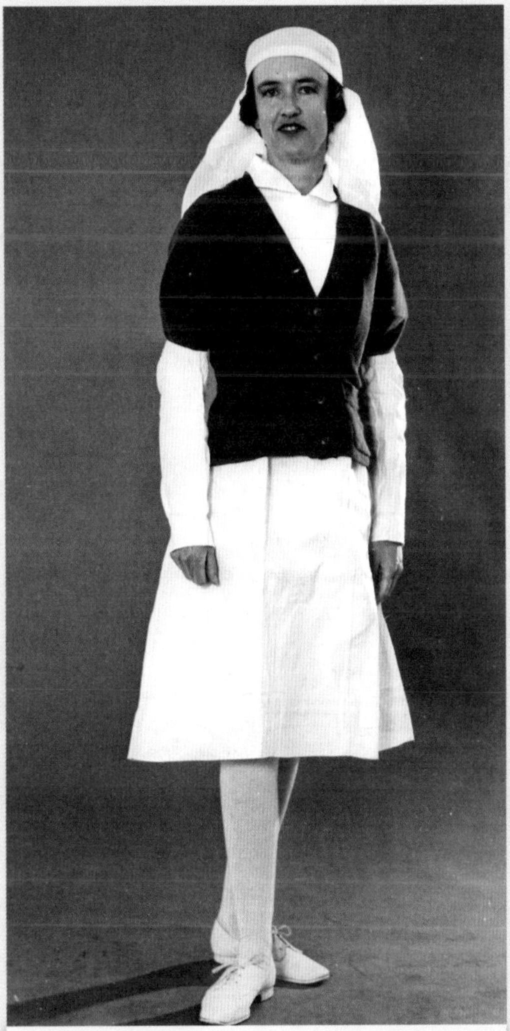

The 1940s

Uniform: Mid-calf length (though worn shorter on model).
Belt: Wide, Service button worn to the side.
Cardigan: Red, with pockets, worn with white cotton half-sleeves.
Veil: Folded with 'wings' at the side. Set low on forehead and a hem turned back.
Stockings: White lisle.
Shoes: White lace-up. No decorative punching or holes. Flat heel.
Dark shade of lipstick.

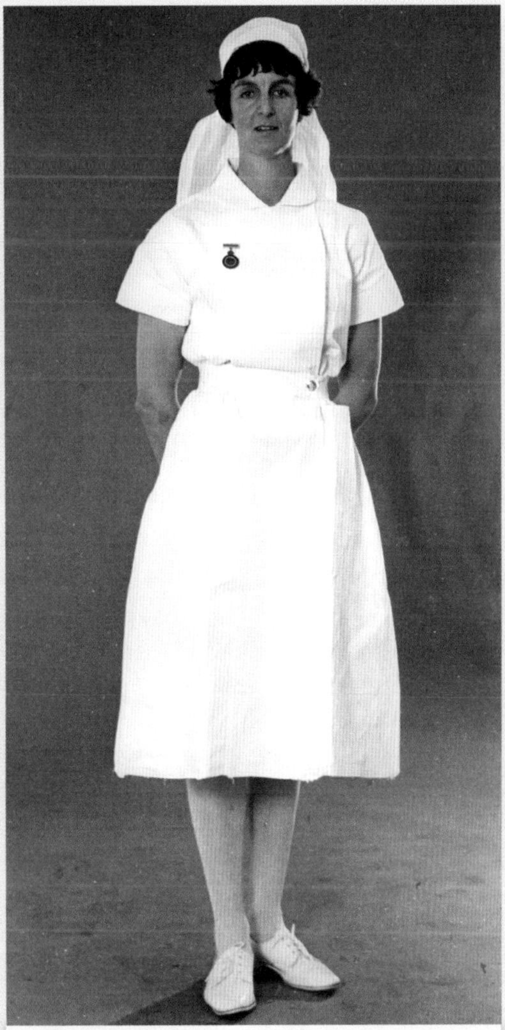

The 1950s

Uniform: Below the knee.
Belt: Narrower. Service button worn to the side.
Veil: Pleated into pin at back. Fairly full on crown.
Stockings: White nylon with seam.
Shoes: White lace-up, rounded toes.
Lipstick, no obvious eye make-up.

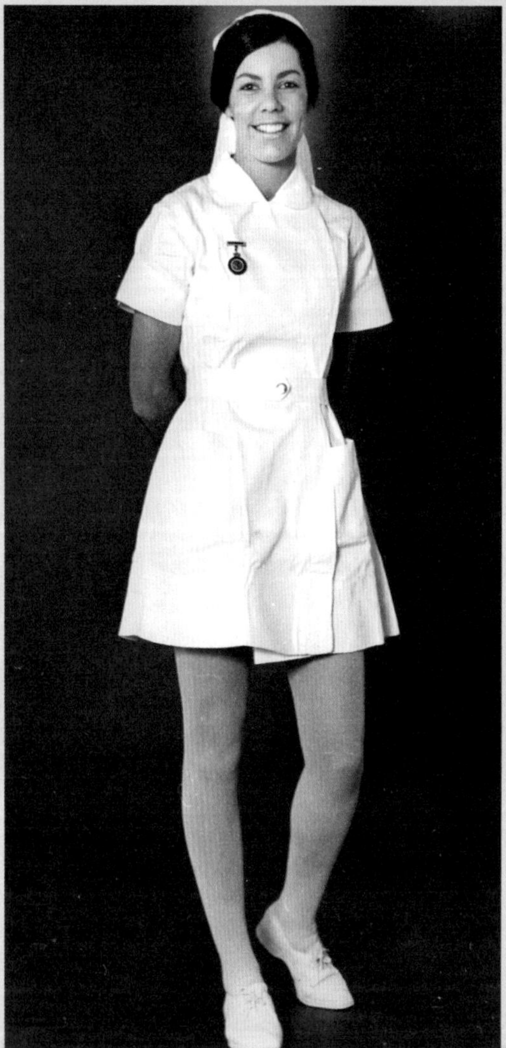

The 1960s

Uniform: Short.
Veil: Small on crown, pleated at back.
Belt: Narrow, tightly buttoned.
Stockings: Nylon, seamless stretch.
Shoes: Lace-up, tapered toes.
Pale lipstick, definite eye make-up.

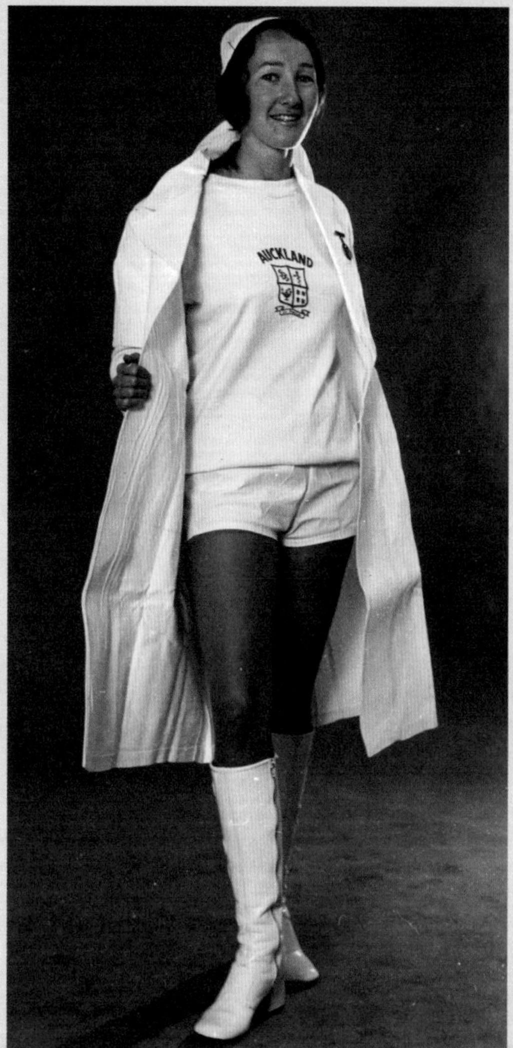

The 1970s

(A playful suggestion for the decade to come)
Midi-coat and hot pants.
Skivvy or Service-monogrammed T-shirt.
Veil with small crown.
Knee-socks and square-toed shoes, or white knee boots.

Months went by. One day in 1973 two nurses, Rhonda Clark and Linda White, were grumbling about their jobs in their school staffroom. One of the male teachers said, 'So why don't you go to your union?' In their naivety about workplace politics, the thought had never occurred to them. Which union represented dental nurses anyway? They discovered it was the Public Service Association (PSA) and contacted an organiser in the Auckland regional office. Could he help sort out their grievances? He would certainly try, and he had some good news for them. They were due a substantial pay increase. For more than two years the PSA had been negotiating a pay claim with the State Services Commission (SSC). The union claimed that school dental nurses should have relativity with teachers: in other words, any pay increase teachers got should be passed on to dental nurses. When the School Dental Service started in 1921, dental nurses were paid the same as teachers because they'd had the same level of training and entry requirements. Over the years, however, teachers' salaries had far outstripped those of dental nurses. The PSA argued that dental nurses were part of the school staff. They were educators and taught oral hygiene in the classroom and provided individual tuition in the subject to schoolchildren.

The negotiations had got nowhere because the SSC did not buy that argument. For more than 30 years dental nurses had had relativity with public health nurses and the SSC could see no reason to change that. If and when public health nurses got a pay rise, the commission would look at dental nurses' pay. Now, the organiser was able to tell them, public health nurses had been awarded a pay increase of $800 per annum ($10,000 in today's money), backdated to 1971. The PSA had therefore immediately lodged a claim for that pay increase to be passed on to dental nurses.

As word spread, dental nurses across the country were jubilant. It was time to crack open a few bottles of Cold Duck.[9] Having not had a pay increase in nearly two decades, they were suddenly coming into money. The back pay would be substantial — enough to fund an overseas trip and still leave money in the bank. You could buy a house in Auckland for $20,000.

The State Service Commission's response to the PSA's claim stunned the dental nurses. The commission now rejected the long-standing relativity between dental nurses and public health nurses. Further, it claimed that any pay increase was now out of the question because the recently introduced Economic Stabilisation Regulations froze public-sector wages.

The sudden reversal of the dental nurses' hopes for a pay rise was caused by a number of disparate events and personalities. The first event occurred in 1972, when the third Labour government swept to power. Dental nurses could have been forgiven for assuming this was a good omen: the first Labour government, led by Michael Joseph Savage, had championed and expanded the School Dental Service and built the Willis Street clinic. Norman Kirk, the new prime minister, seemed to have been cut from the same cloth. Like Savage, one of his first acts as prime minister was to give pensioners, invalids, war veterans and widows a Christmas bonus. Like Savage, Kirk was a self-educated working man, with a strong sense of social justice. Forced to leave school at 12, he'd endured poverty as a child and young man and was keenly aware of how unfair the world could be. Bob Tizard, another figure crucial to the dental nurses' case, had also taken the stage with the Labour victory. Elected to Parliament the same year as Kirk, the former university lecturer believed he was more qualified than Kirk to lead the Labour Party because he was better educated. Abrasive and blunt, he'd been opposition finance spokesperson and expected to be minister of finance in the new government. Instead, Kirk, who'd never warmed to him, appointed him minister of health and minister of state services, the two portfolios under which the School Dental Service operated.

Dental nurses' hopes of a pay rise were tied to the fortunes of the new government. However, despite Kirk's boast 'We're here to govern for 25 years!', things went quickly pear-shaped. On 1 January 1973 Britain joined the European Economic Community, upending trade agreements for New Zealand's exports of lamb, butter and cheese. Inflation sparked demands for higher wages. Worried about a wage/price blowout, the government imposed Economic Stabilisation Regulations. It put a halt to wage negotiations and froze wages, apart from pay rises approved by a new wages tribunal.

Like concert-goers who'd queued for hours only to be confronted with a 'House Full' sign, dental nurses were left deflated by the freeze. In 1953, they'd been denied a rise because it would mean that they were paid more than the public health nurses. Now, because of SSC duplicity and timing, they were being denied a pay rise that would put them on a par with public health nurses. The PSA considered it was a serious anomaly and a delegation went to the prime minister to protest at the unfairness. Kirk, however, was unmoved and refused to make an exception for dental nurses. The SSC also refused to continue pay negotiations while the freeze lasted.

To make matters worse, world events conspired to make it unlikely the wage freeze would be lifted soon. On 6 October 1973, the Jewish holy day of Yom Kippur, Egypt and Syria launched a military attack against Israel to take back the land occupied after the

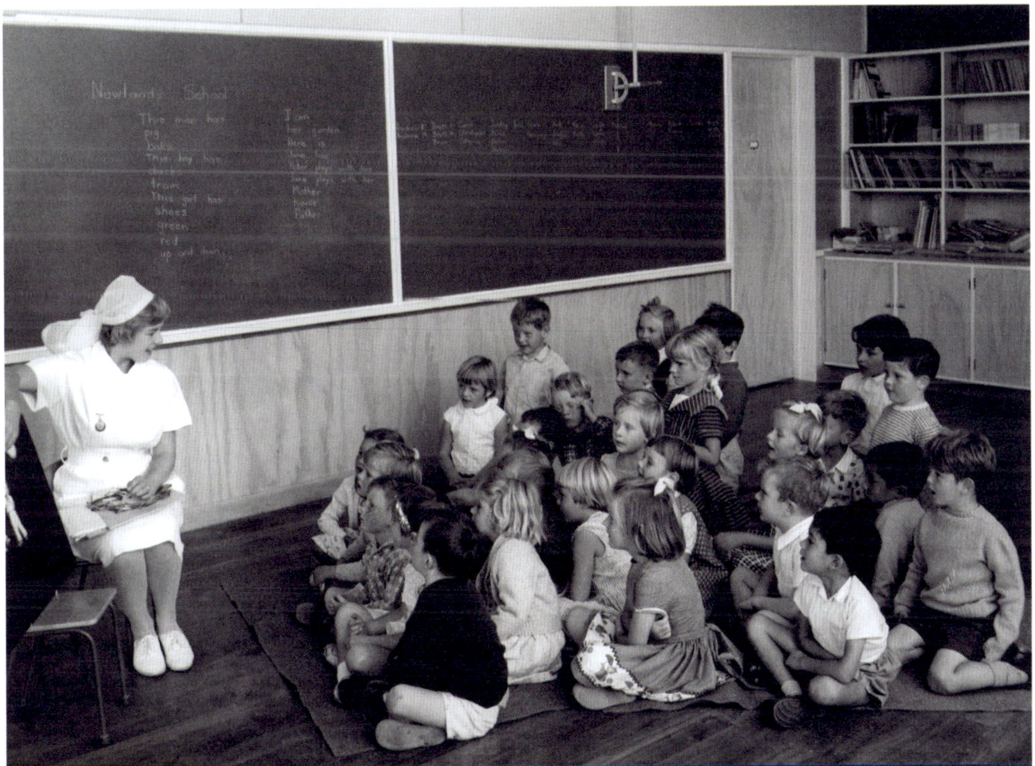

Classroom education was an important part of a dental nurse's work. School dental nurses originally received the same pay as school teachers.

Six-Day War in 1967. The Organization of Petroleum Exporting Countries imposed an oil embargo on countries supporting Israel and the price of crude oil quadrupled. The oil shock pushed many countries, including New Zealand, towards recession.

All that spring and early summer one song dominated the airwaves. Steve Allen's 'Join Together', the promo for the 1974 Commonwealth Games, played endlessly and unmuted on TV (remotes were still a couch potato's dream).[10] In sandwich bars, pubs, hairdressers and shops, the song cajoled patrons: 'We've got to join together.' It was a sentiment that dental nurses needed to take to heart if they were to make any headway with their pay claim. Working alone in clinics up and down the country, they had never jelled as an industrial group, and many weren't union members.

As an all-female workforce, it must have occurred to even the most conventionally minded that gender played a role in how they were being treated. By the early 1970s feminism was beginning to influence ordinary women, making them question their roles in society. Betty Friedan's *The Feminine Mystique* (1963) had shown how the media manipulated women to settle for the role of wife and mother over personal fulfilment.[11] Germaine Greer's brilliant polemic *The Female Eunuch* (1970) urged women to reclaim their sexuality and dismissed the nuclear family as oppressive and antisocial.[12] Women, Greer argued, were complicit in their own subjugation. 'Now as before, women must refuse to be meek and guileful, for truth cannot be served by dissimulation. Women who fancy that they manipulate the world by pussy power and gentle cajolery are fools. It is slavery to have to adopt such tactics.'

If New Zealand women weren't listening they soon got the subversive message when Greer, sans bra and knickers, arrived in Auckland, generating saturation media coverage. Authorities took note. She was charged with saying 'bullshit' at the town hall and 'fuck' at the university and fined $40. Tim Shadbolt, who'd previously been fined for offending public sensibilities with the word 'bullshit', met up with her. He wasn't impressed. As he wrote at the time: 'Perhaps I'm a male chauvinist, but I felt an instinctive dislike of her. She reminded me of Brian Edwards. A highly intelligent person who can brilliantly expose attitudes and prejudices, but who is somehow a cold academic . . . I felt sorry for all us naive kiwis. We turned out in our thousands to welcome our liberation, and all we got was an eccentric beatnik. She slapped us in the face as a country and as a people. She's got all the brains, but so little of the spirit of liberation.'[13]

Ngaire Mune, returning to dental nursing after a 10-year break to bring up her family, found that many of her friends hadn't been taken with Greer's message, either. But Ngaire identified with the feminist movement.

> I never burned my bra but I thought it was a jolly good thing. So I had got this idea in my head that women could now have a choice. They didn't have to stay home and be a wife and mother, they could be a working mother and have a career. But it proved extremely difficult to go back to work. It got so rough at one stage with friends being so critical that my youngest who was six said, 'Mummy, when you go back to work will you love us anymore?'

> That was really hard. It wasn't the men who were so critical, it was my female friends. In their view it was all right if you had to go back to work but if you didn't have to you were neglecting your children. So there was a lot of guilt and I did a lot more round the house than I should have done. You could have eaten off my floor at any time.[14]

She encountered the same attitude at work. 'I rang up the local health department office to rejoin the service and they said I could go way out in the sticks somewhere. So I said, "I really want somewhere around home." And then they asked, "What plans have you got for looking after your children while you're working?"' She got a better reception when she phoned the chief dental officer, John Colquhoun, who offered her work close to home. 'After a while I said, "Are you going to ask what I'm going to do with my kids?" And he said, "That's not my business. You're an intelligent woman, you can look after what needs to be looked after." That was really good.'

When she did start, one older nurse surprised her. 'For the first time since I'd been a mother I got treated like a child. That was probably the only time in my whole career that anybody had ever spoken to me in a way I didn't like.' After 10 years away, Ngaire expected to have to retrain in new methods and techniques. 'I was gobsmacked that there was no change whatsoever. Instead of using the one hypodermic needle over and over again and sterilising it, we now had disposable needles — that was the one change. Everything was still the same, the veils, the uniform, the records, the same supervising dental nurse and principal dental officer and all these endless checks on what you were doing.'

The real changes were happening in the attitudes of the dental nurses. In Auckland, the most militant region, activists Pam Horncy and Maggie Morgan were garnering support for action inside the PSA and among members of the Dental Nurses Institute. With such a scattered workforce, organising was difficult. Without social media, texting or the internet, the telephone was the only means of timely communication, but it was hit-and-miss in the era before answering machines. And rotary dial phones took what would now seem an age to dial a number. Newsletters and flyers took longer, too. Without photocopiers, duplicating involved typing on special waxed paper to be fitted on the drum of a Gestetner machine and cranking out copies by hand amid the heady fumes of methylated spirits.

From the start, the campaign organisers realised their options were limited. 'We set up an action committee through the Dental Nurses Institute to steer the campaign,' says Pam. 'We knew that strike action wasn't going to be a particularly effective way of getting our point across. Number one, the kids certainly wouldn't complain if we were striking. So we had to find a way of bringing this injustice to the eyes of the public.'[15]

A big protest meeting was held in Auckland where there was much condemning and deploring of the State Services Commission's refusal to negotiate. Curious passers-by were handed a leaflet in which Janet and John prose informed them: 'This is a dental nurse. All dental nurses are female. 80% of the work a dentist does is performed by her. Her Matron, New Zealand's top dental nurse, earns only $6558. Most nurses earn little more than half that amount . . . This is a dentist. Nearly all dentists are male. The top dentist in the public service earns $16,204 per year. Many private dentists earn as much as this.'

Pam remembers handing out the leaflets at the Santa parade, but the year was winding down and the public had other things on their minds. When dental nurses returned to work in January the country was gripped by Commonwealth Games fever (and some no doubt were relieved that they'd soon never have to hear that damn song again). People got to see for the first time what the world looked like on colour TV, mostly on sets in shop windows. The games, while a non-event for most of the world, did put New Zealand on the map when Kiwi weightlifter Graham May was instantly inducted into the blooper hall of fame by falling flat on his face holding a 187.5-kilogram barbell over his head.

The *Gazette* saw another reason why the world would take notice of the games. Under the headline 'GOLDEN SMILES FROM GOLDEN KIWIS', it ran a picture of gold medal winners Mark Treffers, Jaynie Parkhouse and Richard Tayler.

> There they were beaming at the camera, obviously still highly elated in their moment of triumph. What was most striking was the broad smile on each youthful face, enhanced to the full by gleaming well-cared-for teeth . . . What an advertisement for New Zealand this turned out to be!
>
> There are many people in the world today who still look on us as a nation of denture wearers. And how wrong they are! . . . Yes, today in this country observers find a positive appreciation of dental fitness and consequent attractiveness in the minds and habits of our young people, and it is not making too bold a claim to assert that the artificial denture once almost a New Zealand dental symbol has now 'had its day' in this far, southern sector of the world [forgetting perhaps that the prime minister had a full set].[16]

Nati●al Provident Fund

s the medium through which tens of thousands of New Zealanders are purchasing retirement pensions. If you wish to supplement your Government Super, why not join the N.P.F. Ensure yourself of an adequate income in retirement.

Write: NATIONAL PROVIDENT FUND
Departmental Buildings,
Box 5022, Wellington.

PUBLIC SERVICE

Journal

THE OFFICIAL ORGAN OF THE N.Z. PUBLIC SERVICE ASSOCIATION INC

)L. SIXTY-ONE, NUMBER ONE — FEBRUARY, 1974

Dental nurses angered by S.S.C.'s performance

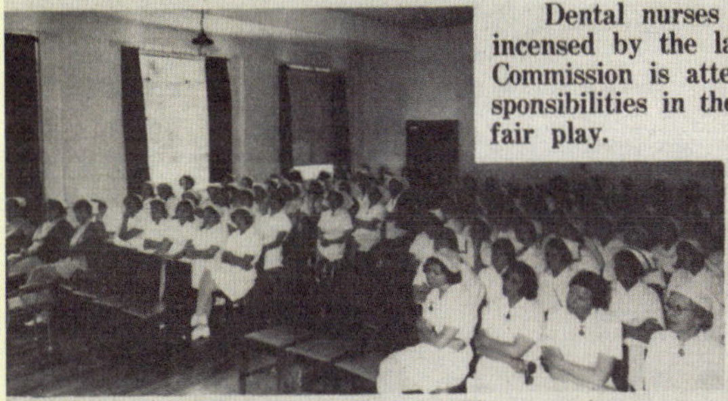

Dental nurses throughout the country are justifiably incensed by the latest indication that the State Services Commission is attempting to absolve itself from its responsibilities in the field of good industrial relations and fair play.

For dental nurses, the suspension of negotiations and the wage freeze occasioned last year by the imposition of the Economic Stabilisation Regulations has meant particular hardship and injustice to the extent that they are hampered in pursuing the historic relativity with public health nurses who gained substantial increases last year.

Of course, these Regulations are like a screen on a set stage for the S.S.C. The Commission can strut on to the centre of the stage, soliloquize along the lines that no wage increase is justified for a group and then retreat behind the safety of the Regulations.

But the groundlings in this current dispute are not like Shakespeare's patrons and prepared to put up with a bad performance for the sake of the diversionary spectacle. They are not grubby illiterate peasants awed by the charade—but dedicated, highly trained intelligent (but underpaid) women who have made the New Zealand School Dental Service the envy of the world. They are, of course, well aware that since 1946 the S.S.C. has consistently applied to them a salary relativity with public health nurses in spite of their own attempts to align themselves with primary school teachers. Claims lodged for dental nurses on this basis since 1946 have been declined or received only trivial increases, as the S.S.C. has insisted that the only relativity is with public health nurses.

It so happens that now that public health nurses have achieved the breakthrough and receive salaries somewhat more commensurate with their value to the community that dental nurses are prevented from following suit by the Commission's interpretation of the Regulations and the convenient abandonment of the "sacred" historic relativity. So much for Commission consistency—or lack of it!

Further action

Dental nurses will contemplate further action at a series of lunch-time and stop-work meetings throughout the country in the weeks ahead.

The S.S.C. will certainly not receive accolades from anyone for its pathetic "performance" in this matter. Moreover, it may find that its feet are pierced with drills rather than rose petals as it flits off the stage to the Economic Stabilisation Regulations screen.

Perhaps that might have a salutary effect, awake the Commission from its torpor and cause it to recognise the serious anomaly that now exists in the salary scales of dental nurses in relation to those applying to public health nurses.

The dental nurses held a luncntime meeting at the Willis Street• Dental Clinic, Wellington, (above) on February 1, and passed the following resolution:

"That this meeting deplores the attiude of the employing authority in its failure to maintain the historic link with the salary scales of Public Health nurses and calls for a general stop-work meeting of all dental nurses in the Wellington area to take place in February, to discuss what further steps should be taken to have what this meeting knows to be a justified claim recognised as such by the employing authority."

Below, one of the student dental nurses under instruction checks the teeth of a young patient at the Willis Street Dental Clinic in Wellington.

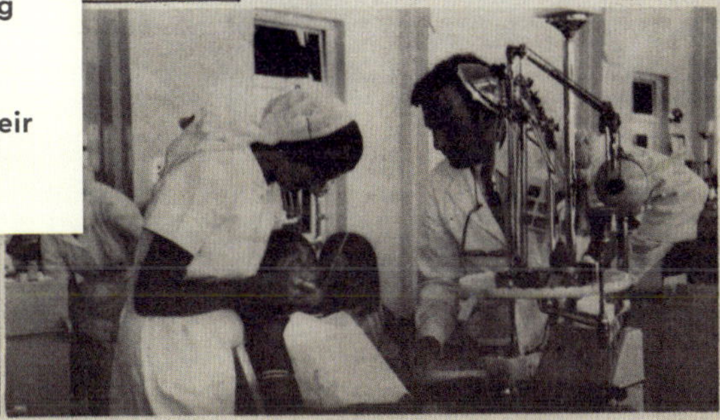

Flexible Working Hours

)URING the last three months of 1973 the Nelson office of the State Advances Cor-oration, the State Fire Insurance Head ffice and the Lower Hutt Branch of the Department of Inland Revenue tested a pilot cheme for flexible working hours in the ervice.

his proved to be a opular and successful in-ovation. The response of tate Insurance and Inland evenue staff who com-leted an Association

social workers with the Social Welfare Department, Invercargill, have conditions of employment that are slightly different from those of clerical workers, and this should also provide some addiitonal ...n.

...oped that at the ... experiment on May ... will be further ex-... roughout the Ser-

From the inclusion of the uckland and Invercargill ffices, information will be ained about the impact of he scheme under differing onditions of geography and limate, and a trading department, the Public Trust Office, as also been included. The

By February 1974 dental nurses were in a fighting mood after the State Services Commission refused to recognise their pay claim.

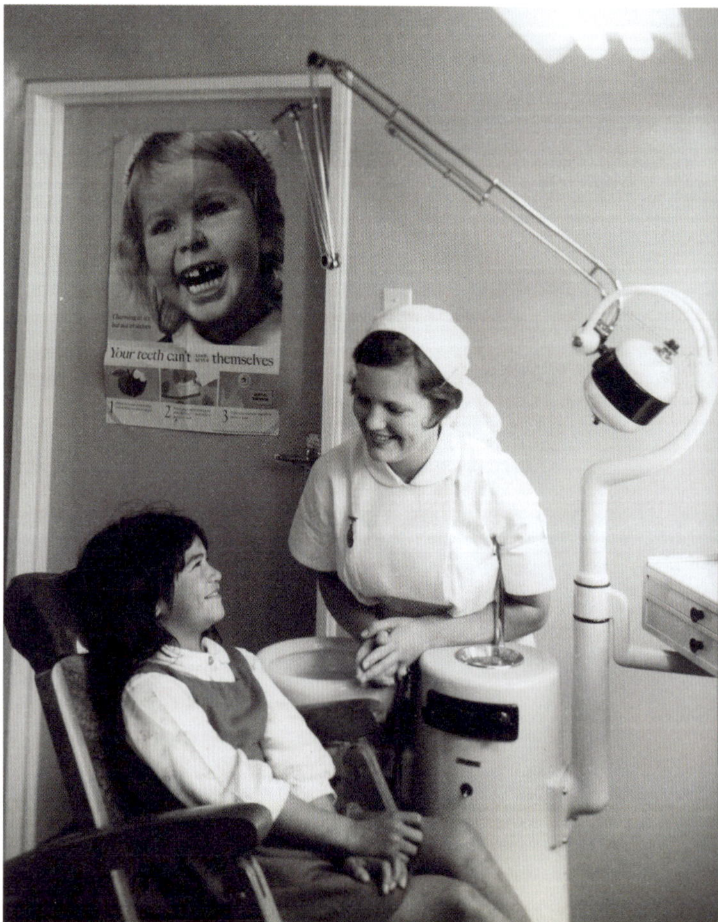

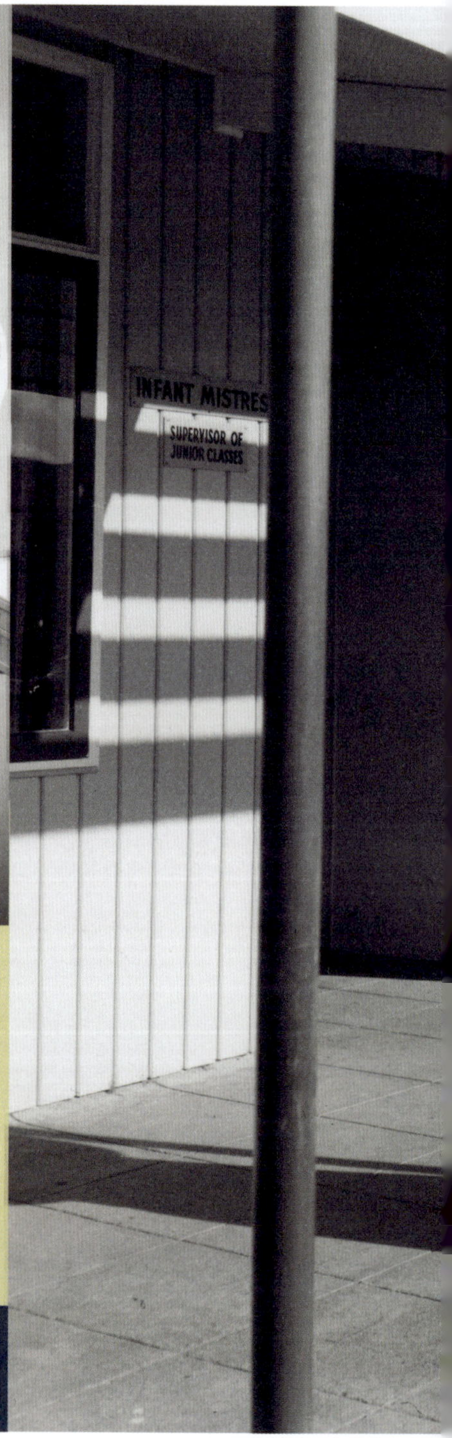

Above: A dental nurse tries to put her patient at ease.

Right: By the 1960s, dental nursing was the profession time forgot. The staid uniform had changed little since the 1940s.

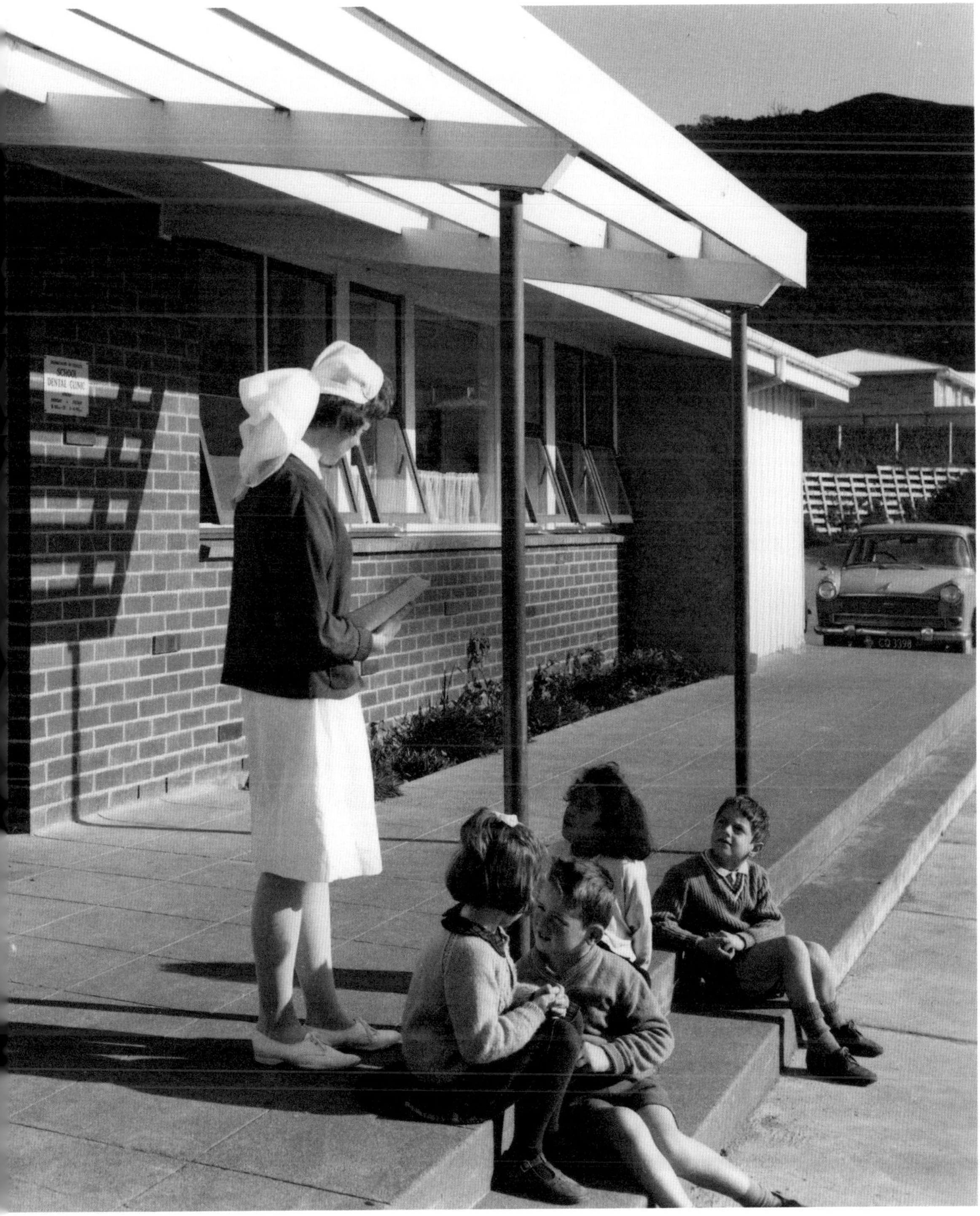
SCHOOL
DENTAL CLINIC

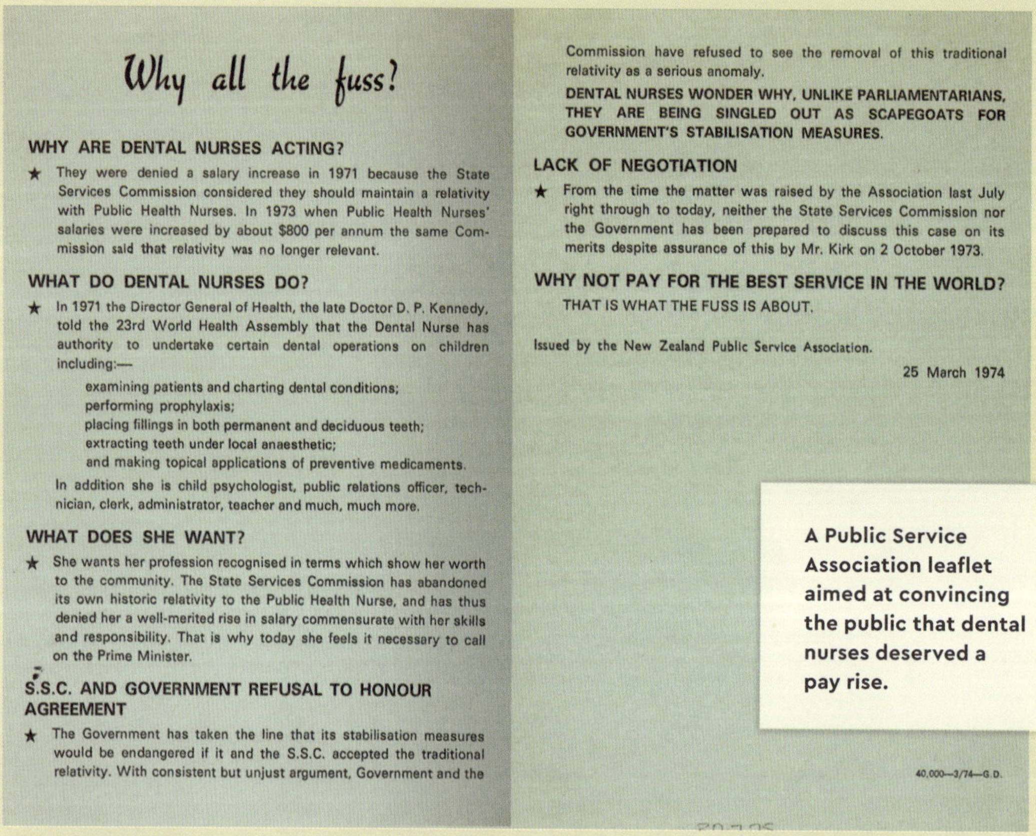

Why all the fuss?

WHY ARE DENTAL NURSES ACTING?

★ They were denied a salary increase in 1971 because the State Services Commission considered they should maintain a relativity with Public Health Nurses. In 1973 when Public Health Nurses' salaries were increased by about $800 per annum the same Commission said that relativity was no longer relevant.

WHAT DO DENTAL NURSES DO?

★ In 1971 the Director General of Health, the late Doctor D. P. Kennedy, told the 23rd World Health Assembly that the Dental Nurse has authority to undertake certain dental operations on children including:—

examining patients and charting dental conditions;
performing prophylaxis;
placing fillings in both permanent and deciduous teeth;
extracting teeth under local anaesthetic;
and making topical applications of preventive medicaments.

In addition she is child psychologist, public relations officer, technician, clerk, administrator, teacher and much, much more.

WHAT DOES SHE WANT?

★ She wants her profession recognised in terms which show her worth to the community. The State Services Commission has abandoned its own historic relativity to the Public Health Nurse, and has thus denied her a well-merited rise in salary commensurate with her skills and responsibility. That is why today she feels it necessary to call on the Prime Minister.

S.S.C. AND GOVERNMENT REFUSAL TO HONOUR AGREEMENT

★ The Government has taken the line that its stabilisation measures would be endangered if it and the S.S.C. accepted the traditional relativity. With consistent but unjust argument, Government and the Commission have refused to see the removal of this traditional relativity as a serious anomaly.

DENTAL NURSES WONDER WHY, UNLIKE PARLIAMENTARIANS, THEY ARE BEING SINGLED OUT AS SCAPEGOATS FOR GOVERNMENT'S STABILISATION MEASURES.

LACK OF NEGOTIATION

★ From the time the matter was raised by the Association last July right through to today, neither the State Services Commission nor the Government has been prepared to discuss this case on its merits despite assurance of this by Mr. Kirk on 2 October 1973.

WHY NOT PAY FOR THE BEST SERVICE IN THE WORLD?

THAT IS WHAT THE FUSS IS ABOUT.

Issued by the New Zealand Public Service Association.

25 March 1974

40,000—3/74—G.D.

A Public Service Association leaflet aimed at convincing the public that dental nurses deserved a pay rise.

By 2 February, the games were over, the fever had passed and dental nurses could get back to campaigning. The media were starting to take notice of the stop-work meetings being held across the country. Dental nurses were at last speaking out. 'Conditions "shocking" Otaki dental nurses say' ran a big headline in the *Dominion*.[17] Apart from the poor pay, the nurses interviewed said they were fed up with the antiquated equipment and disgraceful cramped working conditions. 'We have been the most uncomplaining people for so long that the public has come to take us for granted.' Sensing perhaps that some readers and former patients might be less than sympathetic, they pre-emptively defended themselves. 'We are not trained to be nice — some don't know how to be — and this could ruin a child's attitude for life.' At fault was their training, which didn't cover child development and psychology, they said.

In Auckland, campaigners were trying out new tactics. 'We started visiting MPs and talking to whoever we thought might listen to us,' says Pam. 'Four of us gatecrashed a National Party fundraising barbecue.' They'd guessed correctly that attractive young women in uniform were unlikely to be strong-armed and asked to leave. 'We got talking to Rob Muldoon and George Gair and various others.' Muldoon was wearing white trousers and quaffing gin and tonics, which he offered the nurses. 'Everyone was so sympathetic — "Oh that's not good enough," they said. And of course agreeing with us absolutely because they could, they were in opposition.'

Through the PSA, they secured an unlikely but influential ally: meat inspectors. Meat inspectors had the power to shut down every freezing works in the country and seriously damage the economy. Pam Horncy and Maggie Morgan went to the freezing works to talk to the workers about the dental nurses' case. Pam remembers feeling anxious about venturing into such alien territory. Arriving in their pristine uniforms, the dental nurses found their way blocked.

Ian Baldick, the young and gung-ho chairman of the PSA's meat inspectors national delegates group, was there to greet them. He takes up the story:

> The dental nurses had come to talk to the meat inspectors in our smoko room during the lunch hour. The trouble was the meat managers wouldn't let the dental nurses on to the plant. They wouldn't let them come up the stairs to us. Well, we weren't having that. We decided we would close all the plants down, take the meat inspectors outside the Westfield and have the meeting on the Great South Road. There was an area where we could gather and that's what we did, we closed the plants. The inspectors walked off the chains and we had our meeting with trucks and cars going past beeping their horns.
>
> The meat inspectors passed a resolution that we'd not go back on the chain for the rest of the day and we'd walk off the job. It got passed unanimously. There were lambs, beef hanging on the chain waiting for us to come back and the butchers cheered and everybody was happy because we were going to have a bit of an early finish. The company managers were pissed off, they went through the roof. Our employers didn't know what to do because if they disciplined us we would take more action. It was a breakthrough for the dental nurses because all of a sudden their dispute affected Federated Farmers.[18]

In Wellington the PSA was feeding questions to opposition MPs only too happy to put state services minister Bob Tizard on the spot. Tizard was now arguing that while the relativity between dental nurses and public health nurses had existed, 'such relativities are not permanent. Any assertion that they are implies that no change ever takes place.' Asked on another occasion, he argued that public health nurses had received their pay increase only because it had been difficult to recruit them from the hospital nursing service. Since that recruiting problem did not exist for dental nurses, there was no case for passing that increase on to dental nurses.

Christchurch had never been a hotbed of radicalism, but even there the dental nurses' campaign was intensifying. It was spearheaded by three dental nurse tutors, Kate Hishon, Jackie Humm and Margaret Clarkson. They knew that pay was just one of several issues. 'I was a dental health tutor travelling from Kaikoura down to Stewart Island and I got a lot of confidences from the girls,' says Jackie. 'Dreadful isolation was one of the things. Some of them were living in terrible conditions, in caravans. Some felt there was favouritism in who got salary steps, and some didn't get on with the inspector. There was a lot of frustration building up.'[19]

As tutors they were regarded as management and now they were siding with the rank and file, a stance that bordered on treason in such a hierarchical organisation. 'We were regarded as communists, militants. For a lot of people it was very uncomfortable to be associated with us,' says Margaret Clarkson.[20] It was a period of her life she has tried to forget about; union activist was never a role she had sought. 'It was quite traumatic. Once you've been exposed to the politics of it then you've lost your innocence in a sense and you can't regain it.'

There were weekly meetings of the PSA advisory panel, to which she, Jackie and Kate belonged. Panel members from Auckland flew in and the meetings were usually held in Margaret's apartment, a source of friction in her marriage.

Decades later, seeing the movie *Made in Dagenham*,[21] the story of a group of female Ford machinists who rile union bosses and try their husbands' patience by striking for equal pay, Margaret's anxieties came flooding back. 'I found that film quite distressing because it brought back a lot of the things I'd been through. Even down to Rita, the character who has marital problems because her husband has a certain expectation of what a wife should be, the fifties housewife type. I went through that because my husband was at university at the time and he would come home and find the advisory panel having a meeting and we had a tiny flat. So it did have an effect on us.'

As in the movie, however, they were strongly supported by a local union official, John McKenzie. 'He was like Bob Hoskins, the shop steward character in the movie, a man of great integrity,' says Margaret. McKenzie was regional secretary of the PSA and a give-no-quarter cloth-cap unionist. As a colleague remarked, 'You can relate to John McKenzie like you might relate to a savage guard dog. If he's guarding you it's marvellous, but if you're trying to burgle the union you'd have to give some thought to living in a wheelchair.'[22]

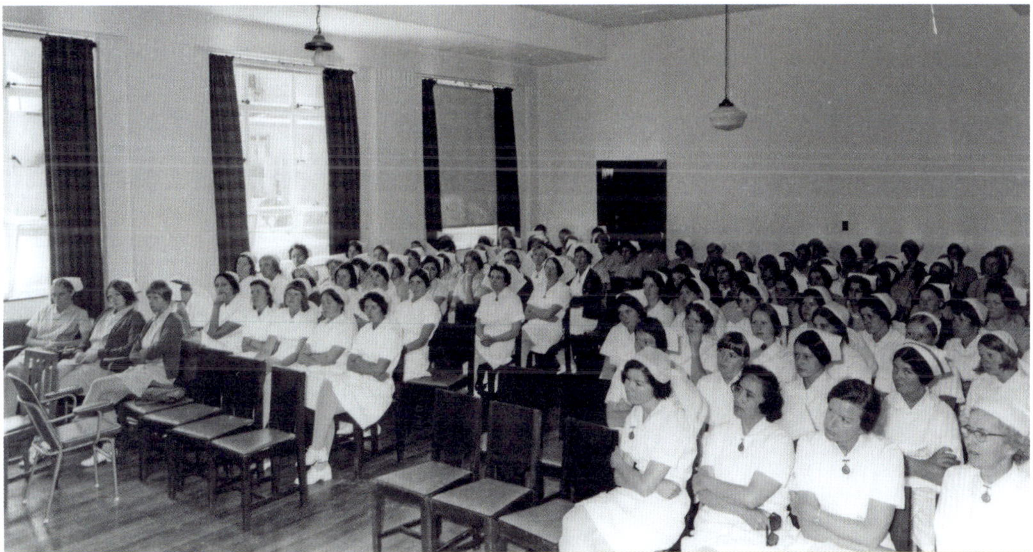

Dental nurses in the Willis Street clinic pass a resolution calling on all dental nurses in the Wellington region to hold a stopwork meeting in support of the pay claim.

Of Greek descent and raised in an Australian orphanage, McKenzie was a staunch unionist but far from a compliant one.[23] Once expelled from the PSA executive for outspokenness, he remained a thorn in the side of union bosses even after becoming the union's Canterbury regional secretary. He was fond of boasting that in the long history of the PSA he remained 'the only person ever appointed to the staff of the PSA on probation. I was too much of a rebel for a permanent appointment at the time.'

McKenzie was frequently at loggerheads with Dan Long, the PSA's general secretary. Presciently, he'd been a vigorous opponent of the occupational classification of members in the PSA, believing separate interest groups would weaken solidarity. As he was to say later, 'When I was chairperson in the 1960s, public service managers would sit next to labourers[;] it was not right wing or left wing, or bosses and workers. Forty thousand public servants were treated the same. But today there is little support from higher paid groups for the Mrs Mopps, the Internal Affairs cleaners. The undoing of that mix is today weakening the PSA.'

A rough diamond himself, he carved greenstone and opal as a hobby. Despite his belligerent manner and tough exterior, he won over the conservative middle-class women who made up most of the School Dental Service in Christchurch. 'We had tremendous admiration for John. We were so politically unaware and he did so much for us,' says Margaret Clarkson. 'He put his heart and soul into our cause. He had wonderful sayings, like "When he hears this, his shirt will go up his back like a roller blind," and "For all he would know about, you could write on the back of a postage stamp with a builder's pencil."'

From McKenzie she learned the rudiments of union negotiations that would later serve her well. One particular lesson stood out.

> Linda Gibson, a colleague, and I went with John to Wellington to negotiate travel allowances. Public servants were getting 10 cents a kilometre and we were getting nothing. We went to the Reserve Bank building and I remember feeling really nervous going up in the lift which was all lined with copper and marble. When we got to the board room there were about six young men in suits looking very sharp. It was quite intimidating. We were in our best clothes and there was John looking like the dishevelled *Columbo* character with his lived-in suit and the mane of black hair that hung over his face. He'd whip it back and when he spoke he lisped because he had a slight speech impediment. He looked like he wouldn't know a thing but he had a very sharp mind.
>
> He carried this old briefcase that was always bursting with papers and thick files. He sat down and took out a couple of files with papers spilling across the table. The other side was looking very superior but suddenly the illusion was broken when in trotted the public service tea lady with her old trolley. She might as well have had carpet slippers on, she looked like she was out of *Coronation Street*. Sipping tea from thick cups we got on with the negotiations. After a while, they said, 'We'll offer you five cents.' John slapped down a file on the table and said, 'This is disgraceful!' He stuffed the file in his briefcase, stood up and said to Linda and I, 'Come on, brothers' and we trotted out after him, our hearts thumping.
>
> When we got to the lift, I said, 'Oh, John, that was dreadful.' 'What do you mean?' he said. 'They only offered us five cents,' I said. 'Don't be stupid, we've only been here half an hour and we have five cents. We'll go and have some lunch and by the afternoon we'll have ten cents like every other public servant.' That was the way he operated — great theatre. And, of course, we got on the plane that afternoon with the same allowance as every other public servant.

But despite the support of union officials like McKenzie, and the push to get parents and the public on their side, the dental nurses' campaign was getting nowhere. On 5 March the *New Zealand Herald* highlighted their plight with a front-page story: 'Pay Rate Toothache for Girls' read the headline. 'For the first time in 53 years dental nurses are protesting publicly about wages. They are furious that after 30 years being on the same pay scale as public health nurses they are well down at $4598 against $5495 for a public health nurse.'

The next day they got a boost when meat inspectors walked off the job for a meeting in support of dental nurses. The stoppage closed three Auckland freezing works, the abattoir and meat-packing plants. The meat inspectors dispatched two telegrams to Tizard demanding that he instruct the State Services Commission to preserve the relativity between dental nurses and public health nurses. Tizard fired back with a terse telegram of his own: 'Do I take from your telegram that nothing ever changes?' Dan Long denounced Tizard's reaction as 'flippant'. Tizard hit back, calling Long 'childish and irresponsible'.

The State Services Commission began a review to investigate 'the duties and responsibilities of dental nurses in order to assess their salary structure'. The PSA saw it for what it was, a delaying tactic, and rejected it. However, it did give Bob Tizard a pretext to ignore the dental nurses until the review was complete.

Then an event on 14 March boosted the dental nurses' case. That morning they picked up their newspapers to read that backbench MPs had been awarded a backdated 45 per cent pay increase and ministers a 30 per cent increase despite the wage freeze. Angry but unsure what to do next, some activists went to see Auckland Labour MP Eddie Isbey, under-secretary to the minister of labour and married to a dental nurse. Might he be able to exert some influence? He proposed a march on Parliament to make their case. It was, on the face of it, a mischievous suggestion for a member of the government to make; it would embarrass the already beleaguered government and enrage Tizard.

Campaign activists latched on to the suggestion. Something had to be done to re-energise the campaign. A march on Parliament would be a bold step and show politicians and the public how determined they were in their fight for wage justice. First, though, two questions had to be settled. Would the PSA support and fund the march? And, crucially, would a workforce of timorous middle-class women be prepared to take to the streets?

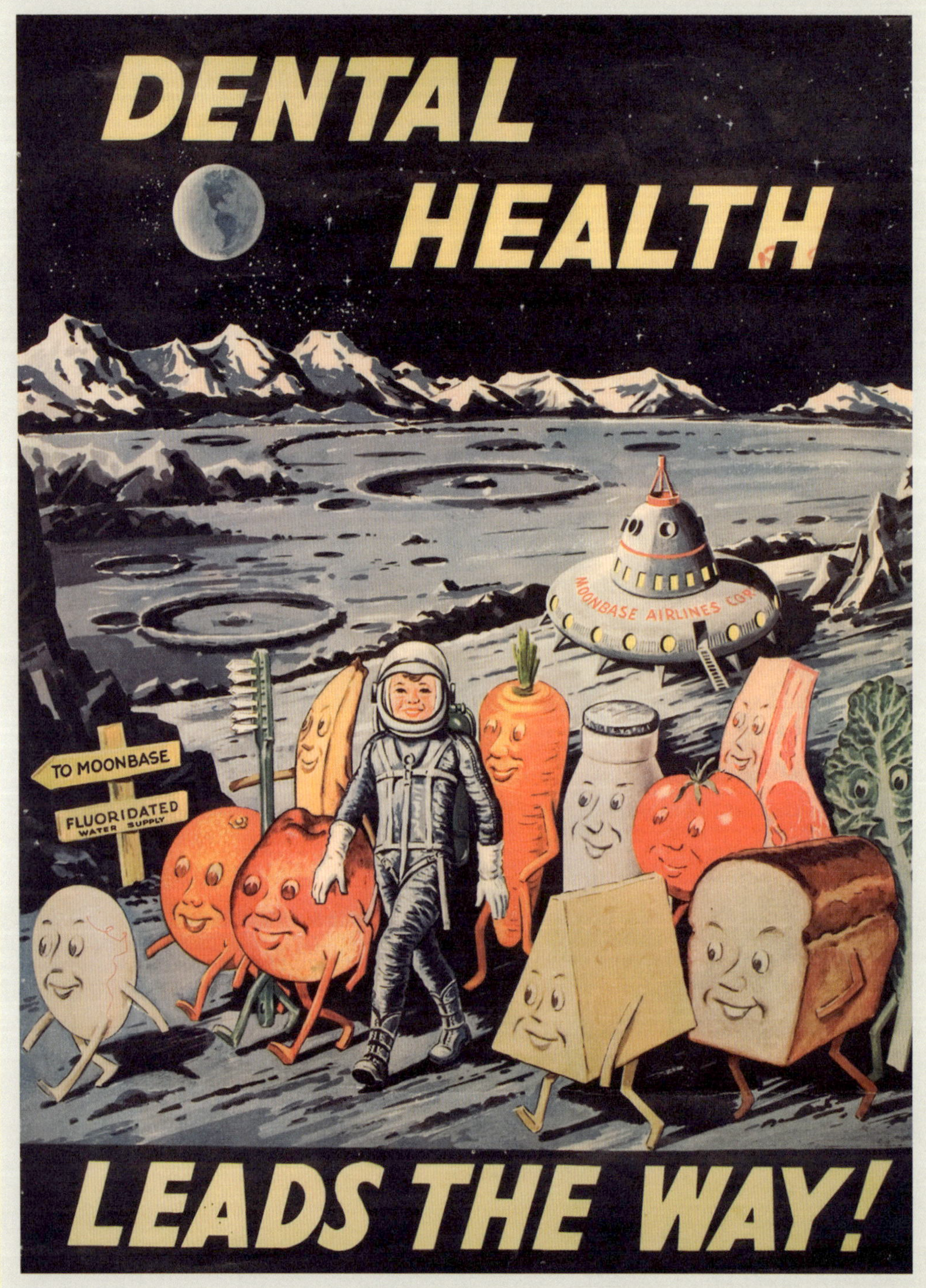
DENTAL HEALTH
MOONBASE AIRLINES COR
TO MOONBASE
FLUORIDATED WATER SUPPLY
LEADS THE WAY!

8

THE MARCH THAT CHANGED EVERYTHING

The fifteenth of March 1974 was not a good day for Norman Kirk. The massive pay increases quietly awarded to MPs were coming under fire from all directions, including the Employers' Federation, the unions and the media. Hadn't the prime minister said, just five months before, that Parliament could not ask other sections of the population to accept wage restraints and allow MPs an increase? In a statement that foreshadowed the defence of fake news, minister of labour Hugh Watt said a transcript of the prime minister's press conference contained no such statement. Why then was the so-called inaccurate report not challenged at the time and steps not taken to correct the impression given? Watt said that was a fair question and he did not have an answer.

There was domestic conflict as well. Kirk's wife, Ruth, was making one of her rare visits to the office. Over the years the marriage had soured and she had a habit of berating and putting him down in front of others. Today was no exception, referring to him as 'His Highness' to office staff and ignoring his requests to come into his private office.[1] The man who was more than a match for parliamentary pitbull Rob Muldoon was at a loss in such situations. Further, at the time of the dental nurses' campaign Kirk was a sick, unhappy man, often in pain. He would die six months later, and his health may well have been a factor in the outcome of that campaign.

Meanwhile, in the cramped PSA offices on the third floor of PSIS House, a short distance from Parliament, Dan Long wasn't having a good day either. The Wellington office was in turmoil as the result of a long-running conflict that had begun when PSA staff had decided they wanted to be represented by the Clerical Workers Union (CWU) instead of the in-house staff association.[2] That morning union staff were holding a hastily arranged meeting to discuss the president and the general secretary's attempt the previous day to persuade some individuals to break the ban that had been placed on certain work duties. They voted to stop work for the day and had advised the bosses that 'any further attempts to intimidate members who have carried out the decisions of the Branch would result in an immediate stop-work meeting being called to decide on further action'.

Late that afternoon, in the near-empty offices, Long had received a letter from the CWU, which claimed to represent PSA staff. It demanded that staff be given three weeks' leave paid at time and a half and work no more than a seven-hour day without the payment of overtime. If the demands were not met within a week, 'a dispute of interests' would exist. In other words: 'See you in court.'

The irony of a union boss not wanting his staff to join a union was entirely lost on Long, though not on the judge of the Arbitration Court, who ruled in favour of the staff's right to join the CWU.

Mark Derby, in his biography of Dan Long, writes: 'The irony continued as the PSA executive refused to recognise the upstart body and insisted on dealing with the remnant of the original staff association. Rivalries between the two camps led at times to absurdly vindictive behaviour. One former staff member related proudly that during a social event at PSA headquarters, he had gone into Dan's unoccupied office and urinated in a drawer of his desk. Others chose to withdraw their services, to the extent of refusing to take part in some of the most inspiring and uplifting campaigns of this period.'[3]

The ban on work duties had extended to the dental nurses' campaign, but the PSA was still pushing ahead with it. PSA president Jack Batt called a number of regional secretaries to Wellington to coordinate the campaign. Noticeably absent from the mix was Canterbury's John McKenzie, perhaps once again in the national office's bad graces. Eddie Isbey's suggestion of a march on Parliament had already been floated within the PSA, and now Batt put a motion to spend $10,000 on bringing the dental nurses to Wellington (a further $2000 was approved later).

With more than 50,000 members, the PSA was in good financial shape, but spending today's equivalent of $136,000 for a single march to raise an issue that affected about one-fiftieth of its members was extraordinary. Unions often hold back their criticism when a Labour government is in office so as not to rock the boat. Staging a major demonstration less than 18 months into Labour's first term seemed poor strategy. All the signals indicated that the government would not budge on the issue, lest it set a precedent for other groups of workers to try to break the wage freeze. Why put so much resource into a march of dental nurses, most of whom had never been union members and, as Annette King believed, were mainly National supporters?

Had they endorsed Isbey's suggestion because they were out of ideas about what to do next and wanted to stick it to the minister of state services? Certainly, they shared Isbey's antipathy towards Bob Tizard and were so incensed by his 'flippant and superficial attitude towards serious questions put before him' that they wanted Kirk to replace him as minister.[4] Tizard made no secret of his belief that the PSA was out to wreck the government's Economic Stabilisation Regulations. To R. K. Logan, director of dental health, the PSA's motives were clear. The union wanted to expand into the health sector where it had few members. 'Its aim,' he wrote to a colleague 'is to increase its membership to about 100,000 in one take-over bid. In pursuit of this objective it is demonstrating its interests in the welfare of health workers. So far it has gained good publicity from the dental nurse group and it intends to hang on to that publicity outlet.'[5]

It is also possible that the men (and it was always men until 1988) who ran the PSA — president Jack Batt and general secretary Dan Long — saw it as a matter of principle to do everything possible to support the dental nurses. Neither was the type to back away from a fight.

Like dental nurses, women in the public service had long been disadvantaged in their careers by a male hierarchy. Their promotion prospects were limited, they were paid less than the junior male colleagues they trained and were required to retire 10 years earlier than men. A great number of women, too, shared the view of politicians and public service heads that men deserved to be paid more because they had a family to support, and that women were not good candidates for promotion because male staff would not work under females.

Dan Long had become the PSA's general secretary in 1960, having stepped down after two terms as president to accept the paid position. In an era when union business was often conducted in smoky backrooms over generous measures of whisky, he stood out as a disapproving teetotaller, though he kept a bottle of whisky in his office to lubricate negotiations. He was sober in dress, too, favouring, winter and summer, the expensive dark suit and tie of a senior public servant.

That evening, as the railcar unit rattled its way from the city to Upper Hutt, Long may have wondered what the odds were that the large bet the PSA had placed on the dental nurses would pay off. An outside chance? A march rarely influenced politicians; more often than not, it got their backs up. It was sure to have been common knowledge in union circles that Norman Kirk had been furious when the Seamen's Union closed down the Port of Auckland and union members marched up Queen Street just days before the 1969 general election, costing Labour victory. Long, however, had never backed down when a principle was at stake, and he was not about to start now.

The logistics of getting more than 600 dental nurses from every part of the country to Wellington on one day by 10 a.m. were daunting. The plan was to airlift them in by chartering Boeing 737s from Auckland and Christchurch and by Vickers Viscounts from Dunedin and Hamilton. Some would also travel on scheduled flights and by bus and train. Provisional dates were 22, 26 or 28 March — in fact none of those worked.

Local organisers like Pam Horncy and Maggie Morgan in Auckland had to provide a list of marchers from their area to the PSA so that airline tickets could be purchased. Without the home phone numbers of members, they had to ring the nurses in their clinics. Many were nervous at the thought of marching. They were being asked to give up a day's pay, defy their superiors and take to the streets, flouting the rule that banned the wearing of uniforms in public. They were to go to Wellington; many had never flown in a plane or been to the capital. 'There were a number of women who were keen to go but you had to spend quite a bit of time on the phone reassuring them, making them feel okay about going,' says Pam.[6] To the likely relief of children, appointments were cancelled and teeth left unfilled. Maggie was reprimanded by her supervisor 'because of my poor output, [which] was decreasing from my activities around the march'.[7]

In some areas senior staff were putting pressure on dental nurses not to go. The PSA advised that 'if steps are taken by local controlling officers or even acting upon the authority of the Health Department head office to refuse leave to Dental Nurses, then the nurses concerned should be told to disregard any prohibition'. Even with the backing of the union, though, it took courage to take a stand and risk being branded a troublemaker in the future.

A glitch occurred when the PSA got word back from the prime minister's office that he could not meet a deputation on the planned march day; Kirk could only meet the marchers on Friday 29 March. 'We had everyone organised,' says Pam, 'and then the PSA rang up and said we're not going on that day. So then we had to ring around everyone again and make sure they were available and some weren't.'

Friday 22 March: With one week to go, dental nurses woke up to a story that had all New Zealanders agog. 'Man charged with attack on Princess' was the banner headline in the *New Zealand Herald*. Princess Anne, who only weeks before had attended the Commonwealth Games with the rest of the royal family, had been the subject of an apparent assassination attempt. A lone gunman, 26-year-old Ian Ball, had swerved into the Bentley carrying Anne and her new husband, Captain Mark Phillips. Ball, armed with a pistol, shot and wounded the bodyguard, chauffeur and a policeman. Bryan McConnell, a Fleet Street journalist, happened to be passing in a taxi and went to the couple's aid. McConnell, serendipitously the author of a book called *Assassination*, which included accounts of attempts on the lives of royalty, confronted the gunman. He told reporters later: 'I ran up to the gunman and stood in front of him. I said, "Look, old man, these people are friends of mine. Don't be silly. Give me the gun."' Ball promptly shot him in the chest. The gunman then fled and was captured soon after. Next day, the princess was literally back on her horse. Ball was committed to Broadmoor mental hospital, to be detained at Her Majesty's pleasure.[8]

It was a riveting story to start the day, but dental nurse campaign organisers were more interested in the story that had been shunted to page two. Under the heading 'Call for Minister to be sacked' it read: 'The Combined State Services Organisation which represents all 150,000 civil servants called yesterday for the Minister of State Services, Mr Tizard, to be given the sack . . . The call for Mr Tizard came originally from the Auckland section of the Public Service Association . . . Earlier this week the call was endorsed by the Public Service Association . . . Now the CSSO has added its weight to the call. It noted in a resolution that civil servants were gravely concerned at the flippant attitude of Mr Tizard to serious questions raised by them.'

The deteriorating relationship with Minister Tizard did not bode well for the success of the march. President Batt appeared to be having doubts about how much difference it would make. His diary entries suggest he was already looking beyond the event:

> Tuesday, 26 March
> At 2pm met PSA secretary organisers and discussed the dental nurses dispute — sorted out the next steps to be taken to have their pay relativity restored.
>
> Wednesday, 27 March
> Meeting of PSA executive officers at 3.30pm — the main problem is the dental nurses dispute and how we can keep up the momentum. We could get the secretary organisers to come to Wellington next week to assess the position.[9]

On that Wednesday, Norman Kirk returned from the South Pacific Forum in the Cook Islands with a bout of dysentery and pain in his legs from varicose veins. In his absence, Rob Muldoon had gone on the attack in the House: '[Kirk's] appearance was built up by a public relations team, but 12 months [in] office has found him out,' Muldoon railed.[10]

There was still fallout from the massive pay increase for MPs announced the week before. Kirk's secretary, Margaret Hayward, recorded in her diary: 'Ever since the Parliamentary wage rise, Brian Edwards on Radio Windy talkback has been vitriolic in his remarks about the Labour Party and Mr K. in particular.'[11]

Kirk, though, was still popular in the country. 'Big Norm', a song by the Wellington duo Ebony, was riding high in the charts with its now familiar chorus:

> A man of great labour is our Big Norm
> A man of social credit is our Big Norm
> A great national favourite is our Big Norm
> The hero of our commune is our Big Norm
> Norman is the fairy on our Christmas tree,
> Handing out goodies to the elderly.'[12]

Thursday 28 March: On the eve of the march, two nurses were interviewed in their clinic for the television news programme *Nationwide*.[13] In the black-and-white TV footage their starched uniforms seem to glow, like teeth in a toothpaste commercial.

> Reporter Guy Salmon: Mr Tizard has made it very, very clear that he doesn't want you to go on this march and be influenced by it. If that's the case, don't you think that by going ahead anyway he'll be put in a position where he can't give in to demands?
> Nurses: Well, we have no alternative now. We've corresponded with him and asked him to negotiate and he's steadfastly refused, so what can we do? This is the only avenue that is left to us. All we've asked for was discussion and he wasn't interested at all. He made the point that the PSA was using us and we really weren't aware of what was going on. He didn't seem to know anything about dental nursing itself and when we left he promised nothing; he didn't even promise to read the correspondence we sent him. We don't mind the PSA using us: we're using the PSA and we don't mind if we get what we want.
> Salmon: What was the impetus for the march? Did it come from your own ranks or the PSA?
> Nurses: I hate to tell you. It was suggested by an MP.
> Salmon: Can you tell me the name of the MP?
> Nurses: No.

Salmon: Can you tell me which party the MP was from?
Nurses: The Labour Party.
Salmon: So he was a member of the government. If your claim is successful how much is it going to cost the country?
Nurses: It's going to be backdated the same as the public health nurses and it will cost the country over a million dollars and this is why Mr Tizard is battening down.
Salmon: I wonder if Mr Tizard is concerned [that] all the other groups whose traditional relativities are threatened are also going to jump onto the bandwagon?
Nurses: Well, Mr Tizard and the State Services Commission made these rules — they made the relativity rules, so if it's good enough to make these rules it's probably good enough to keep them.

In the studio Bob Tizard, in paisley shirt and jacket with far-ranging lapels, answered questions from David Beatson.

Beatson: What will you say to the dental nurses who are marching on Parliament to represent their case to you?
Tizard: There's been a consistent misunderstanding of the situation and the PSA have a large responsibility for this. The commission is quite prepared to discuss a case for changes that have taken place in the dental nurses profession over the years, but they will not accept the relativity argument that linked them to public health nurses.
Beatson: But wouldn't you expect the dental nurses to want more money when they see the public health nurses, to whom they been linked for 30 years in the salary claims, getting more?
Tizard: At the end of the day it didn't come suddenly. There's been discussion about relativities before, not only with dental nurses. The PSA themselves insisted on challenging the meat inspectors' relativity only four years ago. One of the problems with the PSA and other unions is that they take a special case when they feel it's justified and having won that they'll try to add it to the relativity claim. You can have absolute relativity or special cases but you can't pick and choose, go from one to the other as the opportunity arises, otherwise you have galloping inflation.
Beatson: But isn't it true that dental nurses have had claims knocked back in the past because they would have been ahead on public health nurses, who are now in front of them?

> Tizard: They've put in a relativity claim when they could have put in a claim on special grounds. What I'm saying and what the commission has represented to me is that there is a case for the examination of special factors in the dental nurses' case. Many of them stay for far longer than was anticipated when the salaries scale was framed.

In Parliament MPs were working late into the evening. Perhaps stung by property magnate and political gadfly Bob Jones' new book, *The First Twelve Months: A study of the third Labour government's achievements*, which contained only blank pages 'because the Labour Government has done nothing worth recording', Kirk had taken urgency on 10 bills. The House adjourned at 12.41 a.m. Tired and perhaps bruised by another Muldoon attack that would be highlighted in tomorrow's papers, he returned to his office. According to his biographer David Grant, he had a night-time hobby: 'Pigeons roosted across the courtyard on the parapets of the third-floor wing used by foreign affairs. In the evenings when the offices were deserted, Kirk opened the window in his lounge, took aim and shot them with a gas pistol, which made only a slight popping sound before the dead bird dropped into the courtyard three storeys below.'[14]

Friday 29 March: Standing on the southbound platform of Trentham station, Dan Long breathed in the cool morning air. It was going to be a fine day for the march. According to the weather forecast, an anticyclone was slow-moving, extending a ridge of high pressure across the country. When the unit pulled into the station, he found his usual seat and settled down to read the *Dominion*. It was a right-wing rag but there was no alternative and, as PSA general secretary, he had to keep on top of the news.

Scanning the front page, he saw there was no mention of the march, though it would be the biggest thing happening in the capital that day. There was another negative story about Kirk, alleging he was threatening to take away Radio Windy's licence because of Brian Edwards stoking anti-Kirk sentiment on his talkback show. Muldoon, of course, was all over it, calling on the prime minister to 'cease his growing practice of telephoning both privately owned news media and the NZBC when current affairs programmes displeased him and browbeating them in an attempt to relieve pressure on his incompetent administration'.[15] Muldoon's attack on Kirk was no surprise; but Edwards? This was the same man to whom Long had given a temporary

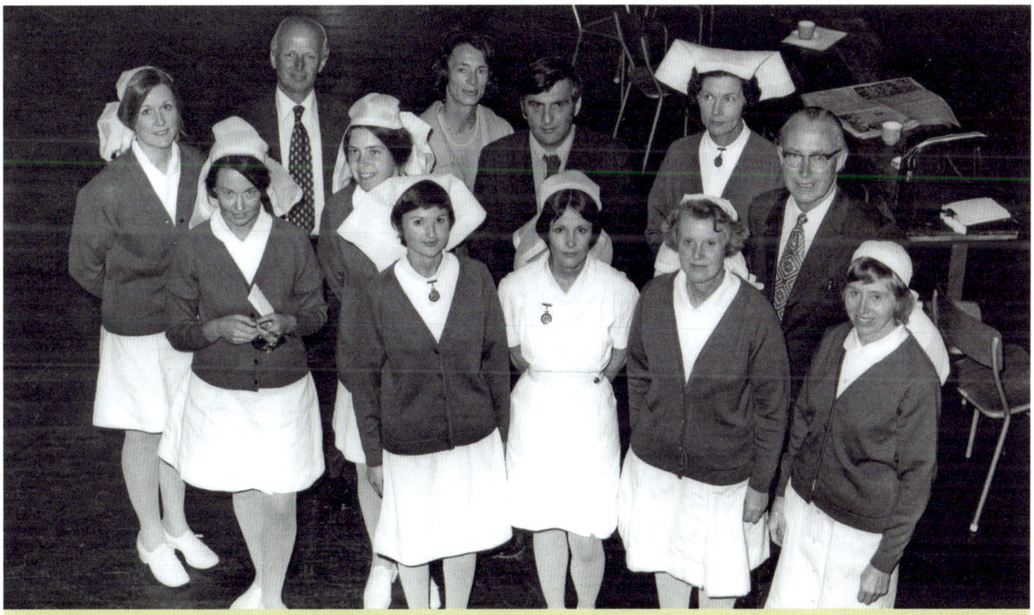

The deputation that met with Prime Minister Norman Kirk. Back row, from left: Nurse Pam Horncy, PSA president Jack Batt, tutor sister Jackie Humm, PSA regional secretary John McKenzie, tutor sister Kate Hishon, PSA general secretary Dan Long. Front row, from left: Nurse Rhonda Clark, nurse Maggie Morgan, tutor sister Margaret Clarkson, nurse Linda Gibbs, nurse Clara Cox and chairperson of the Dental Nurses Advisory Panel Ina Drury.

Dental nurses are briefed before assembling outside the Wellington Town Hall for the march on Parliament.

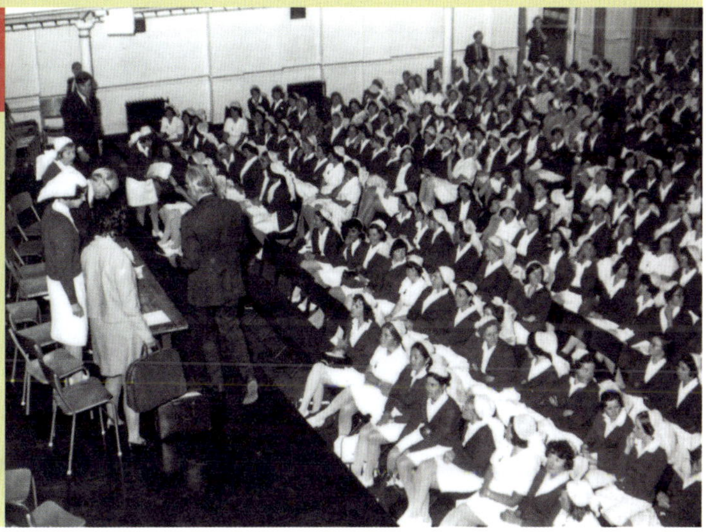

PSA job, partly to provide him with an income when he took time off as a television journalist to contest the Miramar seat for Labour.

He turned to page two and was pleased to see the quarter-page notice the PSA had taken out to make sure the public knew why the dental nurses were marching. The PSA hated to add to the paper's profits, but there was no other way to ensure that the union got its message across. The notice spelled out how the State Services Commission had done a U-turn on relativity to deny the dental nurses the pay rise they were entitled to. In bold capitals it stated: 'Dental nurses wonder why, unlike parliamentarians, they are being singled out as scapegoats for Government's stabilisation measures.' The timing of the MPs' pay rise could not have been better. Would the government have the gall to turn down the dental nurses while MPs scooped up hefty pay rises for themselves?

Long flipped over to page three and another item caught his eye: 'Kirk tackled on public service critics'. It was a report of a meeting he and Jack Batt had the day before with the prime minister and Bob Tizard. Ministers were attacking public servants in public. It was enough that papers like the *Dominion* and *NZ Truth* had been bagging public servants for years, branding them as lazy and inefficient, without ministers reinforcing the stereotype. And more recently, know-nothing first-time Labour MPs Ian Quigley and Mike Moore had jumped on the public service-bashing bandwagon. Where were these people's loyalties?

On the editorial page, Eric Heath had penned a cartoon that looked like a pre-emptive attempt to trivialise the march. It showed a gaggle of young women with placards approaching Parliament. The caption read: 'You're right! It is them — I didn't recognise them out of uniform.'

The racing page was the only thing this rag was good for, Long may have thought. There was only one meet on that day — in Whangarei. Serious punter Long was not swayed by cute or sentimental names, but a horse in the Uretiti Three Thousand Handicap seemed like an omen: March On. What was more, it had form. 'March On has often been disappointing this season but he is very good when in the mood.'

At 10 a.m. in Parliament, weary MPs bowed their heads as the Speaker intoned the prayer. 'Almighty God, Humbly acknowledging our need for Thy guidance in all things, and laying aside all private and personal interests, we beseech Thee to grant that we may conduct the affairs of this House and of our country to the glory of Thy holy name, the maintenance of true religion and justice, the honour of the Queen, and the public welfare, peace, and tranquillity of New Zealand, through Jesus Christ our Lord. Amen.'

It was a prayer with its implicit plea for decorum, to which deputy leader of the opposition Rob Muldoon paid scant attention. Instead, he tried to gain more traction on Kirk's treatment of the media. 'I wish to give notice of my intention to move under Standing Order 88 that the House do now adjourn for the purpose of discussing a matter of urgent public importance, namely, the allegation by Dr Brian Edwards on *Nationwide* television at about 9.20 on 28 March that "this Government not only wants to inhibit free speech but in addition to that is prepared to intimidate the individual journalist in order to prevent him on future occasions from criticising the government"'.[16] The Speaker swatted away Muldoon's request and Parliament continued with its business. The House was sitting until 4 p.m., the last day of the parliamentary session. The prime minister was due to meet the dental nurses' deputation at noon.

Across town, excited dental nurses were already filling the Concert Chamber. Friends who'd worked together, or had shared a hostel and not seen each other since graduation, were catching up. Many had had an early start to catch a plane from all over the country. Margaret Clarkson flew in from Christchurch: 'My job was to hand out all the plane tickets and I remember standing at the front of the aircraft like a hostess, saying welcome aboard, and a man came along and handed me his boarding pass, which caused a huge laugh.'[17]

At the airport, two nurses were on hand to greet arrivals and direct them to buses. Most took the 50-cent ride into the city on the regular NAC bus, which was deviating from its normal route to drop the nurses at the Concert Chamber. The 10.20 from Taupō and the 10.25 from Whanganui were the last flights to arrive. Passengers' heads popped up like meerkats as uniformed dental nurses were disgorged from planes and streamed through the airport lounge, chattering animatedly. 'At the airport people were absolutely intrigued; their mouths were hanging open with all these dental nurses. They'd never seen anything quite like it,' remembers Pam Horncy. Accompanied by Maggie Morgan, a nervous flyer, Pam was on one of the three flights taking the Auckland contingent to Wellington.

Dave Morgan, of the Seafarers Union, was at the airport to greet his wife: 'It was an amazing sight to see all these nurses in red cardigans pouring off the planes and into the airport . . . A little boy next to me said, "Look at all those red, Mum!" I said, "It's all right for you, kid, I'm looking for just one of them."'[18]

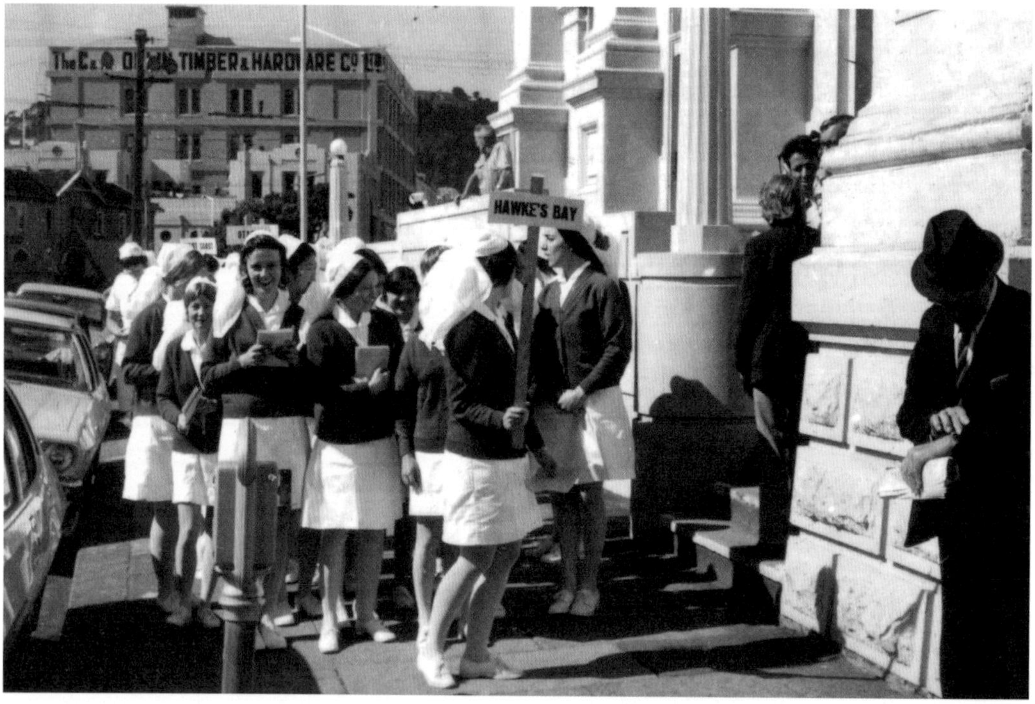

In the Concert Chamber dental nurses were putting on their veils. The tutor sisters wore their distinctive cornette veils reminiscent of nineteenth-century nuns — and an offering to the Wellington wind. Unusually for the capital, the day was calm. On stage, the 23-person deputation to meet the prime minister had taken their seats: three PSA officials in dark suits, Jack Batt, Dan Long and John McKenzie; the chairperson of the Dental Nurses Advisory Panel, Ina Drury; and dental nurses selected proportionally by region.

After speeches from Batt and Long, the 600 dental nurses spilled out onto the pavement, where they were given leaflets to distribute and arranged in geographical sections. PSA staff were still blacklisting the dental nurses' campaign, so there was no one available to help out. However, trained to be orderly and follow commands, the nurses were easy to organise. They lined up, the field nurses in their red cardigans, the tutors in teal cardigans, and student nurses at the end with their blue uniforms and little white caps. The leaders of each group carried a two-by-two-inch garden stake with the sign of their district. At the head, Drury and Kate Hishon were flanked by Long and Batt.

Annette King was made a marshal, given an armband and told to walk on the outside. 'We were scared stiff. It was a huge thing for us to march. We were a bunch

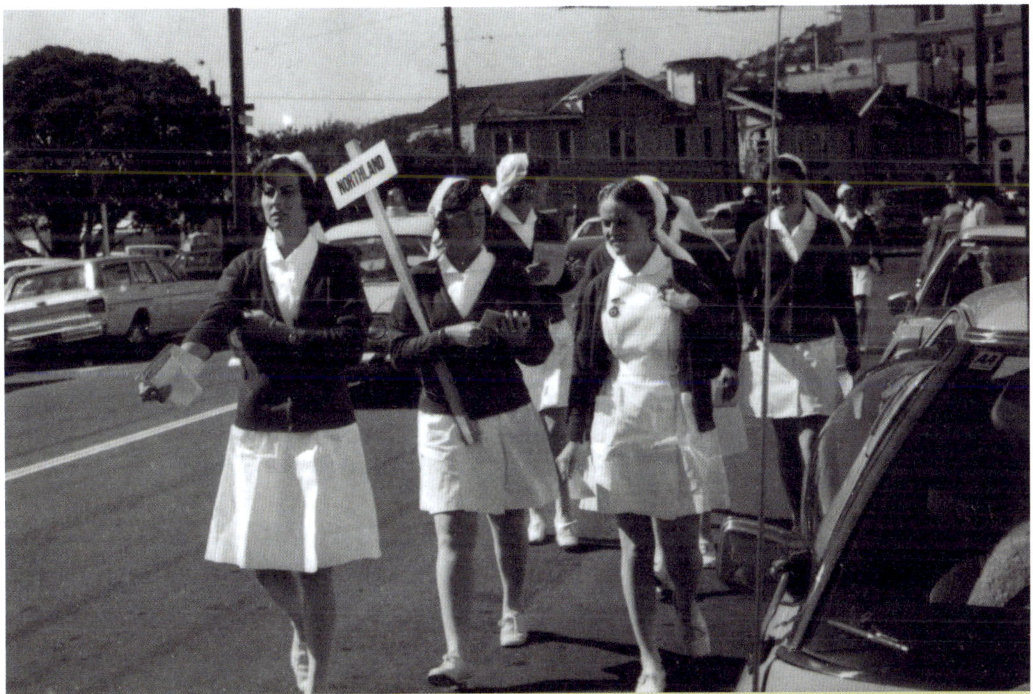

Dental nurses from Hawke's Bay, Northland and Otago get ready to march, some clutching petitions and flyers to give to MPs and members of the public.

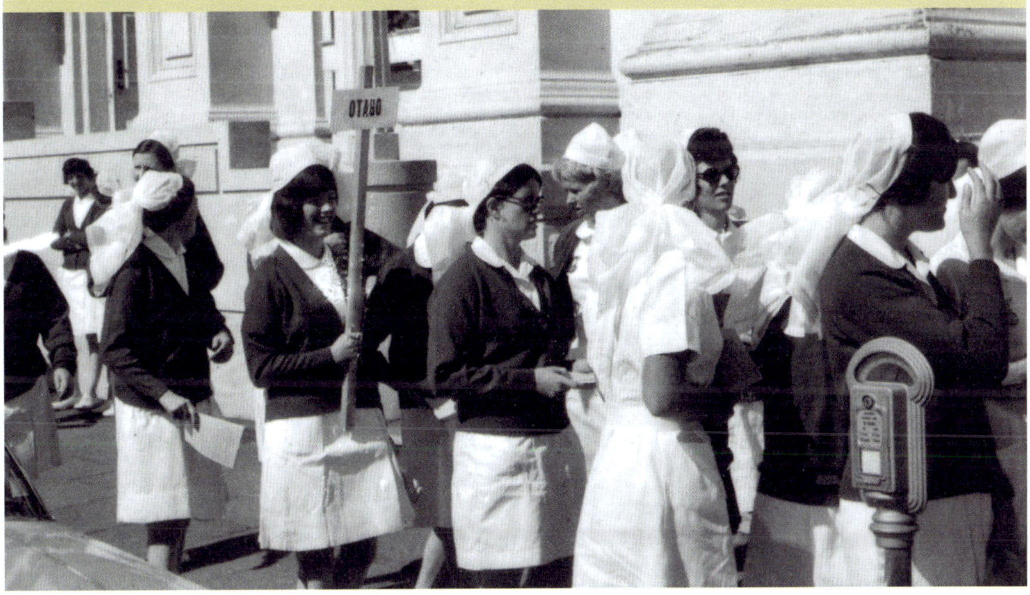

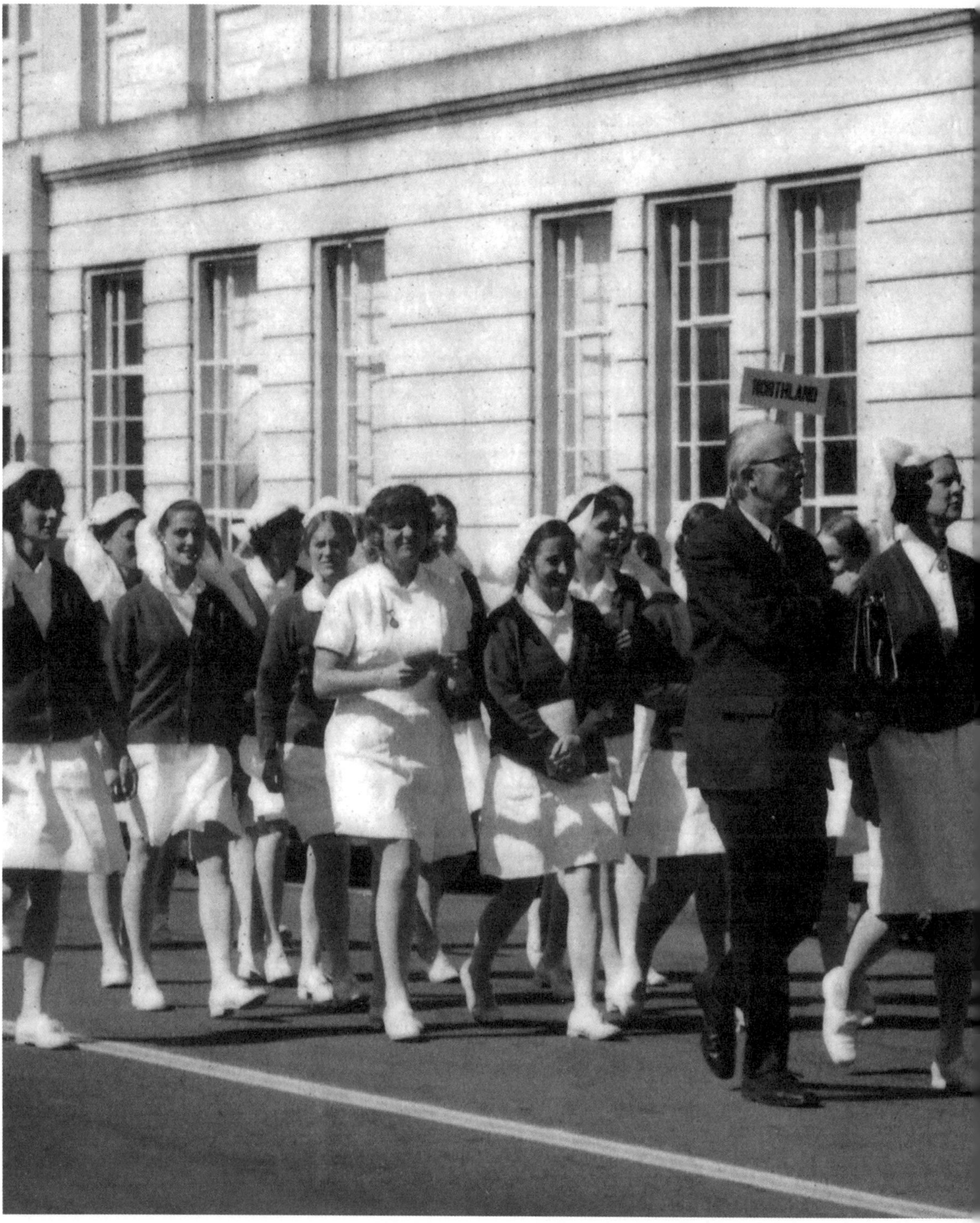
NORTHLAND

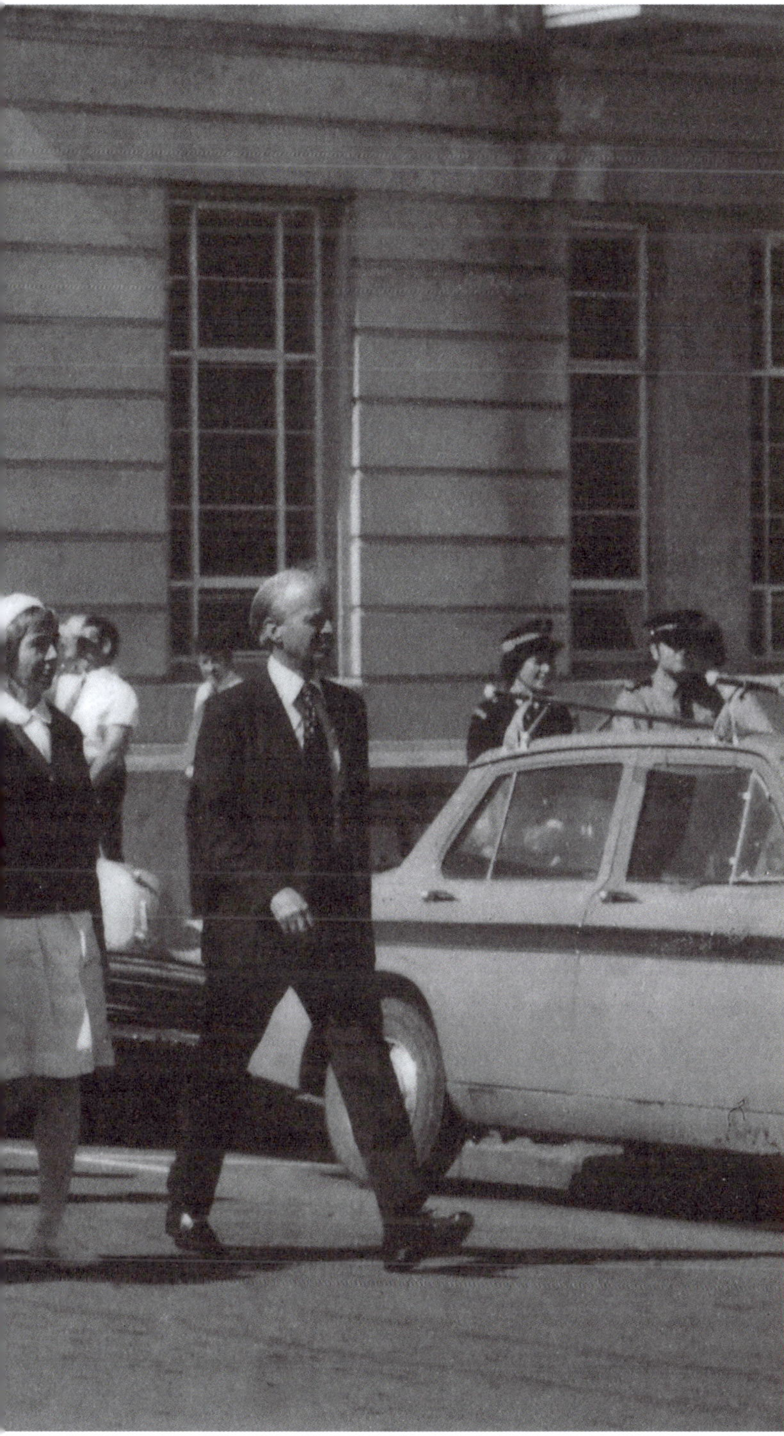

Northland nurses lead the march behind leaders PSA general secretary Dan Long, tutor sister Kate Hishon, chairperson of the Dental Nurses Advisory Panel Ina Drury and PSA president Jack Batt.

of women who had never done anything like that. We were nice girls — that was the sort of label we had. I remember being really, really frightened of it. Because we were going to march up the main street of Wellington — everybody was going to be looking at you. But then group dynamics kicked in, and everybody was talking and we all got excited. And then when we started the march so many people came out on the street, people were hanging out of the windows, yelling out and waving, clapping.'[19]

They walked four abreast in silence, with no placards other than the small signs indicating their region. Annette recalls: 'The other side of the road was open to cars and alongside came this big car, a Zephyr or Kingswood, making that throaty noise and festooned with flags. And as we were walking along, this voice called out, "Hey, hey, you sheilas!" and of course we didn't look, we just kept walking. And the voice called out again, "Hey, you Hamilton sheilas!" And we all swung around and the car was full of young guys with their thumbs up. "Best-looking in the bunch!" And I tell you what, we got a spring in our step after that.'

Dave Morgan, who had followed the marchers, stood clapping as they passed, then he ran ahead up the pavement and clapped again as they approached.

The *Evening Post* reported: 'While the march moved down through Lambton Quay towards the House, W. L. Young, MP for Miramar, gave notice of the following motion: "That this House notes with interest the statement on March 28 by a dental nurse that their proposed march on Parliament was suggested by a Labour member, a clear indication of the impotence of back-bench Labour members to act themselves or influence this Government, and calls on the Minister of Health to at least listen to, or hear the claims of the nurses, whose protests to date have gone unheeded."'[20]

By the time the dental nurses reached Parliament grounds, strong public support along the way had banished their initial anxiety and nervousness. Annette King, though, was suffering: 'I'd bought new white shoes specially for the march, and my feet were bloody killing me!' Photographs taken that day show the dental nurses assembled below the steps of Parliament. They had formed themselves into neat rows, as orderly as a platoon of soldiers. Looking down from Parliament's third-floor balcony it must have appeared as if a flock of exotic birds had landed on the forecourt. Well out of wolf-whistle range, construction workers bringing to life Sir Basil Spence's napkin sketch of a beehive next door had to content themselves with long-distance ogling.[21]

Some dental nurses clapped as a short, roly-poly man made his way down the steps. Rob Muldoon was grinning, which always had the effect of making him appear vaguely menacing, like a Prussian with a duelling scar. Other opposition MPs joined Muldoon on the steps and, as *Listener* parliamentary reporter Tom Scott put

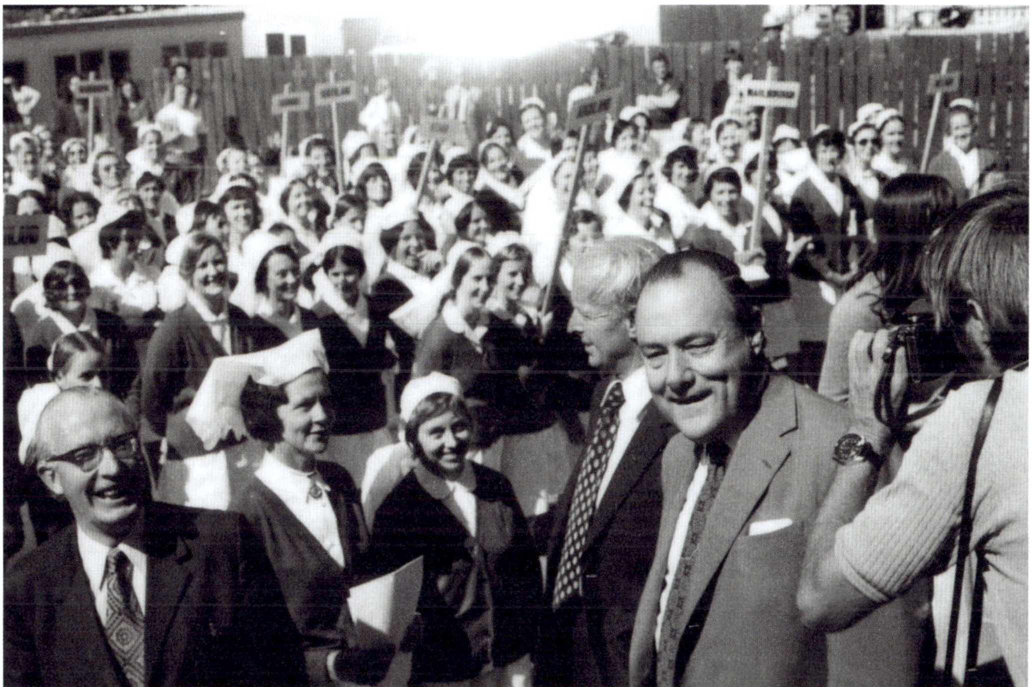

National opposition leader Rob Muldoon, here on the steps of Parliament, was delighted with the dental nurses' protest. Looking on, from left: PSA general secretary Dan Long, tutor sister Kate Hishon, chairperson of the Dental Nurses Advisory Panel Ina Drury and PSA president Jack Batt.

Dental nurses are prevented from entering Parliament by assistant chief messenger Bob Moore.

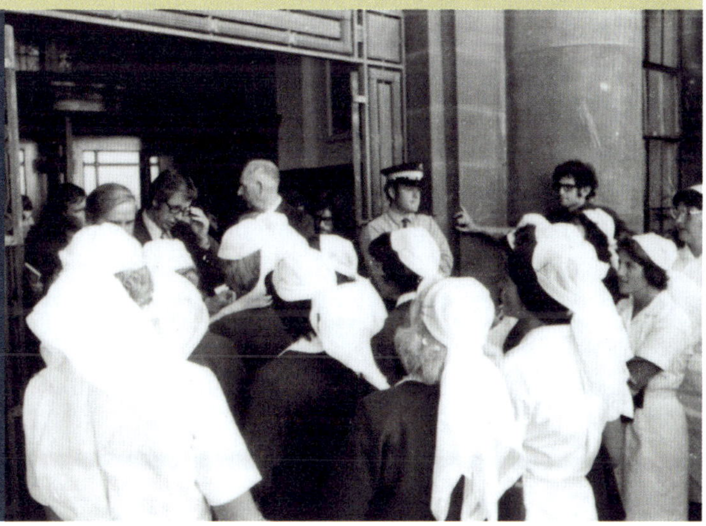

it, 'when not rubbing their hands together, waved to the crowd'. Scott added: 'No way could they be dismissed as an unruly rabble or hysterical women. Difficult to believe also the rumour circulating in certain quarters that they were mere dupes of left-wing agitators in the PSA. The sick person or persons responsible for this improbable lie deserve to have their mouths creosoted and their molars removed without anaesthetic.'[22]

The dental nurses waited in the autumn sunshine while the deputation readied itself to meet the prime minister in his suite. When they had gone in, the nurses surged up the steps to be met by Bob Moore, the elderly assistant chief messenger, and a single embarrassed policeman. 'You can't come in here, ladies,' Moore growled. 'You can't flood Parliament buildings. The House is in session.' He barred the main doors, but the nurses had their orders to seek out and lobby their local MPs and were not for turning. They entered by side doors and were soon swarming throughout the building.

Tom Scott takes up the story: 'A human tidal wave of red and white surged down corridors in search of MPs. They passed [Ruahine MP] Les Gandar on the way. "Hi Mr Gandar." "Gosh, how nice," he smiled, "someone knows me." The Porirua group had come to berate Dr Gerry Wall, but he was busy in the House so they filed into the public gallery. A nervous government gazed up to see itself surrounded on three sides by stern-faced women.' (An opera lover, Dan Long later told Pam Horncy that he imagined the dental nurses as the Jewish slaves in Verdi's *Nabucco*, removing their veils and throwing them onto the politicians below.)

Scott continues: 'Dr Wall eventually appeared to talk to the group from his electorate. In reply to angry queries as to why he had failed to answer their letters he said he disapproved of relativity and although they probably deserved to have their salaries doubled, relativity was not the way to go about it. "I have known," he intoned gravely, "people to die of relativity."'

Meanwhile, the deputation was being ushered into the prime minister's suite. 'What a huge hand he's got!' Pam remembers thinking when Kirk shook everyone's hand. It was undoubtedly a firm handshake. Margaret Hayward wrote later: 'He had a habit of absent-mindedly picking up an empty beer can in one hand and crumpling it into a grotesque shape.'

Tizard was less welcoming. He'd told reporters that while NAC would welcome the extra revenue from transporting the dental nurses to the capital, the way to settle a dispute was by calm discussion, not shouted advice, whether from the steps of Parliament or anywhere else.

Long and McKenzie did most of the talking from the dental nurses' side, with Tizard leading the discussion for the government. Kirk asked a few questions but was mostly quiet. Margaret Clarkson plucked up the courage to speak. 'I remember standing up and saying "Mister Tizard is right" — and the whole room sort of gasped. Then I said, "It wasn't this government who did it — it was the National government." And I looked at the prime minister and said, "But Mr Kirk you are our government now and we're asking you to do the right thing and restore this relativity."'

Jackie Humm was determined to make it clear that it wasn't just pay that dental nurses were concerned about. She had brought along a briefcase full of dental equipment. What people didn't understand, she said, was that children's mouths are different from adults', so the equipment they were supplied with was often not really suitable for children's dentistry.

Maggie Morgan recalls: 'She had a plastic bag of matrix bands, which you put around the tooth when you're packing the filling in. They were a substandard product and she was waving them at Kirk, saying this is the sort of rubbish we have to put up with. And I'm thinking, "Oh my god, put that stuff away, it's not the central issue here."'

The discussion had dragged on for an hour and three quarters as the union leaders and Tizard argued about the minutiae of the dispute. Long had written lengthy submissions to the State Services Commission and could quote Government Service Tribunal judgments going back to 1946. It's likely that eyes glazed over and thoughts wandered. Lunch may have been on the mind of some who'd skipped breakfast to catch the early flight to Wellington. Pam remembers having to pinch herself that she was in the prime minister's office. 'I'd not long been home from my big OE and suddenly I was in the halls of power. What was so exciting was learning how all the wheels within wheels worked and how it operated, so it was a very fast learning curve and it was a real sense of empowerment that you get that knowledge of how it works and what you needed to do to get change.'

Maggie was wondering why the room was so dark. It's likely that the prime minister's office was trying to set an example in conserving power. After a long dry summer, the hydro lakes were at a record low and a couple of cold snaps had sent electricity consumption soaring. After weekends of power cuts, Wellingtonians were bracing themselves for another one that weekend.

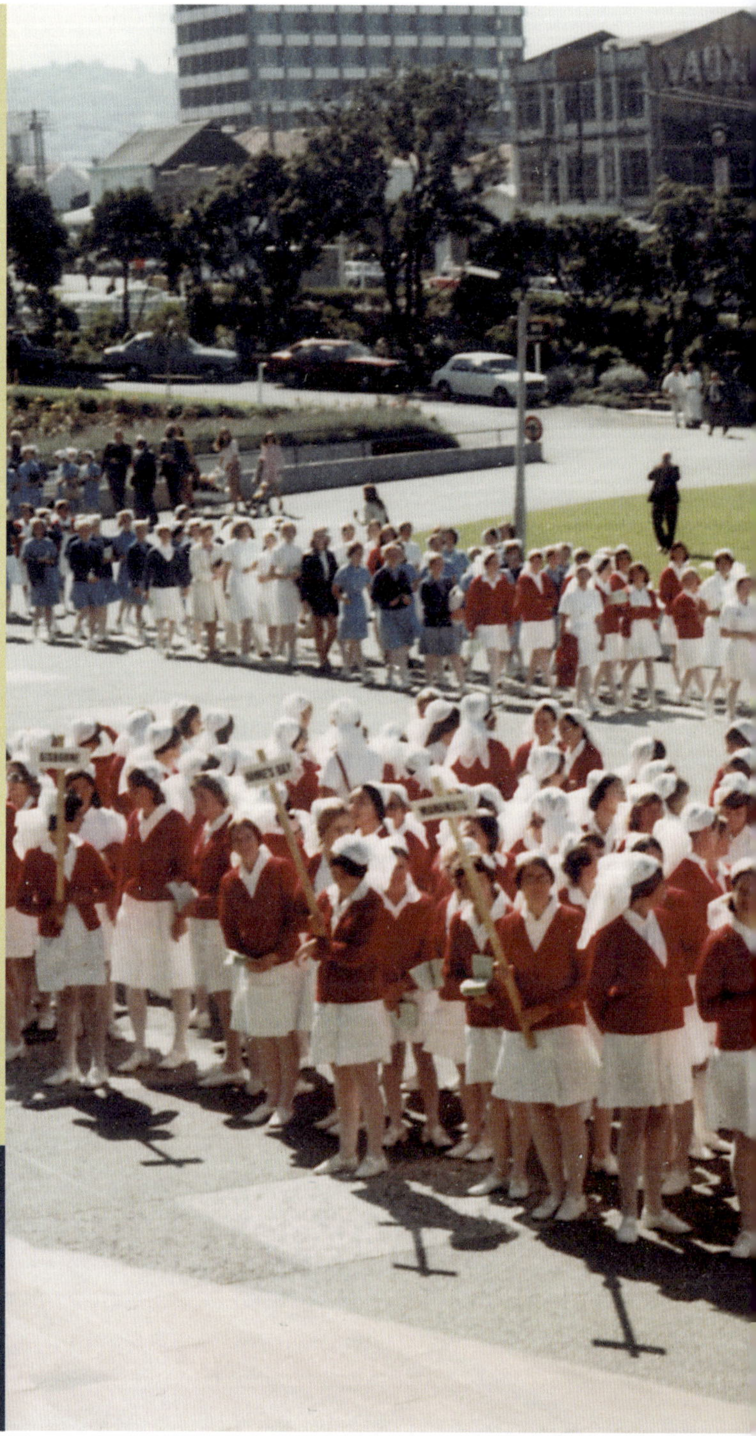

Dental nurses in their red cardigans made a colourful spectacle as they assembled on Parliament's forecourt. Dental nurse trainees in their blue uniforms brought up the rear.

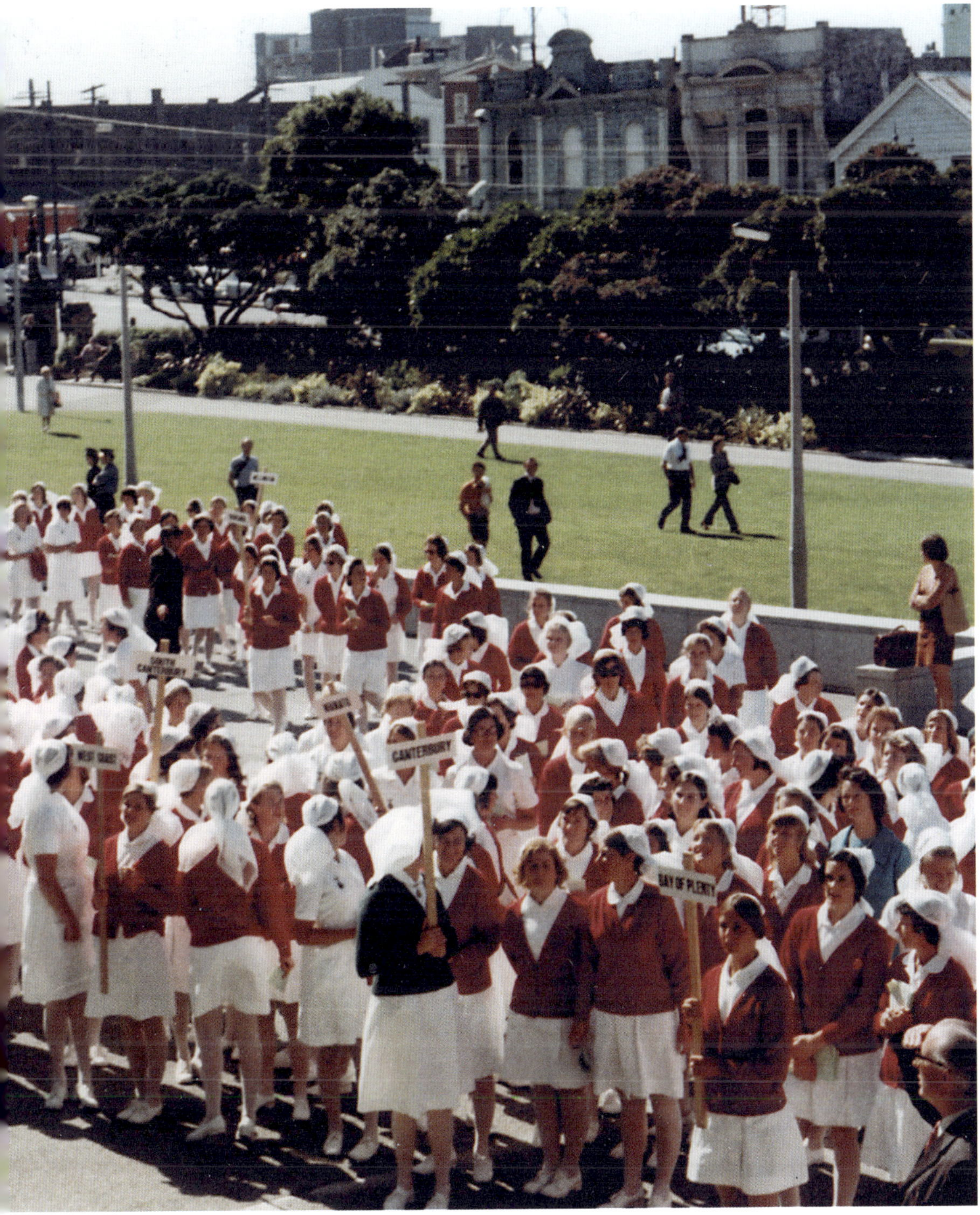
SOUTH CANTERBURY
WEST COAST
CANTERBURY
BAY OF PLENTY

Kirk was probably not following the tedious back and forth. There were plenty of other things to occupy him. The nasty exchange he'd had that morning in the House with Rob Muldoon, who was making hay of the fact Kirk was under attack from 'one of his own Labour candidates in the last election, Dr Brian Edwards'. Then there was a stack of bills still to be dealt with, and Parliament was adjourning that day for two months.

Suddenly Kirk pushed back his chair and got to his feet and all eyes swivelled in his direction. Having taken a back seat for most of the meeting, the big man was instantly a commanding presence in the room. 'I think we can fix this,' he said. 'I'll leave Bob here to tend to the detail.' Maggie recalls: 'I was sitting directly in front of Kirk's desk and Tizard was just off to my right. He looked really cheesed off when Kirk gave him the hairy eyeball.'

Everyone in the room was dumbfounded. Did he need to go to the toilet, still suffering the effects of dysentery? Was he ill? (In fact, a week later he went into hospital for an operation on his varicose veins, and steadily declined after that until his death on 31 August.) Had he just agreed to give the dental nurses all they asked for? Just like that? On the spot? It was unheard of for a group to protest outside Parliament and come away with their grievances righted.

Officials hammered out a short five-clause agreement to request the Wages Tribunal to restore relativity with public health nurses and backdate their claim to July 1972. Jack Batt and Bob Tizard signed the agreement. As the deputation left they were joined by dental nurses who'd remained in Parliament. No need now for the piles of petitions they'd hoped to hand to MPs or the flyers to distribute to the public. It was all so much waste paper.

No sooner had the dental nurses left Parliament grounds than two bus-loads of angry pensioners arrived. 'If it's good enough for the dental nurses to present their grievances to Parliament, it's good enough for us,' Mr H. S. McClaffey, secretary of the Pensioners and Beneficiaries Association, told reporters. Worried about inflation and perhaps Muldoon's remark that housewives would soon have to buy sausages on hire purchase, they wanted an immediate increase of $50 a week. But Christmas was over and there were no goodies. They left empty-handed.

In the green room at the town hall dental nurses, ravenous after their early start and the excitement of the march, were tucking into the catered lunch provided by the

PUBLIC SERVICE
Journal
THE OFFICIAL ORGAN OF THE N.Z. PUBLIC SERVICE ASSOCIATION INC

VOL. SIXTY-ONE, NUMBER THREE — MAY 1974

DENTAL NURSES ACHIEVE VICTORY

In the centre spread of this Journal we carry a display of what was without doubt one of the outstanding achievements by Association members in its 60 year existence.

On 29 March many hundreds of Dental Nurses marched through the main streets to the seat of Government, and placed their case before the Prime Minister, the Rt Hon. N.E. Kirk.

As one of the newspapers described it at the time, it was a "March to Victory".

It was victory at that time in that it achieved all that could possibly have been achieved then.

- it was recognised that a serious anomaly was caused by the failure to maintain a traditional relativity between initial maxima for Dental Nurse and Public Health Nurse;
- it was agreed that the anomaly dated back to 1 July 1972;
- it was accepted that the Government and State Services Commission would join with the P.S.A. in an agreed case asking the Wages Tribunal to decide whether or not a serious anomaly exists and from what date it should be adjusted.

The foregoing agreement came after a 30-strong Association delegation had discussed the matter for an hour and a half with the Prime Minister and Minister of State Services, the Hon. R.J. Tizard. The Association delegation, led by the President, Mr E.J. Batt, included its National Officers and Dental Nurses drawn from throughout the country, including officers of the Advisory Panel, Mrs I. Drury and Miss K. Hishon.

The breakthrough for an agreement — after months of frustration — came from the Prime Minister himself and the terms were recorded in writing and signed by Mr Tizard and the Association's President. (see centre spread)

The Association's application to the Wages Tribunal was lodged on 2 April, two working days after the historic march. Following the Commission's reply to the Tribunal dated 10 April 1974, agreement was reached between the Commission and the Association on all the matters placed before the Tribunal. The Commission conducted a public hearing on the application on Wednesday, 24 April.

STOP PRESS
Application Granted!
Increase effective from?

The 600 dental nurses in orderly rows were an impressive sight. In spite of TV's hospital-dramas, the nurse image is still very potent. They probably constituted the most concentrated assemblage of truth, purity, and selfless devotion to duty ever seen in the grounds of Parliament.

No way could they be dismissed as an unruly rabble or as hysterical women. Difficult to believe also was the rumour circulating in certain quarters that they were mere dupes of left-wing agitators in the PSA. The sick person or persons responsible for this improbable lie deserve to have their mouths washed out with creosote and their molars removed without anaesthetic. The link between dental nursing and Communism is at best a slender contradiction one curing tooth decay and the other causing it.

Opposition MPs came out to greet the nurses and when not rubbing their hands together waved them at the crowd. A special deputation of nurses mounted the steps to see the Prime Minister. They were followed by the others, but an embarrassed policeman and an elderly messenger blocked their path. "You can't come in here ladies". To the cry of "Let's try the side doors", large numbers, led by the Porirua Group, made for the old legislative chamber. A human tidal wave of red and white surged down corridors in search of MPs.

They passed Les Gandar on the way. "Hi, Mr Gandar".

"Gosh, how nice," he smiled. "Someone know Me."

The Porirua group had come to berate Dr Gerry Wall, but he was busy in the House so they filed into the public gallery. A nervous Government gazed up to see itself surrounded on three sides by stern-faced women.

Dr Wall eventually appeared to talk to the group from his electorate. In reply to angry queries as to why he had failed to answer their letters, he said he disapproved of relativity, and although they probably deserved to have their salaries doubled, relativity was not the way to go about it. "I have known," he intoned gravely, "people to die of relativity."

One always hesitates to challenge a doctor in these matters, but I thought the only way you could die from relativity was to travel at the speed of light without the proper clothing.

Courtesy of the New Zealand Listener, April 20, issue, Tom Scott's Parliament

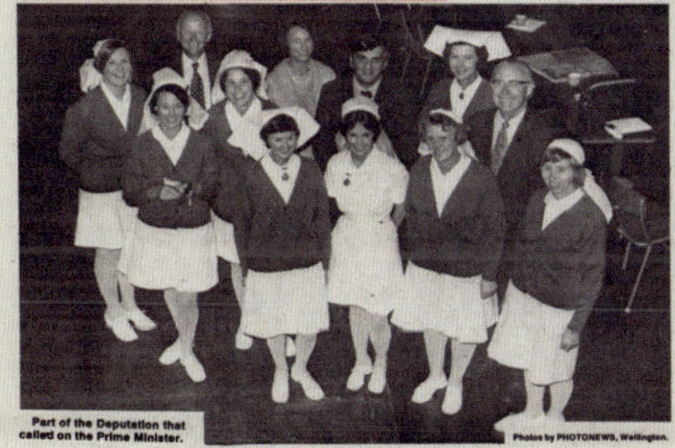

Part of the Deputation that called on the Prime Minister.

Photos by PHOTONEWS, Wellington.

State Services after 1 July

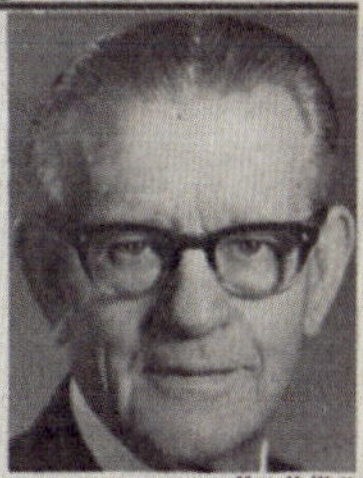

Hon. H. Watt

"State servants will be bound by the same rules as the private sector," said the Deputy Prime Minister, Hon H. Watt.

"They will all receive the 9 percent general increase from July 1, 1974, and any future general adjustments. Increases of up to one-quarter of the general wage adjustment will be able to be negotiated for individual occupational classes with the appropriate employing authority at intervals of not less than 12 months."

"The State Services Tribunal or the appropriate single service tribunal will decide any claims where an increase of more than one-quarter of the general wage adjustment is agreed in negotiations, or where no agreement can be reached," added Mr Watt.

"In considering such applications, the tribunals will also be required to have regard — where appropriate — to the effect of any wage increase on prices, and on economic stability."

"As with the Industrial Commission, the tribunals will not be able to take account of the criteria used in determining General Wage Orders," the Minister said.

"Ruling rates surveys will continue to be taken at annual intervals can be used as guidelines in negotiations in the ruling rates survey area."

"Half-yearly surveys will also continue to be taken, but will revert to their role as a statistical series. Their direct application to State Service wage rates will cease," he added.

Curbs on Salaries, Wages

In a policy statement released on the 19th April the Deputy Prime Minister and Minister of Labour, the Hon. H. Watt, announced the general lines of the Government's proposals to follow the expiration of the present Economic Stabilisation Regulations on the 30th June 1974.

The statement was offered as a "stabilisation package" intended to cover prices and incomes.

Noteworthy was the fact, its attention being d... the CSSO, ... Government's pr... dealt at much ... length and more de... wage restraints th... did with restraints o... and profits. The ... elements of the p... policy as it was ann... by the Deputy ... Minister were:

- a 9 percent gen... increase from July ...
- the restoration of t... negotiate improv... wages and conditi... one-quarter of th... increase with ... beyond this, subj... determination of th... Commission, o... appropriate wag... tribunal
- the same genera... apply to the State S...
- the establishment ... Salaries Commission to fix top salaries in the public and local body sector
- higher pensions and social

... requires to be approved by the particular Wage Tribunal having jurisdiction in that area.

The CSSO is now deep in negotiations with SSCC and

Continued on page 3

The PSA's *Public Service Journal* hails what it describes as 'without doubt one of the outstanding achievements by Association members in its 60 year existence'.

PSA. Afterwards, when all were assembled, President Batt went on stage. He recorded in his diary: 'I told them the result of the deputation — it was pandemonium. I have never seen a more excited group of people. It was exhilarating and very moving. Probably one of the great moments in the PSA's history.'[23]

Afterwards the dental nurses dispersed by plane, train and bus. Their famous victory was all over the news. The *Evening Post* ran a large picture of the marching nurses with the headline 'Parliament invaded by Dental Nurses'. Pam flew back with the Auckland contingent. 'We had a lovely reception, the group that I was with, husbands and boyfriends and friends who were out at the airport to meet us because they'd seen the evening news.' Annette was with her Waikato colleagues. 'We were walking down Lambton Quay and it was on the news on a television set in a shop window so we all crowded round.' They were on the way to the railway station to catch the overnight train to Hamilton. 'I tell you what, we got stuck into the booze, we were all pissed by the time we got back to Hamilton.' McWilliams, the 'sweet sherry for all occasions', came in handy flagons. 'We hardly slept a wink, we were so excited.'

Visiting the TAB on his way home Dan Long noted that in the Uretiti Three Thousand Handicap March On had paid off with a third placing.

Michael Bassett, historian and one of Kirk's ministers, considers that Bob Tizard had made a serious miscalculation in not taking the dental nurses more seriously:

> Without approaching the State Services Commission or Bob Tizard, who was the Minister of State Services, the P.S.A. and the dental nurses launched a public campaign to get wage rises which most of us felt were legitimate. Bob, however, felt such rises might open up a Pandora's box of problems. Others within the State Services would undoubtedly want similar treatment. All of us could see Bob's predicament. On the other hand fighting the Kawerau site committee [an earlier dispute] and fighting the local dental nurses were two different things. Some of us felt that Bob let the dental nurses wait far too long, and the telegenic invasion of Parliament that took place a few weeks later, with the nurses all in their uniforms, seemed rather unnecessary. The inevitable happened and the nurses got their extra pay.[24]

Reflecting from the union side, John McKenzie said:

> I'd never in my wildest dreams have believed that dental nurses would march on the Government. The Association fought their case over relativity with public health nurses, but to most of the women in the march it was something else. For one dental nurse it was a rebellion against the oppressive system of having to wear a veil. For another it was against the system of having to stand with her hands behind her back when the principal nurse came to check her books. For another it was against the practice whereby nurses were simply told that they had to go to a different location. For another it might have been in protest against being transferred from Auckland to relieve in Haast, where she was put in a caravan which seemed really beautiful until she found she was sharing it with four fisheries inspectors.
>
> Workers like the dental nurses and typists and so on are the most dangerous of all for an employer, and for that matter us as well. I organised that march but we never knew what the next step would be. Other groups, with a more militant history, have a pattern of action which you can follow hour by hour. But with previously non-militant groups they're unpredictable. We didn't know what the dental nurses would accept. When they got on the plane we said, 'Don't let anybody intimidate you. Don't come back until you've got the money in your pocket.' But we couldn't get them money in their pockets and we didn't know how they would respond. We had to go through a tortuous bureaucratic path to get there and it took time. As it happened they responded well. They knew they'd had their hour on the stage and they knew it had made a real impact. I can always remember telling Mr Tizard that dental nursing would never be the same again. They could never turn the clock back and be able to get those nurses to think as they had before.[25]

He was to be proved right.

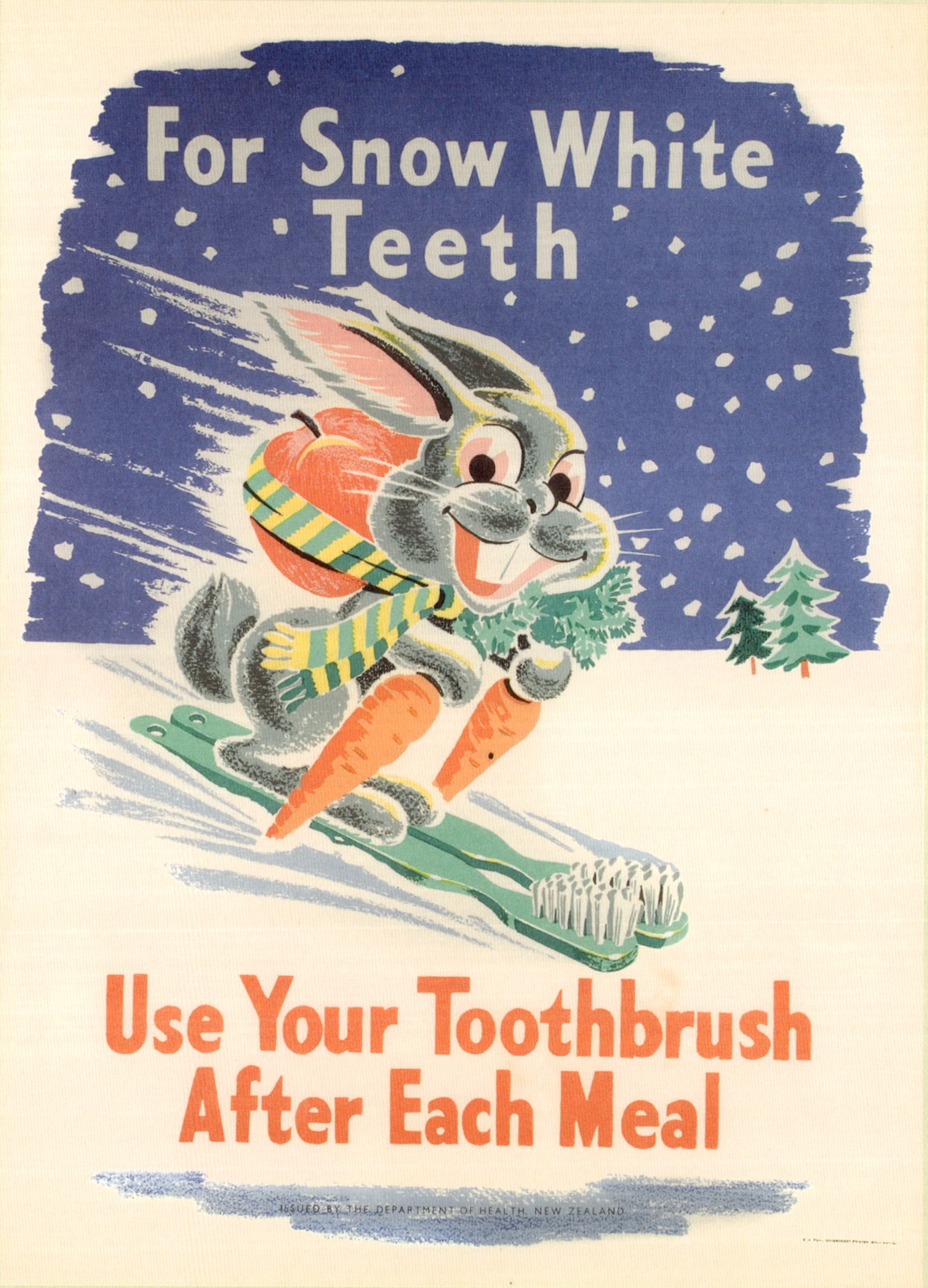
For Snow White
Teeth
Use Your Toothbrush
After Each Meal
ISSUED BY THE DEPARTMENT OF HEALTH, NEW ZEALAND

9

DECLINE AND FALL

As John McKenzie had predicted, the dental nurses' march changed the profession and many individuals within it. Annette King was to say later: 'Afterwards we became a much stroppier organisation. The more experienced you became, the less you got inspected. You were treated as an adult. It was a fantastic progression to watch. That march built up a sisterhood of school dental nurses. I've always been an outspoken person, but until then I never saw myself in a political role. I felt so encouraged after that march that I became more and more involved in the Dental Nurses Institute and the PSA.'[1] Ten years after the march, Annette was elected to Parliament, and five years later she was sitting round the same Cabinet table as Bob Tizard.

Like Annette King, the dental nurses who marched were mostly young — but not all. Auckland nurse Maynie Thompson was 55 when she took part. She began her training in 1935 when the service was less than two decades old. Dental nursing hadn't been her first choice. 'I would have quite liked to have been a teacher but I hadn't taken the mathematical course and you couldn't train as a teacher unless you had [taken it]. But I wanted something that would be a profession and where I would work with children. As I was leaving one of the teachers said, "What are you going to do?" I said, "I'm going to be a school dental nurse," and she said, "What a waste of a good brain!" And I went back to my seat and I said to myself, "Now you tell me in the sixth form that I have a good brain."'[2]

Still, she found the training demanding. 'We were trained in perfection. Nothing was passed; they would come around and examine the work we'd done and it had to be perfect, otherwise it wasn't accepted.' She was proud to be a dental nurse. 'During the depression free dentistry was something that was very much needed.'

She'd had to leave when she got married. She had just had her fifth child when her husband walked out. 'I had to bring up his five children on my own.' When the youngest child was five Maynie returned to her work. 'I needed a good job so I was really pleased to return to dental nursing.' It was a job on top of the one she already had. 'I have a clear picture in my mind of coming home through the front door, straight to the kitchen to peel the potatoes for dinner while the children were watching television. It was a very difficult time but I was pretty healthy and I managed the work. The children had to be fed and looked after. That was the time I was very pleased to have a good profession.'

The dental clinic, though, was not the limit of her horizons. 'I was involved in prison reform in those days and used to go out to visit prisons and I was shocked at the lack of education they had, and I worked hard with the government to improve prisoners' conditions.' As an activist, Maynie became something of a mentor to Pam Horncy and Maggie Morgan.

Ten years after the dental nurses' march, Maynie would be back marching to Parliament. Inspired by Australian anti-nuclear advocate Helen Caldicott, she joined the Waiheke Island 'Mum's Army' on a two-month trek to Wellington to urge the government to go nuclear free. That year, Maynie also travelled to the Greenham Common US Air Force Base in England to protest against the nuclear cruise missiles being deployed there. This was just the start of Maynie's international protests: in 1986 she took part in the 'Great Peace March for Global Nuclear Disarmament' across the United States and, 10 years later, the Women's Peace Flight to Tahiti to protest against the French government's resumed nuclear testing at Mururoa Atoll. Twenty years later, at 97, she turned up for her last peace march in Auckland in 2016.

There were other, less public transformations. Pam Horncy had seen at first-hand how politics works and how lives could be transformed through political action. In 1975, the PSA sent her to the United Women's Convention in Wellington. Dr Margaret Mead told the 2200 women present that men's and women's roles had been established by tradition, rather than by any real differences between the sexes. It was International Women's Year and its official anthem was Helen Reddy's stirring, inspiring paean *I Am Woman*.

Pam threw herself into union activities, now with a filter of feminism. 'It was the coming together of a feminist analysis and a labour analysis that showed me the union as a model for reaching your aims and aspirations.'[3]

School dental nurses were determined to build on the success of the march. Pam became part of the PSA advisory panel that started to investigate occupational health and safety issues, such as the toxicity of the mercury used widely in fillings. 'It was everywhere and I got very ill,' recalls Marjorie Orchiston. 'It was due to mercury poisoning. I'd been in the field about a year or so. The symptoms were chronic diarrhoea. I had an operation. Quite a lot of nurses had miscarriages or malformed babies.'[4] The health department was at first dismissive of the dangers posed by mercury, but quickly capitulated, testing mercury levels in all dental nurses and decontaminating clinics.

Funding & Fillings

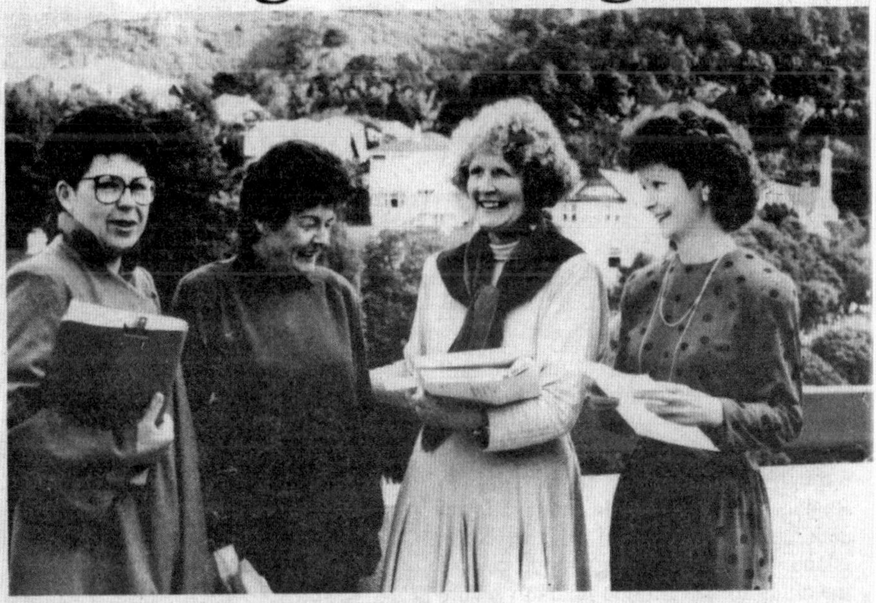

The establishment of Area Health Boards has resulted in a number of changes for School Dental Nurses. PSA members have been checking these out.

PSA activists Maggie Morgan, Sheila Brown and Kathryn Lanyon pictured with PSA Industrial Officer Pam Horncy (second from right) after a recent meeting with Health Department Management.

School Dental Nurses are concerned to ensure that adequate funding arrangements are retained when Area Health Boards take over responsibility for the service.

"The funding lines have not been clear and we were also concerned to clarify training and management issues" l
Journal.

The PSA represents
service employed in th
primary health care t

When area health boards were set up in 1983 it spelled the end of the School Dental Service as a national service.

(The full story of mercury poisoning is told in the next chapter.)

Other successes followed. Perhaps more than any other group, dental nurses were potentially exposed to the full range of infectious diseases, from measles and mumps to hepatitis and tuberculosis. 'I actually got shingles off a child, because chickenpox becomes adult shingles,' says Annette King. 'Chickenpox went through the school when I was working on the kids. But the good side was you built up huge immunity to

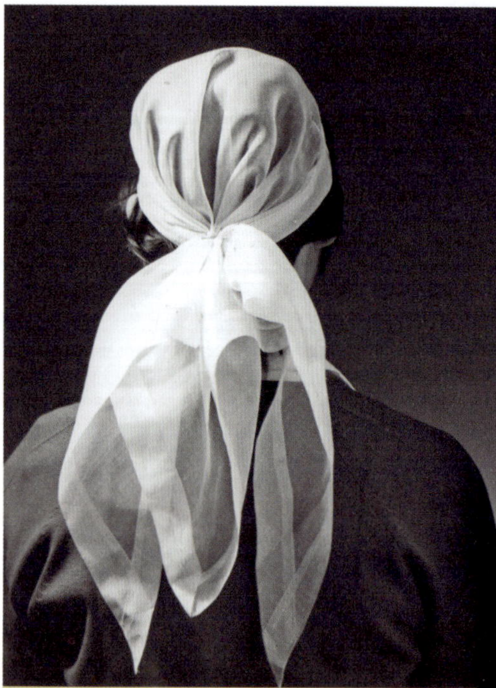

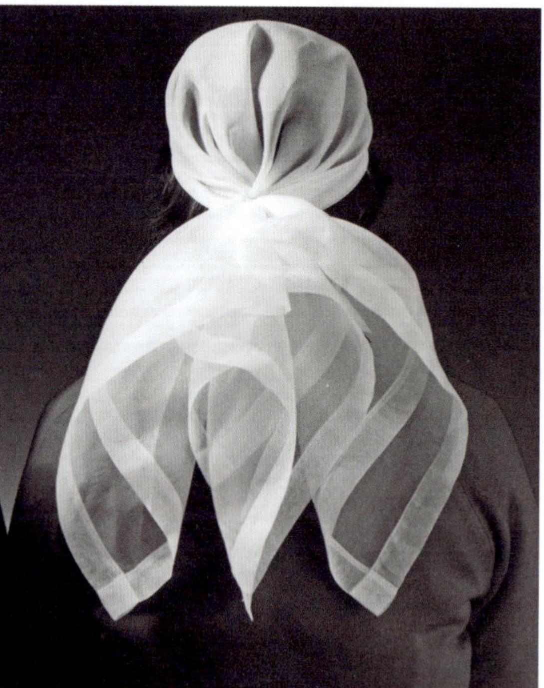

'What religious order do you belong to?' an overseas visitor once enquired of a dental nurse. In a concession to the times, a lighter half veil (above left) was introduced in 1974 to replace the cumbersome full veil (above right). Veils made a mess of hair and were a health and safety risk; more than one nurse had the experience of her veil accidentally catching fire as she prepared a filling over a Bunsen burner. The veils were eventually phased out in the 1980s.

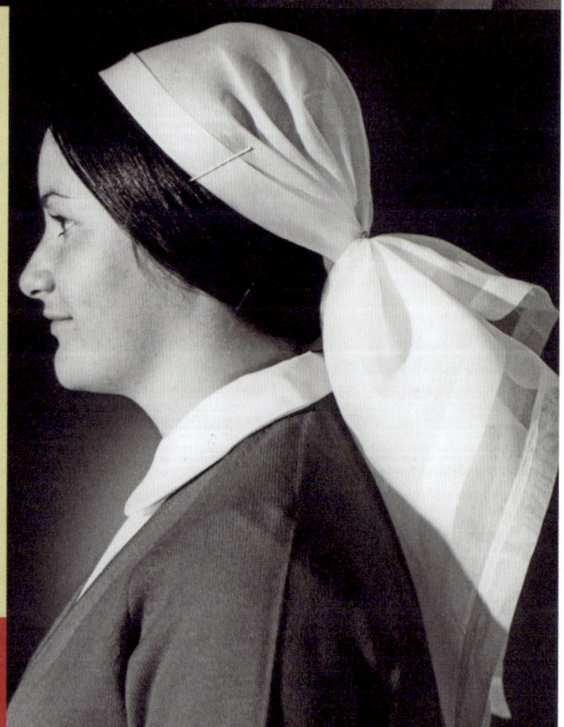

things. I've had great immunity to things that have lasted me most of my life. Every snotty nose, every cold and flu, you had your hands in it.'

Dental nurses were granted 'epidemic leave', but only if they could prove that 'the particular patient was suffering from the complaint at the time the dental attention was given or that the officer rendering treatment developed the same complaint within the usual incubation period or has been isolated because of her contact with the patient'.[5] What they'd never been given were masks and surgical gloves to reduce the chances of being infected in the first place. The PSA argued successfully that these items should be standard issue for workers who spent their day poking around in people's mouths.

Head lice were harder to deal with. 'You were so close to kids, the likelihood of getting head lice was huge,' says Annette. 'There were head covers that went on the back of the chair, which we wiped down each time with methylated spirits. I just put the plastic cover on the kid's head so I would work with them. You could see head lice moving.'

The starched uniforms and veils had not changed since the 1930s. Polyester uniforms were introduced and lighter half-veils. However, the health department was at pains to point out that this was not a licence to be casual and warned that 'uniforms should be worn in the specified way and not according to the whims of the individual'. The *Gazette* devoted two full pages with photos to uniform instructions, including the reminder that 'the new material is more transparent than the former cottons and suitable underclothing is necessary'.

But dental nurses wanted more changes, and put their request in verse:

> With stocking off and sandals white
> We'd be transformed to help the fight
> of tooth decay and all that rot,
> But at the moment we're too hot!
> Please can we take our stockings off?
> Inspectors, dears, you must not scoff
> We really could be more at ease
> Our hairy legs to catch the breeze.
> Our little toes to move around,
> in cooling air that's near the ground,
> our veils are also in the way,
> Can we move them from today?[6]

The *Gazette*'s reply was uncharacteristically playful:

> The starchy look has gone its way
> The drip-dry type has come to stay
> And now the nurses wish to pose
> A question that concerns their hose.
> 'To be or not to be' they ask
> To answer that is quite a task
> It's quite beyond the normal male
> At every point his face turned pale.
> As for veils, while nurse is drilling
> Would not hair drop in the filling
> If vagrant locks weren't kept in place
> And stopped from falling round the face?
> As for sandals ousting shoes
> Toenails would come in varying hues![7]

In the 1980s the veils eventually went. 'It was good when they got rid of veils: you looked a mess when you got home; your hair was flat every day, you'd have to wash it,' says Annette.

Holidays were another issue dental nurses wanted addressed. Taking your child to the dental clinic was not a popular school holiday activity. 'So in January,' says Pam Horncy, 'we'd often go to the back of the clinic and sunbathe; many of us also brought our sewing machines along. There was nothing to do. That was such a dead period, it used to be a great area of aggravation and after our march on Parliament the nurses would often ask us at union meetings, "Why can't you get us the school holidays right through with the school teachers?" We wanted six weeks' holidays at a time when the maximum you could get was three weeks. The PSA wasn't particularly sympathetic. They could see the difficulty they would have negotiating that.'

It wasn't just that they had nothing to do; it was also a security issue: dental nurses were often on their own in empty school grounds, as Pam explains:

> There were some occasions where the nurses were raped in their clinic. One was almost strangled. She used to wear a scarf around her neck for quite a while afterwards because she had really bad bruising. By that stage we were quite active collectively and the health department must have decided that

> was quite a liability to carry. They didn't change our holidays, but in our terms and conditions there was just a sentence that said dental nurses were not required to be at the clinic when school teachers weren't there, when the school wasn't opened.
>
> Our hours were shortened a bit, too, because in those days teachers tended to work until three o'clock and were out the door by ten past. So you'd be working in quite often an isolated clinic, a long way from the main buildings. I had a young high school kid come into my clinic one evening. I was doing something and I looked around and there he was in the door. It gave me a hell of a fright and I said, 'What are you doing?' And he sort of mumbled something and I said, 'Go away!' Anyway he did and I immediately locked my door. After that we got fish eyes into the doors so we could lock the doors when we were the only ones in the school grounds.

The most ambitious of the PSA advisory panel's claims were proposed in its 1977 report *School Dental Nurses: A blueprint for the future.*[8] It was a declaration of independence, an assertion that dental nurses were professionals in their own right, not dental auxiliaries. It stated: 'Upon graduating, dental nurses are proficient in 90 per cent of routine operative procedures carried out by a graduate dentist.' The term 'dental nurse' was a misnomer, it added, and graduates should be called 'school dentist'. It demanded a new curriculum, career paths and pay relativity with dentists.

R. K. Logan, director of dental health, seemingly could not believe what he was hearing. He raved to a colleague about 'the so-called "Women's Lib" group which is not sure what it wants but is determined to remove the restrictions that stop dental nurses from practising dentistry in the full sense of the term. It claims that dental nurses are already as highly qualified as dentists and are doing 90% of the work of dentists.'[9]

It was too much even for some dental nurses. A major rift developed between the PSA's reformist advisory panel and the conservative Christchurch-based School Dental Nurses' Institute. The institute's president, Kate Hishon, sided with the PSA while most of the executive were enraged by the union's militancy and lack of consultation. Accusations flew back and forth. The executive committee fumed that the advisory panel and the PSA were 'maintaining a state of running hostility with the Health Department and the State Services Commission'.[10] In November 1974 the PSA held a dental nurses' conference; not to be outdone, the institute held its own conference the following February. Kate was deposed for aligning herself with the PSA.

The bitterness spread to the rank and file. This letter from a dental nurse to the institute executive still smoulders in the National Archives:

> Dear Ladies of the Executive, I am not sure how you got where you are but I do know I never voted for you and what is more I have never been given the opportunity to vote for an Executive since my graduation in 1960.
>
> From your letter you sound very typical of the petty squabbling women who we have unfortunately come to associate with Dental Nurses — unable to formulate constructive thought and with no power or knowledge of negotiation . . . As the Auckland girls have obviously a far better grasp of this general situation I cannot understand why the whole Executive is not in Auckland where it would represent a far greater number of field nurses.
>
> Also I seem to recall that the Executive was working on salary claims from when I graduated till I left NZ and it was not until the PSA and the abovementioned Auckland girls emerged that we made any progress.
>
> You are the coffee, cake and chatter ladies and you don't make progress with that sort of attitude.
>
> And the only vote I have for you is one of no confidence — you were not even able to rid us of that ghastly headgear.
>
> The Advisory Panel — as it now stands — represents my case and probably most other thinking nurses as well. You have had your chance and do not have much to show for it.[11]

Despite the infighting, dental nurses may have felt they were on a roll, and that the march on Parliament would be the trigger to propel them to a bright new professional era. In fact, the march was their zenith and the descent thereafter was swift. Just six years later, in 1980, a headline in the *PSA Journal* read: 'Dental nurses fight for survival'.[12]

Five months after the march, Norman Kirk died, setting off a series of events that would have dire consequences for dental nurses. In 1975, National won the election with a scaremongering television ad featuring Cossacks dancing through the New Zealand landscape. The country would, it claimed, turn into a communist state if Labour's compulsory superannuation scheme, the KiwiSaver of its time, was allowed to continue. In 1976, on another ides of March, Dan Long, who'd championed the dental nurses' cause, died of a heart attack in Melbourne, where he'd been attending a union conference. The general secretary of the PSA was only 53. As with Kirk, overwork had been a major contributor to his death. The change of government had put the PSA on a collision course with the government and it was a time of intense pressure for the union.

There were also darkening clouds on the professional front. During the 1950s and '60s the School Dental Service had been stretched as the baby-boom children flooded into the schools. At the same time, the service faced a recruitment crisis. Now in the 1970s, with school rolls falling, there were fewer teeth to fill and the government refused to utilise the spare capacity by allowing dental nurses to treat secondary school students.

In 1973 the World Health Organization (WHO) had published a study that threw into question dental nurses' role and its usefulness. The New Zealand section of the report, focused on the Canterbury region, showed that the average 14-year-old had 37 restorations since they enrolled in the service aged five. The most shocking finding: 36 per cent of New Zealanders aged 35–44 were 'fully edentulous' — they had no natural teeth at all. Of all the countries surveyed, New Zealand had the highest percentage of people in this age group with no teeth.[13]

New Zealand prided itself on its dentistry. It had pioneered free dental care for children and been lauded for its School Dental Service. Now it ranked bottom. The boast in the *Gazette* that New Zealand was now a land of 'gleaming well-cared-for teeth' was not borne out by the facts. As Susan Moffat wrote later: 'The Editor of the *New Zealand Dental Journal* claimed that before the survey, "New Zealand dentistry tended to be rather smug" and had boasted to the rest of the world that they had "the greatest SDS the world had ever seen". "The alarmingly high level of edentulousness in New Zealand shook [them] all out of [their] smugness."'[14]

In 1976 the New Zealand Dental Research Foundation conducted its own Survey of Adult Oral Health and Attitudes to Dentistry. It confirmed the WHO findings: 20-year-olds had half of their teeth decayed, missing or filled. By 40 years, this figure had risen to 75 per cent and by 65 years, to 96 per cent. A third of those over 20 did not have their own natural teeth.[15] Further analysis of the surveys showed that the poor and those who lived in rural areas were the worst affected by the decline in dental health.

The surveys were a wake-up call for dentistry in New Zealand. In 1978, a Dental Health Workshop involving all the key players was held in Rotorua. It marked a radical shift in how dental nurses operated. Instead of drill and fill, which the service had insisted they do, they were now instructed to reach for the drill only as a last resort; they were to spend more time detecting early signs of disease, and apply direct fluoride treatment to any lesions they found. The new method resulted in a 64 per cent reduction in fillings. The 'murder house' was no longer so murderous.

While dental nurses had less to do as school rolls declined, the oral health survey had shown there was a desperate need in the community for more affordable dental care. The PSA proposed deploying dental nurses in other areas such as public hospitals, and treating secondary school children, the handicapped and the impoverished. The union's priority was to protect dental nurse jobs, but it would also 'maximise their skills and resources in the interests of community dental health'.[16] However, a government that had ridden to victory on the backs of dancing Cossacks was never going to agree with such expansion of state care, no matter how much sense it made.

By 1979, New Zealand was well into recession and government departments were ordered to cut spending. The School Dental Service became a target. Minister of health George Gair ordered a review of dental nurse training. At the Dental Nurses Institute's conference in 1980 he dropped a bombshell: trainee intake would be cut to 30 in 1981 and thereafter would never exceed 55. The Auckland and Christchurch training schools would close. Gair argued that there were already enough dental nurses to keep the service going. The *Gazette* had reported that there were 111 dental nurses on special leave without pay and another 300 former dental nurses ready to return to the service.

Maggie Morgan, then chairperson of the PSA's dental nurses' central committee, hit back: 'It's just a tactic to make us accept the closures. We believe that most of the ex-dental nurses are in the main centres and that is not where the jobs are. We believe that in the long run the service will become so understaffed that it will either be closed down altogether or its work will be farmed out to dentists in private practice.'[17]

But there wasn't going to be a long run. Dental nurses once again took to the streets, marching in Wellington and Auckland. The *PSA Journal* was upbeat about their protests:

> It looks as though the Government has seriously miscalculated. The protest has been impressively supported by both the nurses and the public. In Auckland and Wellington, for example, nearly all the available nurses participated in the marches. They attracted ripples of applause from lunchtime pedestrians — the only group so favourably accepted. When the Government adds the votes of the nurses themselves and all the disgruntled parents who will have to pay for their children's dental treatment, the political wisdom of the closures looks very doubtful.[18]

However, when dental nurses presented a petition with 34,000 signatures to Parliament, they were incensed by MPs' indifference. The *PSA Journal* reported: 'A select committee of Government and Opposition MPs heard submissions on the

Dental nurses fight for survival

On 6 and 7 November school dental nurses gave massive support to a nationwide series of meetings and marches to protest against the Government's decision to close dental nurses' training schools at Auckland and Christchurch.

The dental nurses are not a militant group and their protest was all the more impressive because of that. They see the Government's decision as a major attack on the school dental service and they accepted that a vigorous public response was essential.

It is no exaggeration to say that the service will rapidly fade away if the present pattern of recruitment continues. In 1970 there were 200 trainees admitted to the service. Last year this had dwindled to an intake of 90 and next year the Government hopes to cut it back to 25.

The PSA responded to the decline some time ago. In 1977 it lobbied the Government with two major papers suggesting ways in which the service could expand into new areas so that its resources would not be wasted. There is a huge public investment in training, equipment and buildings and it would be irresponsible to squander this in the interest of short term saving.

As Rae Blomfield told the Wellington meeting on 7 November, we are witnessing yet another example of "contracting out". She said the Government seems hell-bent on dismantling the school dental service so that the work can be passed over to its friends in the private sector. The cost will be carried by the parents of young children.

The Government's motives were indicated by the fact that they made a \$3.5 million grant to the Otago dental school at at the same time as the two closures were announced. The Otago school trains dentists for private practice.

The PSA has identified a number of areas where school dental nurses could usefully participate. Among these are pre-school dental care, secondary schools and public hospitals. They could also expand their programme of preventative care in primary schools.

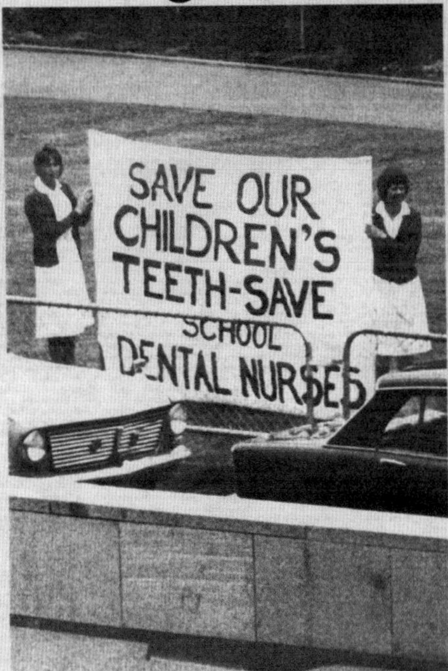

FREEZE DECISION

The nurses through the PSA, have called on the Government to freeze its decision until there has been a proper opportunity to explore the alternatives. John Swinburn, acting president of the PSA, said that the Government's secrecy over information which led to the closure implies that the decision would not stand up to public scrutiny.

Maggie Morgan, chairperson of the group's central committee, told a Wellington meeting that dental nurses in the field knew that workloads were increasing. She contested the Government's figures that several hundred ex-dental nurses were waiting in the wings ready to snap up any vacancies. "It's just a tactic to make us

The PSA was optimistic that dental nurses' protests and public support would force the government to back down on its decision to close the Auckland and Christchurch training schools. Its confidence proved to be misplaced.

COUNTING VOTES

It looks as though the Government has seriously miscalculated. The protest has been impressively supported by both nurses and the public. In Auckland and Wellington, for example, nearly all the available nurses participated in marches. They attracted ripples of applause from lunch-time pedestrians – the only group to be so favourably accepted.

When the Government adds up the votes of the nurses themselves and all the disgruntled parents who will have to pay ...heir children's dental treatment, the ...cal wisdom of the closures looks very ...ful.

...e Wellington march obviously shook ...Government's confidence. Before it ...ned National Party MPs decided they ...ln't see the nurses because the march ... form of strike action. One of those ... cancelled appointments was the ...L. Adams-Schneider.

...ter a deputation tried to see the ... Minister, Adams-Schneider was dele... to stand in for him. Other National ...verlooked the original plan to ignore ...march. Marilyn Waring, apparently ... sympathetic than some of her col..., is understood to have been dis...nted that she wasn't invited to ...s the marchers along with numerous ...r MPs.

...e Wellington march turned out to be ...tensely political experience. It coin... with a royal visit and security forces ...rliament were so twitchy that the ... were kept behind barricades. There ... large numbers of police on hand and ...urses were suddenly able to see for ...elves the aggressive aloofness that has ... trademark of this Government.

...ey also saw numerous Labour MPs who not only relished the chance to do some unopposed politicking but delivered promises which were largely in line with what the nurses have been asking for since 1977. Marchers who were not Labour supporters were left to consider whether the promises were good enough to earn a vote.

Other victims join dental nurses in Auckland rally

An Auckland rally on 6 November linked the closures of the dental nurses' training schools with the run-down of the Housing Corporation and the closures of the North Shore Teachers' College, Lopdell House, part of State Insurance and the Southdown Freezing Works.

Auckland section chairperson Alan Hughes said that in addition to these sudden panic actions there has been a drop of 1000 permanent staff positions in the Ministry of Works and Development. "Over the next seven years 500 dental nurses' positions will be lost and thousands of other jobs will be cut from social services, health and education.

Barbara Drinkall said, "Once again career opportunities for women have been slashed. Free dental care for the nation's 700,000 pre-school, primary and intermediate children is in jeopardy.

"How can 25 trainees a year possibly ensure the continuation of the unique service that dental nurses have provided for the last 60 years? Their service has a proven record of success and is often cited as an example overseas."

Drinkall expressed concern about the drop-out rate from dental treatment in secondary schools. "There are 35,000 children who do not even enrol with a dentist when they leave.

"We do not believe the bland assurances of the Minister of Health that the role of school dental nurses will be maintained."

HOUSING CORP RUN-DOWN

Graham Roberts, speaking on behalf of Housing Corporation workers, told the meeting that on 14 August staff in the Construction Division were called together ad told that 75% of them were no longer required. These are the people who have designed, built and administered state rental housing. There are about 200 of them throughout New Zealand and this number will be cut to 50 in three years.

There was no consultation and no detailed study. The Housing Division has been a political sacrifice. It is naive and economically bad. A staff of 50 will not be capable of doing the job.

TEACHERS' COLLEGE CLOSURE

Brenda Knight said that on 19 September the Principal was summoned to meet the Minister of Education. "When he came back he called us together to tell us that Mr Wellington had decided that over the next two years the North Shore Teachers' College would be phased out and the Auckland Technical Institute would take over the site for their health sciences programmes.

"The gist of this made the headlines in the New Zealand Herald the next day.

"When this bombshell began to wear off anger began to set in. This decision had been made without any consultation whatsoever with the key people involved.

"It was all planned in secret and the Minister refused to make public the report on which he made his decision. No one knows how it was compiled, what figures were used, nor since those who know most about the situation were not involved, how accurate the report was.

"PSA members at the college in the office library and a/v department read their fates in the lines from the Minister's press statement 'some administration staff will transfer to Epsom, some could be absorbed in the health sciences faculty and in-service training centre. That was seven weeks ago and we are still awaiting further details. Will we be able to stay on the site? Will some of us be asked to work at Auckland Teachers' College or will there be nowhere for us to go and should we be looking for other jobs? This is not helping our mental health."

MEAT INSPECTORS SUDDENLY HIT

Ian Baldick, chairperson of the Meat Inspectors' Group, said that he and his colleagues had considered themselves relatively safe until this year. A series of events, including the closure of Southdown, have destroyed that sense of security.

"We have joined with other unions to try and keep Southdown open. Should this fail we are faced with the dispersal of 54 meat inspectors. Thirty of these could be forced to transfer out of the district or lose their jobs. As this is a large group of members to be transferred in a short time a serious confrontation could develop."

LOPDELL HOUSE

George Gebbie added yet another chapter to the meeting when he reported the closure of Lopdell House. He said, "I know how the staff of North Shore Teachers' College and the dental nurses feel, as on 25 September we were called into the staffroom by an officer of the Education Department who was phoned evidently two hours before and told of the closure of Lopdell House.

"We were told that Lopdell House would shift to North Shore Teachers' College to utilise space even though it is completely unsuitable for in-service training.

"Most of our staff who have worked most of their working life at Lopdell House for obvious reasons could not make a daily journey across to the Shore even if we were offered the job.

"We feel that if the Government can close Lopdell House which has operated as such for the past 19 years, who are going to be the next victims?"

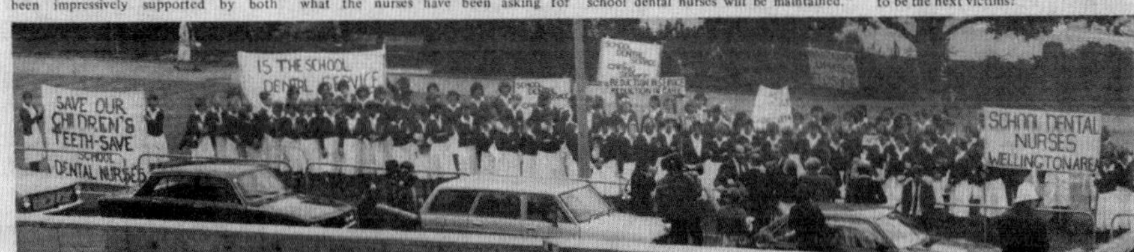

WELLINGTON DENTAL NURSES behind the barricades at Parliament on 7 November.

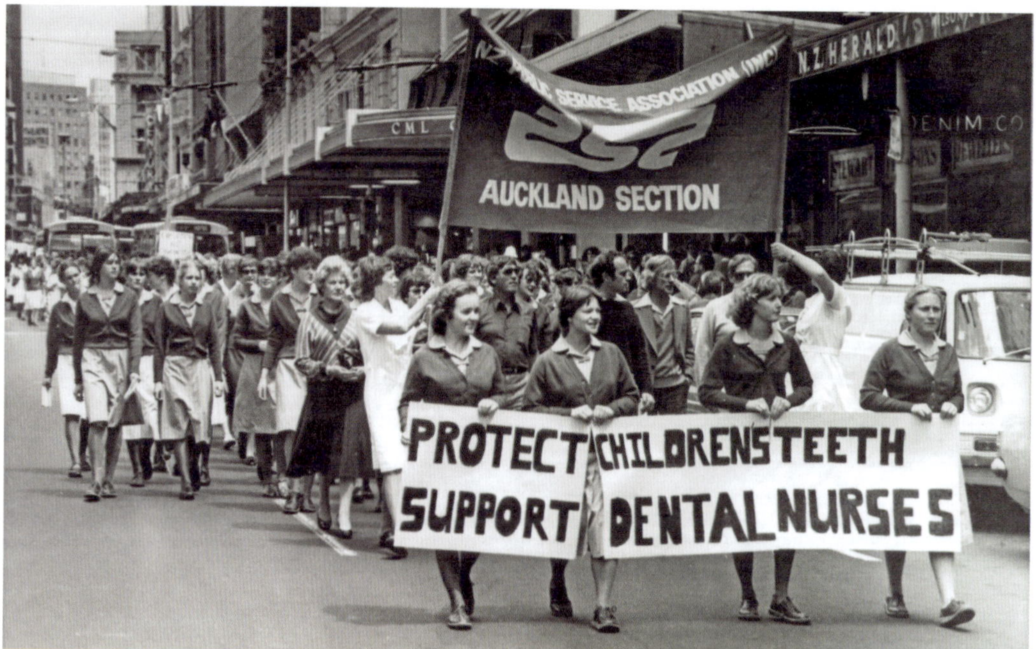

Protests against training school closures and cutbacks took place across the country, but were to no avail. The Auckland and Christchurch training schools closed in February 1982.

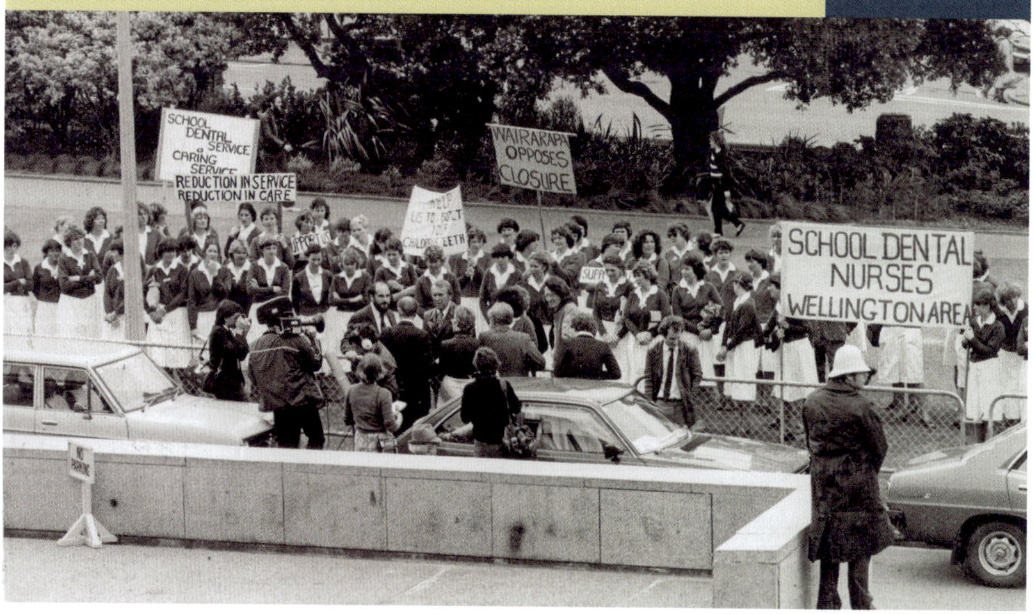
SCHOOL DENTAL SERVICE a CARING SERVICE
REDUCTION IN SERVICE
REDUCTION IN CARE
WAIRARAPA OPPOSES CLOSURE
SCHOOL DENTAL NURSES WELLINGTON AREA

petition on 24 March 1981. The way the meeting was conducted was an insult to dental nurses. The most vocal MP was D. C. McKinnon (National Albany) and the PSA delegates found his behaviour the most offensive. He asked questions and promptly began talking with a colleague. He also stretched back in his chair with his arms stretched behind his head as if to say, "Ho hum, this is all a big yawn".'[19]

PSA assistant secretary Mike Coleman said, 'We were really treated as the peasantry. It was a crass performance even by the standards we've grown used to at Parliament. The dental nurse on the delegation was intensely offended. It was just a naked display of power — they wanted to make us grovel. They were listening to us purely as a matter of form and asking as few questions as possible. They treated the whole procedure in a very offhand manner. I thought that petitions had a place in our democratic system but I would never recommend one again after our experience on this one.'

The protest marches and the petition were to no avail. The Auckland and Christchurch training schools closed as planned on 19 February 1982. A year later the School Dental Service received another blow when the government passed legislation to create 14 area health boards, which would effectively mean dental nurses would no longer be part of a national service. For a brief moment a reprieve seemed possible. On 14 June 1984, Prime Minister Rob Muldoon, eschewing his usual whisky for too many brandies, announced a snap election, to be held within one month. 'It doesn't give my opponents much time to run up to an election, does it?' he slurred.

It proved to be a boon for Labour candidate Annette King. 'I was going to take June to November off to campaign, though I didn't know how I was going to live.' The snap election resolved that dilemma. 'One day I was drilling teeth, the next day I was a member of Parliament [for Horowhenua]. It happened so fast.' Muldoon said she had put the horror into Horowhenua.

Like his grandiose Think Big projects, Muldoon's early election was a massive miscalculation: Labour, under the charismatic David Lange, surged back into power. Unfortunately for dental nurses, Labour continued with National's plan for area health boards. Worse, the raison d'être of the School Dental Service was now under question. Like big hair and shoulder pads, certain ideas took hold in the 1980s. Words like 'national' and 'state' started to be used pejoratively. They became bywords for bureaucratic, slow and inefficient. Business speculators were lauded for their acumen and afforded the respect once reserved for pioneering heart surgeons. Such was the skill and competence of the average business executive, it was claimed, that they could run any public-sector organisation more effectively than public servants who'd spent their careers acquiring expertise.

Governments, like some overbearing nanny, needed to stop interfering in people's lives, neoliberals argued. The fairy dust of market forces would transform society, making every enterprise more efficient and cost-effective, generating wealth for all so they could buy the services they needed, from housing to health. Faced with the financial mess left by the Muldoon government, the Labour government partially adopted that philosophy, selling off state assets at fire-sale prices and commercialising government entities by turning them into state-owned enterprises.

In 1990, the National government, after slashing welfare benefits, sought to build on Labour's state sell-offs by creating a framework for the privatisation of the health system. It engaged the Chicago accounting firm Arthur Andersen to investigate the efficiency of the public health system. The accountants reported that costs could be reduced by more than 30 per cent if the health system was run like a business. The government lost no time in acting on the report, which it refused to make public. Shunning any input from the health department or health professionals to avoid 'professional capture', it reconfigured the 14 area health boards into 23 Crown health enterprises, structured as for-profit companies. There were now 23 competing health organisations in a country with a population half the size of London's.

Janet Quigley was a Christchurch dental nurse caught up in the restructuring. Reflecting on that time on the PSA's centenary website in 2013, she said:

> The health reformers didn't know where to put dental nurses. They based us in a Crown Health Enterprise (CHE) called Health Link South, attached to Princess Margaret Hospital. But that CHE was mostly concerned with mental health and older persons' health, so it didn't suit us. At one stage they were going to sell us off to the University of Otago, but that fell through. Then came the restructuring.
>
> I was very heavily involved as the PSA spokesperson on the restructuring committee. We had a huge fight about the fact that it came down to costings. It was the young ones who had to go because they were cheaper to pay out. Totally bizarre! We lost those in their early–mid-20s, those with their whole career in front of them, a generation of dental nurses. There were about 30 redundancies from our CHE and I chose not to see the names till the job was done. They were very hurt, they wouldn't even answer calls. There were a lot of older ones who were happy to go, but the CHE wouldn't part with the necessary money.[20]

All the gains dental nurses had made, along with the respect they'd won with the march on Parliament, were quickly eroded. Janet was able to observe it up close:

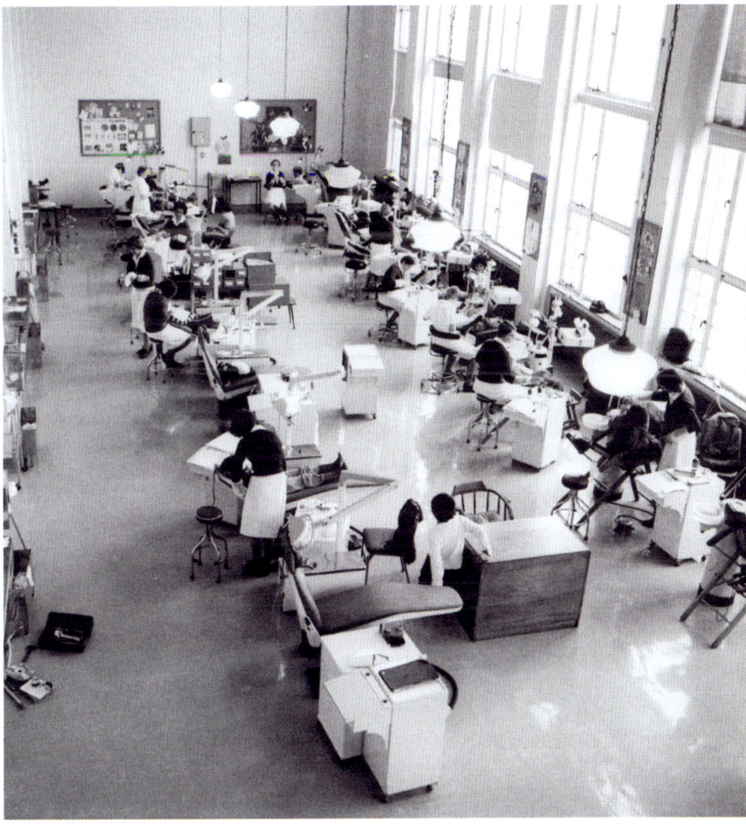

By the early 1980s the Wellington training school was a shadow of its former self. Only 29 trainees graduated in 1984. In 1999, the school was closed.

Being at the bargaining table was a frustrating experience. We had almost no training; we were simply told how to behave. The PSA organisers did most of the talking, though many were new and at the mercy of the CEO and his management or HR team. We didn't win anything; they just kept chipping away at all the things we'd fought hard for. The CEOs that came from health, they might have been more sympathetic but they still had to do what they had to do. There were people on the CHE from the Ministry to make sure everyone was toeing the party line.

Being a PSA delegate and bargainer was part and parcel of what I did. Sometimes it was very tricky for my job, but I challenged anyone who held it against me. I wasn't there to make life easy for them, I was there to make life better for our members. I remember things being thrown at us, being sworn at. But you had to rise above it.

Different terms and conditions had to be negotiated with each CHE, which was competing with all the others. 'If you developed something,' recalled Janet, 'you weren't able to share it with your colleagues in other places because we might have been able to sell it to them.' Dental nurses were losing pay and conditions and few were now entering the service. 'No one negotiating for the CHEs understood our role or our worth. All they knew was that they hated going to the dental nurse at school and based the rubbish they threw across the table at us on that. Salary movements were zilch for 14–15 years.'

In December 1999 the Willis Street Dental Clinic held an open day before closing its doors for good. Hundreds of former dental nurses who'd trained there turned up for the wake. They walked up the wide entrance steps and passed through the swinging glass doors, something they'd never been allowed to do as students. They had not only studied here, they had also skivvied — cleaning, polishing, washing dishes. Climbing the stairs to the second floor they entered again the training room with its six-metre-high windows, in its heyday a bustling dental production line. Visiting dignitaries, dentists and even royalty had marvelled over its efficiency, so many that a little balcony had been constructed, enabling them to observe the busy scene from above. The Dominion School for Dental Nurses had been the symbol of the School Dental Service for nearly 60 years, but now the jewel in the crown was a relic of a bygone era. It was losing Massey University, which used the building for its dental therapists' course, $250,000 a year.

In 1999 Labour was voted back into power and Annette King, the dental nurse who marched on Parliament in 1974, was appointed minister of health. But it was too late to reverse the cuts and training school closures that had taken place under National's George Gair. 'I had a real vision of what I wanted to do with the School Dental Service, only to have it all dumped when the training schools closed,' Annette reflected later. 'When I was minister I made some big changes in the training, making it a degree. I also made it a registered profession.'[21]

There were no longer school dental nurses: the name was changed to 'dental therapists' in 1991, and a year later the training of dental nurses was transferred from the Department of Health to the Department of Education. During Annette King's six years as minister of health, Otago University and Auckland University of Technology took over dental nurse training, offering diplomas and bachelor of oral health degree courses.

The 'hub and spoke' model of dental care introduced in 2006 introduced fixed hubs with the latest technology and equipment and mobile clinics visiting schools to carry out regular dental check-ups. Today, if treatment is required, parents usually have to make an appointment at their nearest community hub. 'You can imagine what happens,' says Annette. 'Say you've got three fillings. Mum or Dad has to take time off work to bring their child to the dental hub; that's if they have a car. They've ruined the model in my view.'

Thomas Hunter would be disappointed. In 2011 the *New Zealand Herald* reported: 'The dental health of young children continues to be among the worst in the developed world, figures reveal. Forty-four per cent of 5-year-olds have at least one decayed, missing or filled tooth, a school dental services report has found. The Government has spent $417 million on the problem since 2007 but the figures have shown little improvement. In 2000, 48 per cent of 5-year-olds had cavities, and the

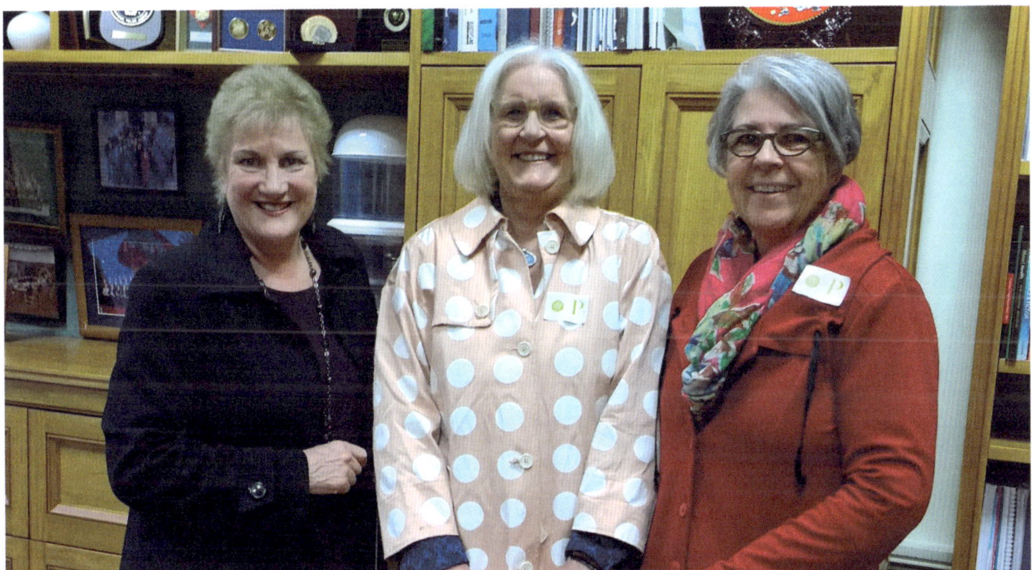

Annette King, Pam Horncy and Maggie Morgan reunite in 2016 in King's parliamentary office to reminisce about their careers as school dental nurses.

figure has not dropped below 43 per cent since. New Zealand rates are worse than the UK, US and Australia.'[22]

The redundancies of young, cheaper to pay out dental nurses as part of the restructuring in the 1990s, and the ongoing closure of rundown dental clinics attached to schools, have produced an unusual sound in many communities: the flapping of wings as chickens come home to roost. In 2017 Radio New Zealand reported that children now have to wait more than a year for treatment.

> Dunedin has three community hubs in Mosgiel, South Dunedin and the University of Otago Dental School, as well as mobile dental clinics in Port Chalmers, Portobello, Abbotsford and Wakari.
>
> Green Island School principal Steve Hayward, who is the former president of the Otago Primary Principals' Association, said he warned the DHB there would be problems when it closed school dental clinics and replaced them with the hubs and mobile clinics. 'I'm disappointed and disturbed because they promised us a number of things a few years ago when they revised the School Dental Service.' One of those promises was that there would be a 100 per cent student attendance at the new hubs and clinics, he said.
>
> Mr Hayward said parents often ended up taking a child out of class for a whole day to get to the nearest mobile clinic at another school for a quick screening check-up and it was hard for families to access the mobile clinics, let alone the hubs, if they didn't have their own transport.
>
> The DHB's oral health director, Tim Mackay, said in a statement the DHB aimed to provide annual check-ups for primary school children but some were waiting for more than 12 months. 'The main reason for overdue appointments is staffing,' he said. 'Southern DHB has a workforce of dental therapists who are steadily retiring and the competition to attract new graduates and experienced therapists is high, making it difficult to fill dental therapy roles.'[23]

The Ministry of Health admits that 'dental decay remains the most prevalent chronic (and irreversible) disease in New Zealand'. And it is likely to remain so as dental treatment is well beyond the means of many adults who struggle to pay rent and buy food for their families. Lack of regular treatment is compounded by consumption of sugary drinks, junk food and poor dental hygiene. Up to a third of children miss out on dental treatment because of the barriers of time and transport their parents face to take their children to a dental hub.

In 2018 Bill O'Connor, president of the New Zealand Dental Association, told its annual conference that school dental services were 'underfunded, understaffed, overwhelmed'.[24] More than 96,000 children were up to two years overdue for checkups with a dental therapist, 29,000 children had teeth extracted in 2017, and 7000 required hospital dental treatment under general anaesthetic. 'None of what I have outlined is a negative comment regarding the dental therapists — they have a hard job, they are our colleagues. We all know how hard their job is. The system has failed these children and their parents. The system has failed those who work in it, trying to deliver the best outcomes for their patients.'

When the School Dental Service began in 1921, the situation was dire for children: 90 per cent needed treatment. In her thesis on the history of the service, Susan Moffat writes: 'There was no doubt, however, that in its early years the Service did much to alleviate pain and suffering in children by treating dental caries. Success in treating dental emergencies and reducing them through regular care was monitored by changes in the extraction-to-filling ratio. This ratio was reduced rapidly at first from 78.6 extractions per 100 restorations in 1923 to 17.4 extractions in 1933. There was a more gradual fall until 1967 when the extraction ratio was only 3.17.[25]

School dental nurses treated children in the remotest and poorest parts of New Zealand. They worked alone with poor equipment and little support. They benefited generations of children and reduced disparities between rich and poor. They were seldom thanked for their work and few remember them with affection. Indeed, former patients often vie for who can tell the most horrendous story about a visit to the school dental nurse.

But at least one patient was able to keep a sense of perspective. Angela Fitchett in the *Nelson Mail* wrote: 'Looking back at mid-20th century school dental treatment from the careful present, where reassurance and comfort is an expected part of any dental or medical treatment a child receives, it's easy to be horrified . . . But in defence of the treatment, it was free, it was regular and we children couldn't avoid it because it was compulsory. And I still have all of my teeth, even if some of them are now more the creation of my dentist than of my maker. Despite the fear and the pain, I really am truly grateful to those dedicated young women in their crisply starched white uniforms who cared for the teeth of New Zealand's school children.'[26]

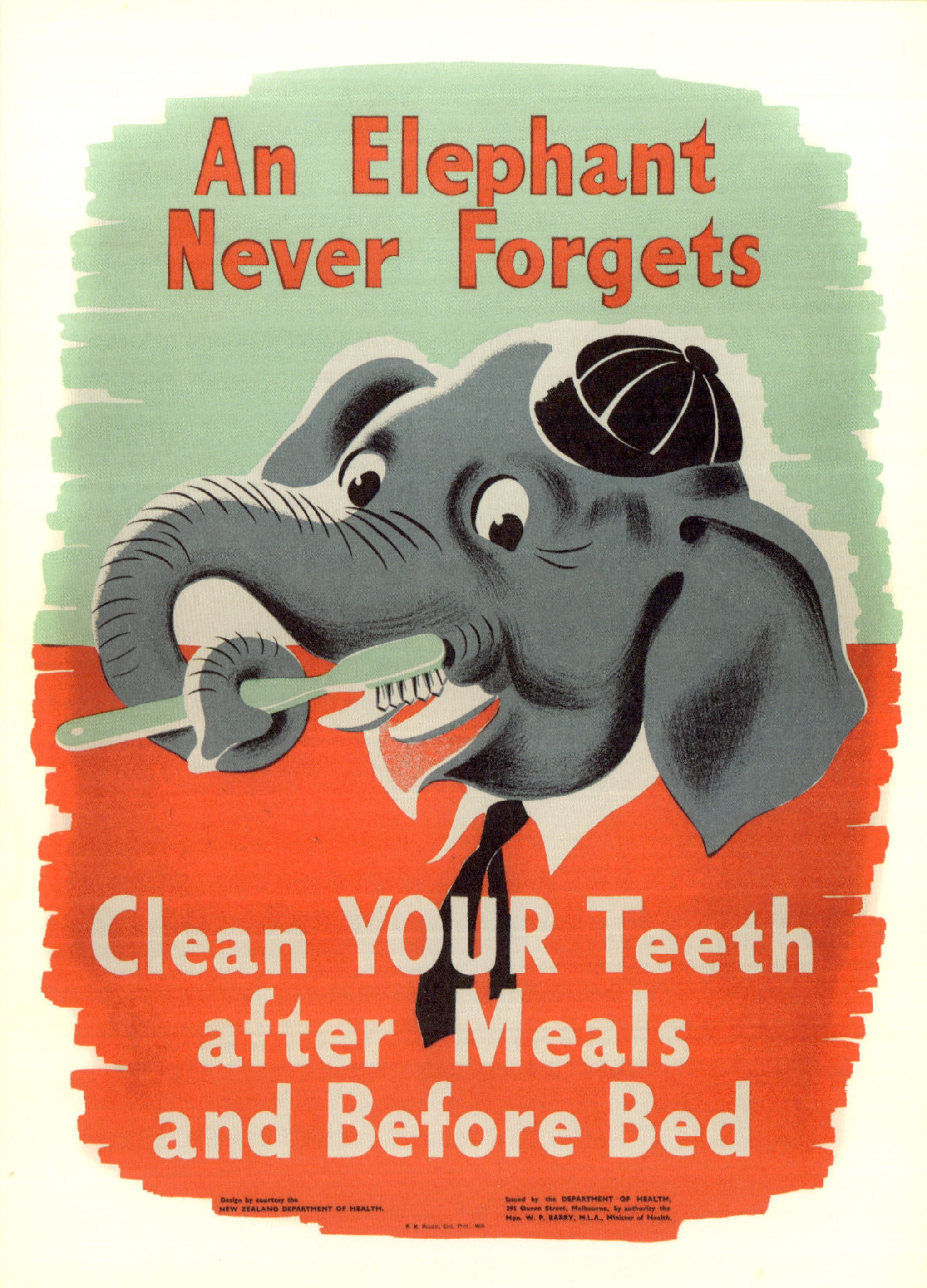
An Elephant
Never Forgets
Clean YOUR Teeth
after Meals
and Before Bed
Design by courtesy the
NEW ZEALAND DEPARTMENT OF HEALTH.
Issued by the DEPARTMENT OF HEALTH,
295 Queen Street, Melbourne, by authority the
Hon. W. P. BARRY, M.L.A., Minister of Health.

10

EVERYDAY MERCURY POISONING

On the morning of 6 March 2017, three fire engines, their sirens wailing, raced to Camberley School in Hastings.[1] They'd been alerted to a chemical spill and the school had been evacuated.

Firefighters donned orange hazmat suits, strapped on oxygen tanks and entered the building. A toxic smell had been reported when the school opened after the weekend. Pupils were quickly evacuated to the school hall and teachers notified parents to collect their children in case the wind spread the toxicants. Sixteen people, teachers and pupils, had felt unwell and were taken to hospital. The cause of the chemical hazard: an old-fashioned thermometer in the science area had broken on the Friday afternoon. The mess was cleaned up, but some mercury soaked into the carpet. With temperatures in the 30s over the weekend, the mercury reacted with solvents in the carpet and vaporised, creating the chemical hazard emergency. The thermometer had contained between 0.5 and 3 grams of mercury, less than a quarter of a teaspoon.

Rewind to 1974. In a school dental clinic, a dental nurse is preparing a filling for a young child. She takes a square copper pellet and places it on miniature scales. From a small wooden bottle, befitting its exotic contents, she pours mercury on the other side of the scale. It's important to get the correct ratio of copper to mercury, and hard to keep the slithery quicksilver from spilling over the lip. She combines the two and heats them over a Bunsen burner until the mercury bubbles to the top, then grinds the mixture in a mortar and pestle. The amalgam is nearly ready to use. She places it in a gauze cloth, squeezing out the excess mercury with her fingers, sometimes dropping the silver beads into her patient's hand: it never fails to fascinate. Inevitably, it ends up on the floor, splattering like a silver raindrop on the lino. Mixing amalgam is an operation school dental nurses performed up to 10 times a day over a working lifetime.

Dental nurses had never been warned about the dangers of working with mercury — second only to radium in its toxicity — and it must have seemed unlikely that the odourless liquid silver element, used in both copper and silver amalgams, posed any danger. Poisons came in bottles with skull and crossbones and warnings in capital type, not in elegant wooden vessels. Yet the toxic effects of mercury have been known since ancient times. According to science writer Julie Sloane, 'The Romans used their mercury mines as penal institutions for criminals, slaves, and other undesirables. The warders were among the first to recognise that there was a high likelihood that the prisoners would become poisoned and spare the keepers the need for formal executions . . . The lifespan of a worker in those mines was tragically brief.'[2]

The mystique of mercury has intrigued civilisations for millennia, from Hindu and Chinese to Greek and Roman. Alchemists believed it could be used to convert base metals such as lead into noble metals like gold. Despite its known toxicity, mercury was used as a medicine. (The term 'quack' to describe a medical charlatan is derived from the German word for quicksilver, *Quecksilber*.) Arabs used mercury ointments for skin diseases in the eleventh century, and the ointments and pills were touted as a cure for syphilis and were used right up until the introduction of penicillin in the 1940s.

Such treatments led indirectly to the use of mercury in the manufacture of felt. In Turkey, camel hair was compressed to produce felt, and moistening the fibres with camel urine was found to speed up the process. Without a ready supply of camel urine to hand, French felt workers experimented by urinating on the fibres themselves. One worker was able to produce a consistently finer felt with his urine. What set him apart was that he was a syphilitic, being treated with mercury. The connection was made, and using a mercury solution to make better felt soon became standard practice. And this, in turn, led to mercury poisoning among hatters.

'Hatters' shakes' was a widely used term to describe the tremors developed among workers in the industry. In Danbury in Connecticut, 'the hat city of the world', locals referred to it as 'the Danbury shakes'.[3] You could spot a Danbury hat-maker by his hand tremors. Other symptoms were less obvious — slurred speech, dizziness, and mental confusion. A study in 1925 reported that out of 100 Danbury hatters, 43 had mercury poisoning: 'Boys 20 and 21 years old are already so badly poisoned that their hands shake continually, while many of the men who have served longer at the trade cannot even feed themselves.'

Hat industry manufacturers and their insurers refused to accept the findings, and sought instead to blame the hatters' symptoms on excessive alcohol and smoking. Finally in 1941 the use of mercury in hat-making was banned in America, though the

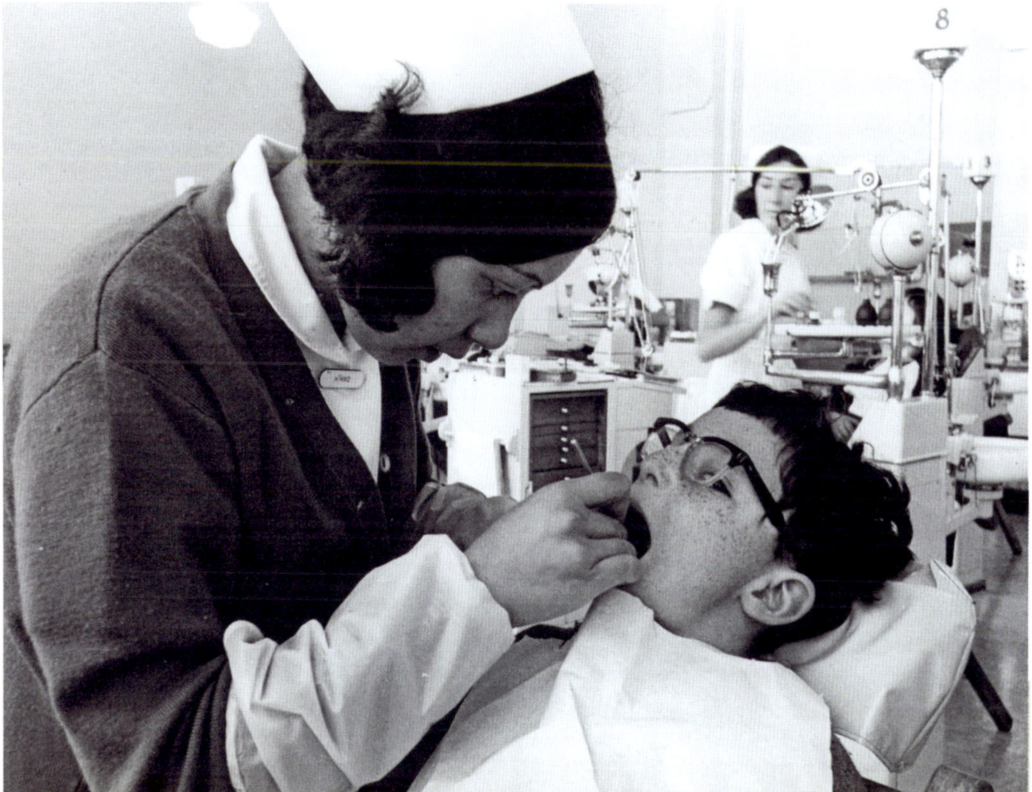

A dental nurse probes for decay. Up until the 1970s dental nurses were unaware that their jobs were hazardous to their health due to continual exposure to highly toxic mercury vapour.

sites where the factories stood are still polluted with mercury residue.

Mercury has been used in dentistry for more than 190 years. Dental amalgam fillings came into general use in 1826, but not without controversy. In 1840 the American Society of Dental Surgeons, worried about mercury poisoning, banned its members from using mercury amalgam fillings. They considered that placing a known toxin like mercury in the mouths of patients was 'malpractice' and they were determined to 'rid the profession of charlatans and their obnoxious materials'.[4] Nonetheless, dentists continued to use mercury amalgam because it was cheaper and easier to use than the standard gold fillings, in which gold foil was pressed into a cavity.

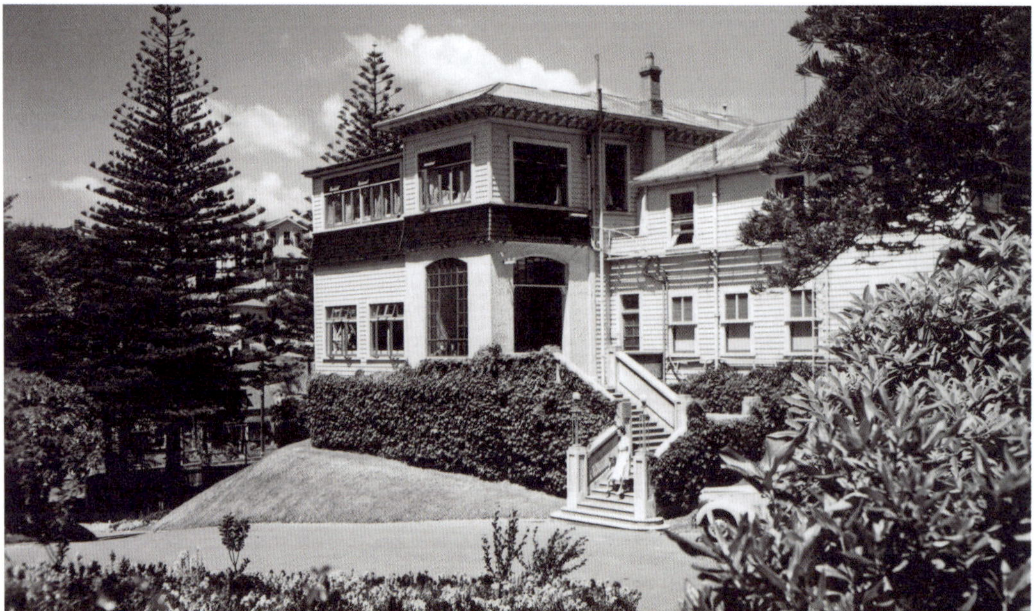

Premier House, once the official residence of prime ministers in Thorndon, Wellington, served as the dental annexe from the 1930s to the 1970s. It was widely known as 'The Murder House', an epithet later used to describe all dental clinics. It was highly contaminated with mercury.

What became known as the 'First Amalgam War' broke out between the anti- and pro-mercury amalgam factions. By 1859 the pro faction had won and formed the American Dental Association. In the 1920s the 'Second Amalgam War' erupted when a German chemist, Alfred Stock, began publicising the dangers of using mercury in dentistry. Stock, who had suffered from chronic mercury poisoning himself, was concerned about all those who worked with mercury, as he pointed out in a 1928 paper: 'No one can doubt the ubiquitous spread of chronic poisoning by mercury vapour among the professionally employed chemists, physicists, physicians, dentists and school teachers teaching subjects in the natural sciences, etc. Wherever mercury is used it is unavoidable, even with the greatest care, that liquid metal is occasionally being scattered; it divides itself as tiny dust everywhere and evaporates only slowly, taking months and years without being noticed. That is what the special dangerousness of this poison is based on.'[5] Stock advised taking the greatest care when working with mercury, and using good ventilation, hoods and extractor fans. Debate about Stock's work raged in Germany in the 1930s, only to be forgotten amid the upheaval of the Second World War.

During the postwar era, mercury's notoriety continued to spread. In 1956, in the Japanese city of Minamata, 900 people died and 2265 became seriously ill after eating fish contaminated with mercury from chemical plant waste. In Iraq in 1971, 459 people died and 6530 were admitted to hospital after consuming seed grain that had been treated with a mercury-based fungicide. In both these cases it was the more highly toxic methylmercury that had caused the tragedies, not the elemental mercury used in dental fillings. Still, it was a reminder that mercury was a substance that needed to be treated with great care. By then, new technology, such as mass spectrophotometry and the portable mercury vapour detector, made it possible to detect trace amounts of mercury, spurring the 'Third Amalgam War'. It became clear that mercury could pass through the blood–brain barrier, through the placenta and into tissues and organs.

The mercury-related tragedies prompted the *Gazette* to publish an editorial in 1971. It read:

> School Dental Service procedures for manipulating amalgam and for disposing of mercury residues in the form of amalgam wastes have been adopted after careful consideration of available knowledge of the human body's response to exposure to mercury vapour and metallic mercury.
>
> Obviously our first concern must be for our young patients. Does the placement of an amalgam restoration constitute a hazard to the health of children? The answer is an unqualified 'no'. Research has shown that the patient is under no risk whatsoever. His encounter with mercury vapour is too brief and the total amount involved is too small. Even an accidental swallowing of a small amount of filling material would be no cause for alarm.
>
> Our thoughts then focus on ourselves — the dental personnel. Will exposure to the risk of contamination over a long period of time constitute a danger to health? There can be no unqualified 'no' to this question. *The determining factors are controlled by the individual operator* [emphasis added] and the observance of a few simple rules of mercury hygiene will to all intents and purposes eliminate that risk.[6]

A cynic might conclude from the above that this was an attempt to blame a dental nurse for her own misuse of mercury should she ever suffer any mercury-related illness. The same cynic might ask why there was not a single mention of mercury handling in the dental nurse's bible, *Standing Instructions*, when it was so prescriptive on, for example, the correct wearing of uniform.

The editorial was vague about why dental nurses needed to pay 'meticulous' attention to mercury hygiene: 'It is important to realise that metallic (liquid) mercury is a source of harmful vapour, which if inhaled in sufficient concentration over a long period of time could prove injurious to health.' What constituted a 'sufficient concentration'? 'Over a long period of time' — was that hours or years? And exactly how was it 'injurious to health': was the injury likely to be life-threatening, or prolonged, or temporary like a cold?

Given that dental nurses were exposed every day to mercury vapour, they surely deserved to know how it might affect them and what symptoms to look out for. The risks had already been identified and papers published when the School Dental Service was founded in 1921. Alfred Stock had already observed many symptoms among those exposed to mercury: mental fatigue, inner restlessness, bad mood, irritability, diminished memory, drowsiness, headache, restless sleep, lack of desire to live, shyness, salivation, chronic nose cold, diarrhoea.

The Ministry for the Environment website today summarises the main dangers of working with mercury thus:

> Inhaled elemental mercury vapour easily crosses from the lung into the blood stream. Approximately 80% of inhaled mercury is absorbed into the blood stream, while only 0.01% of elemental mercury is absorbed through the gastrointestinal tract. Once in the blood stream, elemental mercury readily crosses the placental barrier and the developing foetus can be exposed to mercury (WHO, 2003).
>
> The main effects of chronic toxicity of mercury inhalation are tremors and psychological disturbances. *The principal psychological symptoms include excessive timidity, diffidence, increasing shyness, loss of self confidence, anxiety, and a desire to remain unobserved and unobtrusive* [emphasis added] . . . Moderate and repeated exposures (lower than a few mg/m^3, but higher than 0.05 mg/m^3) causes tremors in hands, gingivitis (bleeding from the gums), excessive salivation and mercurial erethism. Mercurial erethism is a term to describe the classic neurological symptoms associated with mercury poisoning.[7]

The psychological symptoms are striking given the unusual docility of the dental nurse workforce over decades. Was that in part because they were inhaling mercury vapour every day or simply a reflection of an era when women were more submissive?

Not only were dental nurses putting themselves at greater risk preparing copper amalgam fillings (which they used for baby teeth), but they may also have been endangering the health of their young patients. The use of copper amalgam fillings had been condemned by the scientific community since the 1920s. Stock didn't even feel the need to address the issue in 1928, so unanimous was scientific opinion: 'We do not have to dwell much on copper amalgam fillings. Even though only 1 and ½ years ago they were still defended and even praised for their qualities to disinfect the mouth, they are nowadays pretty much dropped. The fact that they may cause severe health damage cannot be denied any longer.'[8]

The news that copper amalgam fillings were dangerous had reached New Zealand the year before. On 7 September 1927 the *Otago Daily Times* reported: 'According to a congress of German dentists, patients throughout the world are suffering slow poisoning due to the use of cheap composition in stopping teeth. Professor Fleischmann says that there is no danger in expensive compositions containing platinum or gold. The commonest composition, containing copper, is likely to admit mercury, poisoning the system. The congress decided not to use cheap composition pending the discovery of protective measures.'[9]

The New Zealand Dental Association was quick to respond:

> The secretary of the Otago branch of the New Zealand Dental Association informed a reporter that the main fillings used in New Zealand were gold and amalgam, and that amalgam fillings [for adult teeth] contained no copper. Another common filling was porcelain cement, which was free from metal. In Germany evidently they were using cheaper materials than those in New Zealand.
>
> As the result of an inquiry at the dental school, information was supplied that this particular question had cropped up from time to time, but throughout the profession in New Zealand no known material used for filling teeth was likely to cause poisoning. The alloys in common use were all high-grade and were subjected to severe tests before being supplied to dentists . . . The president of the local branch of the New Zealand Dental Association stated that as far as New Zealand was concerned, copper alloys were unknown, and, as the fillings were all high-grade, there was no chance of patients being poisoned.[10]

While that might have been true for some dentists, it seems unlikely that unregulated dentists were not opting for the cheapest materials they could find and even less likely that the fledging School Dental Service, which was so under-resourced it had to rely on used army equipment, was not using copper amalgams. In fact, dental nurses had been instructed to use copper amalgams for baby teeth fillings and to use the more expensive silver amalgam only for permanent teeth.

The fact that only young children were given copper fillings was both a positive and a negative. On the one hand, their baby teeth would soon fall out; on the other, their young age made it more likely they would be affected by the mercury. Copper amalgam fillings were composed of 70 per cent mercury and 30 per cent copper and they were prone to corrosion. Even silver amalgam fillings, generally considered safe, have now been banned in Europe for use on children under 15 years old and in pregnant and breastfeeding women.

Dental nurses were never informed of controversy surrounding copper amalgam, much less of the risks they were taking working each day in a contaminated clinic preparing the fillings. In clinics with two dental nurses the exposure was doubled. And yet, when in 1971 the *Gazette* finally acknowledged that mercury was 'injurious to health', they were told they were in no danger provided they followed a 'few simple rules'.

That changed in 1974. A technician who made the rounds of clinics maintaining equipment happened to remark to two dental nurses on Auckland's North Shore: 'You know, you people are working with a highly toxic chemical.' The nurses were alarmed and started to do some research. What they found was enough to bring their concerns to the PSA. Emboldened with the success of their march on Parliament months before, they wanted action.

The PSA engaged the services of an occupational health consultant, Dr Bill Glass, to investigate the claims. Within the health department and even among some dental nurses, the issue was being dismissed as 'scare-mongering'. To Logan, director of dental health, it was no doubt another example of the PSA wanting to be seen as the champion of healthcare workers and absorb them into the union.

Margaret Clarkson was on the dental nurses' advisory panel and was involved in the discussions about mercury. 'I and John McKenzie went on the mercury negotiation and there was the director-general of health, the director of public health and director of dental health present. Our argument was that the mechanism we used for handling mercury was very unsatisfactory. You had to be extremely careful not to spill any. I'd taken along the little balance and little bottle of mercury we used to demonstrate how careful you had to be that it didn't spill over the lip. And one of the directors said, "You girls would drink the stuff if you got publicity." That was the attitude. They weren't interested at all in the issue. They were interested in the fact that they would get adverse publicity. They wouldn't take any responsibility.'[11]

Margaret was concerned enough to have a urine test to check her own mercury levels. 'And I was walking down the corridor at work and the principal of the dental school was walking the other way and he said, "Oh Mrs Clarkson, it's good that your mercury levels weren't high." And I said, "I beg your pardon?" And he said, "Your test results show your mercury levels weren't high." And I said, "I haven't had my test results." They'd been sent to him, not to me. So he flushed and disappeared into his office. I was really cross because I'd done the test privately and yet the results had gone to him.'

The Department of Health deployed its own experts to counter Dr Glass, but the matter was surprisingly quickly settled. As the *PSA Journal* put it, 'The Association, after taking the advice of one of the medical experts in occupational health in New Zealand, Dr. W. Glass, can take considerable satisfaction in the adoption by the Health Department, almost in toto, of the proposals put forward by the Association and its consultant for safeguarding the health of Dental Nurses; for de-contaminating clinics which may at present be impregnated with mercury[;] and for developing procedures designed to ensure the safe use of mercury in the future.'[12]

The quick capitulation of the Department of Health may have had more to do with adverse publicity, as Margaret Clarkson says, than concern for the safety of dental nurses, because the mercury contamination had been there for decades. Dental nurses remember that the dental annexe in Premier House in Wellington was one of the worst sites. 'When I worked at Tinakori Clinic,' Margaret McLean recalled, 'you'd get to work early in the morning and on the metal parts of the stairs you'd see all these little stalagmites sitting up on the stairs from people's shoes. The mercury had grown up. We had it on our shoes everywhere. They used to bring the Geiger counter round and it just about put it off the dial. When they lifted the lino there were gallons of mercury that had got into the cracks.'[13]

'They never told us what they found,' says Ngaire Mune, 'but I think they found a lot of mercury because we were told you can't wear your duty shoes outside the building.'[14]

The department began a programme of clinic air monitoring and replacing old lino. 'They gave us bags of flower of sulphur to put on mercury spills,' remembers Maggie Morgan. 'I took it home to put on my rose bushes.'[15]

Nurses were given a flagon and funnel for a 24-hour urine test to check the level of mercury in their system. 'It had to be done on a particular day and we were having a school party that day,' recalls Annette King. 'You had to collect every drop, so they gave me a big flagon. Well, about nine o'clock that night I had filled it, and somebody at the house where the party was gave me a plastic bottle so I had to give them two, the official one and the other plastic one. I'm sure they must have decided that it was almost pure alcohol!'

'Nurses were put off work until the levels of mercury dropped down to a satisfactory level,' says Pam Horncy. 'Some dental nurses were off work for over a year. I was really envious of them because mine was okay.'[16]

The copper amalgam pellets that exposed dental nurses to the greatest risk of inhaling mercury vapour were withdrawn, and silver amalgam capsules prepared in a factory were introduced. Dental nurses were advised to keep their clinics well ventilated and to minimise the use of electric bar heaters. However, the *Gazette* made clear where the buck stopped: 'In the final analysis it is the action of the individuals, both dentist and dental nurse, that will determine the effectiveness of safety programmes.'[17] But was it?

As Dr Linda Jones has pointed out in her 2005 thesis on the effects of mercury in dentistry, 'School Dental Clinics did not have extraction fans or any kind of air conditioning. Variation and fluctuations in New Zealand's seasonal temperatures meant that the instructions were impossible to follow. The manual measurement of liquid mercury for silver fillings, the naked-hand expression of excess mercury from amalgam mixes, and the naked-hand clean-up of accidental spills, in the absence of any protective clothing, demonstrates that even the most conscientious woman would still be at risk of mercury poisoning.'[18]

Dental nurses were never told the results of their urine tests unless mercury exceeded a safe level and they were put off work. Those who were off work were monitored until their mercury levels dropped and they were able to return to work. Nine hundred and thirteen women were urine-tested, and three per cent of them were off work for varying periods.

Was a single urine test enough, though, to establish that dental nurses had suffered no ill effects from, in some cases, decades of exposure to mercury vapour? It was an issue Jones explored in her thesis.

> For any individual, their proclivity to store or excrete cannot be known except from autopsy. A urine test measures mercury excreted by the kidneys. A blood

> test shows what level of mercury is circulating. Hence, what tests do is confirm exposure has occurred with an excretion level at one point in time, not what level of mercury is causing an adverse response. Test results become an aid to diagnosis, but are a poor measure of individual body burden and an unreliable indicator of symptoms . . . High excretion may mean high storage and hence high risk; but it could result from low storage if a person has a metabolism that is efficient at excreting toxins, and hence low risk. Low excretion may mean low storage and hence low risk; but it may also result from high storage if a person has a metabolism that is inefficient at excreting toxins, hence indicating high risk.

In other words, urine-testing alone was not enough. Were some dental nurses displaying symptoms of mercury poisoning? Would there be any long-term effects of their exposure to mercury vapour? The health department chose to ignore these possibilities.

Fast-forward 24 years to 1998. Linda Jones, now a lecturer in psychology at Massey University, gets a letter from a former dental nurse, who'd attended a reunion of dental nurses who graduated, like her, in 1968. 'The concern expressed in the letter arose because, when they compared their lives, over one-third of their class talked of reproductive problems: difficulty conceiving; miscarriage; congenital abnormalities; children with learning difficulties; and sudden infant death.'[19]

Jones was already familiar with the issue of mercury study, having just completed a study of dental patients who'd been diagnosed with mercury poisoning from amalgam fillings. The patients displayed the key symptoms of erethism: depression, anxiety and emotional fragility. Some had considered suicide because their symptoms were dismissed as psychosomatic or they were labelled hypochondriacs by their doctor.

Jones was intrigued by the dental nurses' stories. Could there be long-term damage to health caused by chronic exposure to mercury that had not been investigated? Why was there no follow-up on the nurses who'd had high mercury readings in 1974? She found that not only was there no attempt to track the ongoing health of those who'd been tested but there was also no documentation she could use as a starting point. It was a cold case, but, unlike a police investigation, there was no box of files marked 'Dental Nurses' Mercury Poisoning' to be dusted off in the basement. 'Establishing the facts required persistence, and I spent prolonged periods at National Archives. There was no single location for documentation. Anything from 1970–1979 relating to the school dental service was searched.' She pored over copies of the *School Dental Service*

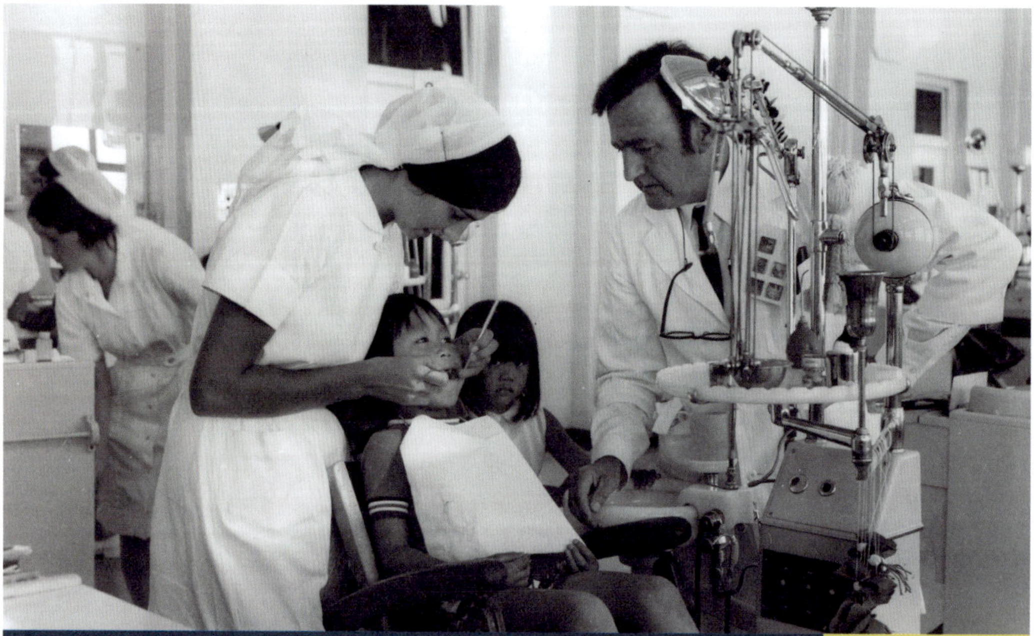

By the 1980s dental clinics had been decontaminated and dental nurses had been tested for mercury poisoning, but no studies were conducted to ascertain whether or not there had been any long-term effects of mercury exposure.

Gazette, correspondence between officials, minutes of meetings. She found the names of some dental nurses and their urinary test results but others were anonymous.[20]

The trail was about to grow colder. The Willis Street Dental Clinic was closing its doors and files were destined for the tip. 'I was asked to go through all the files remaining after all of the dental staff had left, to locate anything that should be archived rather than destroyed. There were several rooms stacked floor to ceiling with files literally tied in red tape!'

Jones was able to locate and interview a number of dental nurses who'd been working when mercury testing was carried out in 1974.[21] They said they'd never been told mercury was toxic when they were training. Mercury went everywhere in the clinic, the nurses told her. 'Mercury spills often happened in the course of the day and were light-heartedly dealt with. Corners of the clinic often had small 'balls' of mercury in them through inadequate cleaners, children were often given balls of mercury to play with.'

They'd been told to store amalgam scraps for collection, but they often lay around for years. One nurse recalled: 'I was at a sub-base and discovered in the cupboard an open shoebox full of AgAm scraps which should have been sent off to Dominion Gold Waihi for reprocessing. I tipped it into the provided canvas bag and took it to the local post office — I handed it across the counter and before I could explain, the young man undid the string and the tag and emptied it across the counter! Well, we both gasped! He had chunks of old filling material and beads of mercury spread everywhere and onto the floor! He said, "I thought it was money." It was very heavy.'

Their casual attitude to mercury, born of ignorance, came at a high personal cost for some. Jones writes: 'Conception difficulties and spontaneous abortion were experienced by many although never connected to mercury.' When they compared notes when they got together at work seminars, they found that many had experienced mood problems and were taking Valium. Dr Bill Glass had documented mood effects in his 1974 study, but 'general and reproductive problems seemed not to have been assessed'.

In the course of her investigations Jones discovered perhaps the real reason the dental nurses' mercury poisoning claims had not been taken more seriously. Before beginning her mercury studies she'd been told that in the 1970s, 'the Department of Health and the NZDA executive considered that the real reason that some women in the School Dental Service had high urine-mercury levels was not their occupational exposure, but their overuse of spermicidal jelly and blue eye shadow'.[22] For her study Jones conducted a battery of tests, both psychological and psychomotor skill assessments, on the nurses and on a control group of women of similar age who had never been dental nurses. They were also questioned about their past health. There were significant differences in their reproductive health. Twenty-five per cent of the dental nurses had had hysterectomies, compared with just 6.6 per cent of the control group.

Dental nurses were more likely to have repetitive strain injury or occupational overuse syndrome (35.5 per cent, versus 6.6 per cent of the control group) but it was unclear whether this was caused by nerve damage from exposure to mercury vapour or the fact they'd spent years working with vibrating dental drills. Similarly they displayed hand tremor, but again dental drill vibration could not be ruled out as the cause.

Dry skin and eczema were common complaints among the dental nurses in the past and are consistent with the effects of mercury poisoning. The dental nurses also reported significantly more thyroid symptoms than the control group.

All the dental nurses who elected to take part in the study reported that they enjoyed good health, but did that fact skew the results? 'If symptoms of erethism have endured,' writes Jones, 'there may well have been among the non-responding women some clinically depressed, highly anxious, or shy women who would be very unlikely to volunteer for something the information sheet called neuro-behavioural testing taking up to two hours.'[23]

A Norwegian study of dental nurses went further than Jones' conclusions. It found that 25 per cent of the dental nurses reported having neurological problems; 36 per cent of the dental nurses had tremors compared to 8 per cent in the control group; 14 per cent of the dental nurses had problems with memory, though the control group had no memory problems. Eighteen per cent of the dental nurses were depressed, compared to 4 per cent in the control group, and 21 per cent of the dental nurses had heart and lung problems, compared to 5 per cent of the control group.[24]

In 2005 a Norwegian Broadcasting Company documentary, *Mercury Girls*, about dental nurses with high levels of mercury, drew a huge response from viewers. Nearly four hundred women who'd worked with mercury while pregnant or breastfeeding reported children born with birth defects, learning difficulties, immunological issues and muscular/skeletal problems. The mothers had severe bleedings and multiple late spontaneous abortions.

While the dental industry disputes the level of damage caused by inhaling mercury vapour, there seems to be consensus among doctors. The World Health Organization states:

> Mercury is highly toxic, especially when metabolised into methylmercury. It may be fatal if inhaled and harmful if absorbed through the skin. Around 80% of the inhaled mercury vapour is absorbed in the blood through the lungs. It may cause harmful effects to the nervous, digestive, respiratory [and] immune systems and to the kidneys, besides causing lung damage. Adverse health effects from mercury exposure can be: tremors, impaired vision and hearing, paralysis, insomnia, emotional instability, developmental deficits during foetal development, and attention deficit and developmental delays during childhood. *Recent studies suggest that mercury may have no threshold below which some adverse effects do not occur* [emphasis added].[25]

It will never be known how dental nurses were affected by mercury poisoning; how many suffered infertility or spontaneous abortions or had children with birth defects or developmental difficulties; who suffered from depression or other mental health issues or other symptoms wrongly attributed by their doctors to hormonal changes. And what of long-term damage in old age? The PSA and the New Zealand Dental Therapists Association are now sponsoring a study to follow up on Linda Jones' work, seeking women who were working as dental nurses in 1974 and who were told their mercury levels were high or whose clinics needed detoxification. There is some evidence linking mercury with Alzheimer's disease.[26] Some autopsy studies have found increased mercury levels in brain tissues of Alzheimer's patients. Whatever the findings of a follow-up study, it is already too late.

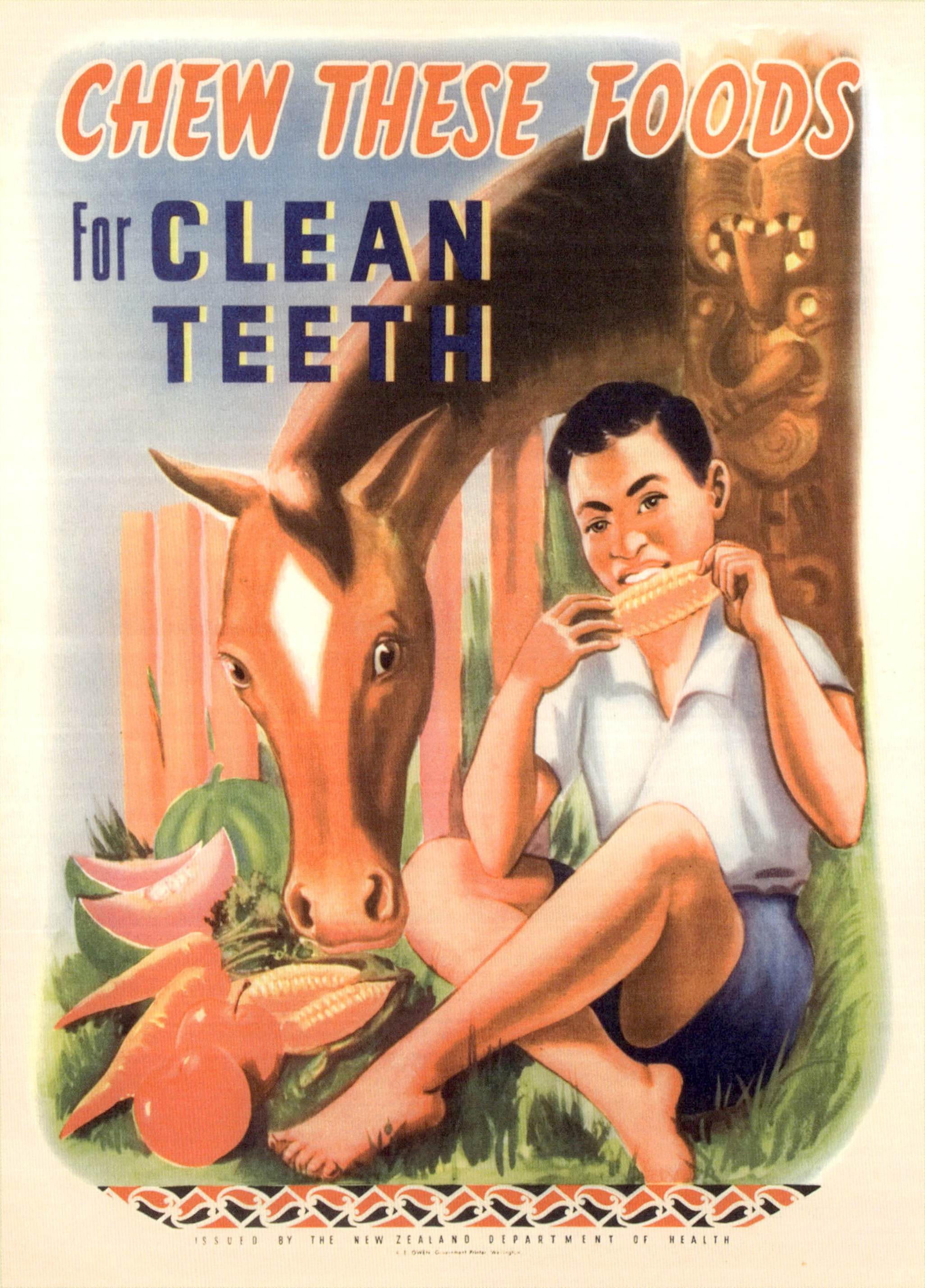
CHEW THESE FOODS
for CLEAN
TEETH
ISSUED BY THE NEW ZEALAND DEPARTMENT OF HEALTH

11

PAIN AND POLICY

When I was beginning this book, a short article about my project appeared on the Stuff website.[1] Reading the posted comments, I was shocked by the level of hostility towards dental nurses.

> These women inflicted untold much pain and distress on very young children, with impunity. If this were to happen today the 'service' would be shut down and people fired. An entire generation of adults have been harmed by their childhood experiences, and many have had their teeth ruined needlessly.

> I remember getting my teeth drilled out and it being like smoke like taste. I told someone how the dental nurse drilled my tongue, which she did, when I went back she said are you telling people I drilled your tongue. I said dam straight and I ain't retracting!!! Shuddddeerrr

> I had all my old fillings removed 8 years ago and discovered that majority should never have been put there in the first place as there was no decay to begin with, some teeth had drill marks that were far deeper than they needed to be, apparently this happened a lot that kids were 'experimented on' and a lot of unnecessary work was performed. The nurse was not very tolerant and would get angry if I moved or flinched, horrible lady, still can't stand the smell of those places and the sound of those drills send shivers up my spine. And sitting on those chairs while she mixed up the filling mixtures in those machines that shook back and forward, they were horrible frightening place for a child.

> Ah yes the school 'Murder House'. The memories of waiting for your name to be called when they came to visit your school. That smell, the chair of fear, the belt driven drill that sometimes slowed so much it stopped in your mouth in the massive hole that they had drilled removing way too much tooth

> enamel that in years to come would cost us dearly in tooth re-repairs. One of my school friends held the record for the most fillings in one sitting — 11!!
>
> Took me years to get over the fear of the school dental nurse to actually go and see a dentist . . . and when I did the dentist said 'Ah . . . school dental nurse has been in here'. I said 'how can you tell?' He said by the amount of amalgam that was in my mouth :) Please . . . why didn't they pay them more rather than take it out on us little folk . . .

Of course, online comments have become so negative and abrasive that many news sites no longer allow them. So were the comments my story generated just the work of the permanently disgruntled, the views of a minority? In 2010, dentist Susan Cartwright completed a thesis on dental anxiety. She wrote of her personal experience:

> Many adult dental patients were anxious or fearful and on questioning frequently referred to their unpleasant experiences as children at the school dental clinic. The stories often told included reference to the treadle drill, so that even those patients, who were too young to have received treatment with this particular drill, talked about it as though they did experience it first-hand. Being called up from the classroom to attend the dental clinic seemed to have caused much anxiety, perhaps because of a lack of parental support in such a potentially frightening situation. Another common story told by this group of patients was that unnecessary fillings were placed so that the dental nurse could practise upon them. Whether these memories had been directly acquired from personal experience or were a result of stories that had been heard, or a combination of both, was hard to assess. Nevertheless, it appeared that a large proportion of adult patients harboured unpleasant memories of school dental service treatment.[2]

However, as Cartwright points out, dental anxiety is common throughout the world. Studies estimate that 50–80 per cent of people experience some level of dental anxiety and for 5–20 per cent it is severe and debilitating.

So-called painless dentistry is a very recent phenomenon, but it remains a grossly invasive procedure, with fingers and sharp instruments probing an important and sensitive orifice. The dentistry of the past has left an indelible mark on our collective memory, argues Joanna Bourke, author of *Fear: A cultural history*.[3] Certainly a cursory

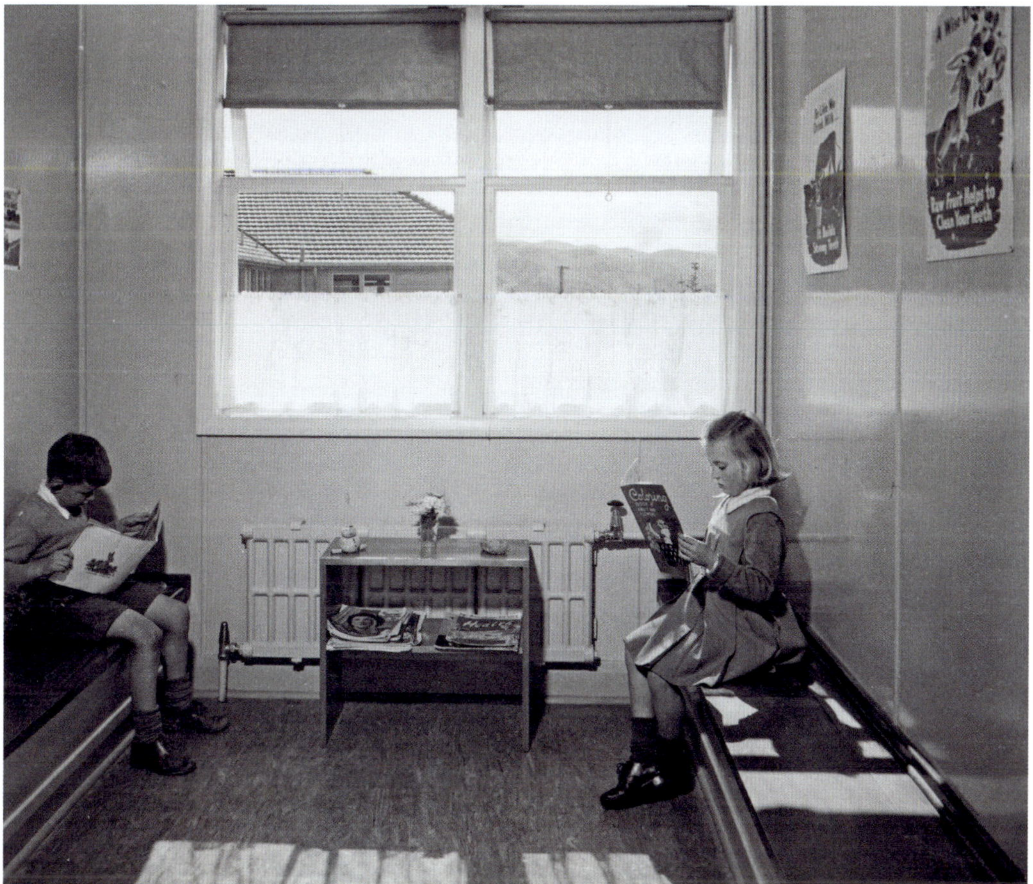

Children await their turn in the chair.

survey of dentistry through the ages is enough to make anyone thankful they live in the twenty-first century (see box, page 235).

Is it possible that the accumulated stress and trauma of visiting a toothpuller or dentist has been passed down the generations? Scientists are now exploring the phenomenon of epigenetic inheritance. Recently a study found that the trauma of Holocaust survivors could be passed on to their children through their genes.[4] A region of the gene associated with stress hormone regulation was the same in both survivor and their children but was not present in the control group.

If an inherited fear of dentists exists, a visit to the school dental clinic would have done little to dispel it. The lonely walk to the clinic, isolated from the main school buildings — to ensure classes were not unsettled by screams? — would only have increased the fears of a nervous child. The dental nurse in her white uniform and blood-red cardigan, the steel instruments glinting in a tray, the pungent antiseptic smell, the heavy black treadle drill looming near the seat: all must have created a state of unease hard to counter with a smile and kind words. In some clinics a child had to wait in one chair while the dental nurse worked on the child in the other chair. The 'murder house', that unfortunate nickname first used in the mid-1960s about the dental annexe in Premier House, Wellington, soon became common usage throughout the country, adding to children's anxieties.

All this created a climate of fear that exacerbated any pain experienced when being treated by the school dental nurse. Cartwright notes: 'Anxiety can cause an individual to be hypersensitive to pain so that their pain threshold is lowered and may even cause stimuli that would normally not be painful to be perceived as such. Conversely pain increases anxiety and so a vicious cycle is established.'

Many dental nurses took time to make children, especially younger ones, feel at ease — more so than dentists, who were operating a business where time is money. The butterflies and bees they fashioned out of cotton swabs, paper bibs and dental floss and gave to children are now part of Kiwiana. Unfortunately, the dental equipment they had to use offset any attempts to make treatment a pleasant experience. The treadle machine was the major cause of pain because of its grinding slowness. But even when it was superseded, dental nurses were forced to continue using it because the School Dental Service was slow to update clinics. The high-speed drill that would have made treatment almost pain-free for children was not introduced until the late 1970s.

Inadequate anaesthesia turned what was an uncomfortable procedure into torture. Dental nurses were only permitted to provide anaesthetic injections for extractions, not fillings, a ruling that some described as barbaric and cruel. Children suffered in agony because health officials wanted to cover their backsides in case they might be held responsible for any misuse of anaesthetics. As dental nurse Kath Salter said: 'The anaesthetic supplied was only 1% strength. The department was too scared to issue anything that might cause reactions. It was made up in Wellington and sent out to us.'[5]

Nerve blocks, which would have eliminated pain by anaesthetising the whole lower jaw, were used by dental nurses in Australia, but not in New Zealand. G. H. Leslie, director of dental health, defended that decision: 'I am still of the same mind that any advantage that might accrue from the introduction of regional anaesthesia into

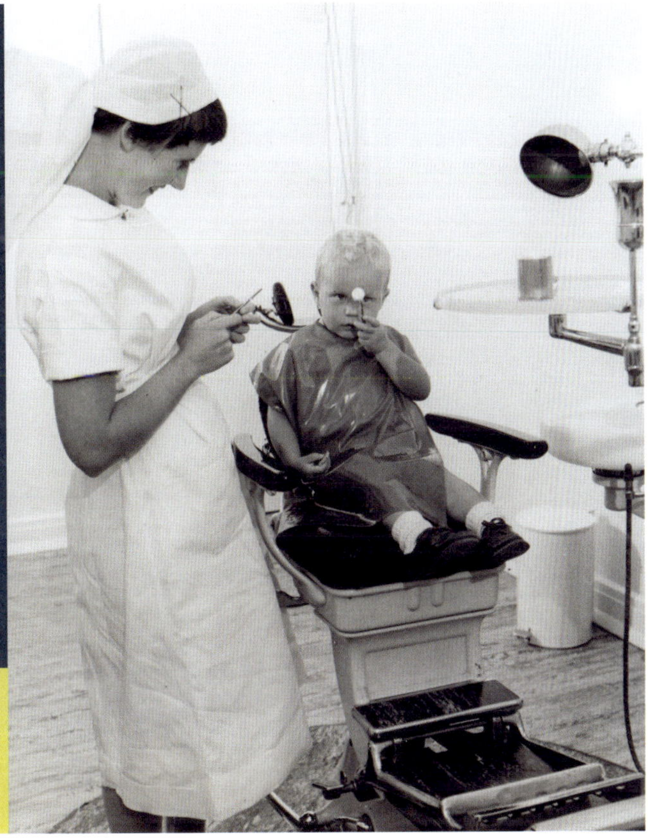

Dental nurses often did their best to calm the fears of young children by taking time to make them comfortable in the clinic.

the scope of work of the New Zealand School Dental Nurse would be outweighed by the risks inherent in entrusting the technique to 1400 operators, none of who have had a sufficient basic education to support our unqualified defence in law should an accident ever occur.'[6] (Ironically, the family pet could have nerve blocks as it was a breach of veterinarians' code of practice to cause unnecessary suffering to animals.)

Dental nurses were frequently accused of practising on children and doing unnecessary fillings. A theme of this book has been the tight control exercised by management over school dental nurses. No one graduated who had not met the exacting standards. During training every aspect of their work was examined with military rigour. In the field they had no need to practise; they were proficient and the work they did was strictly controlled. They were also required to keep meticulous records of the children they treated and they were subject to frequent inspection. Any fillings they did were what they'd been trained to do, and what was demanded by the

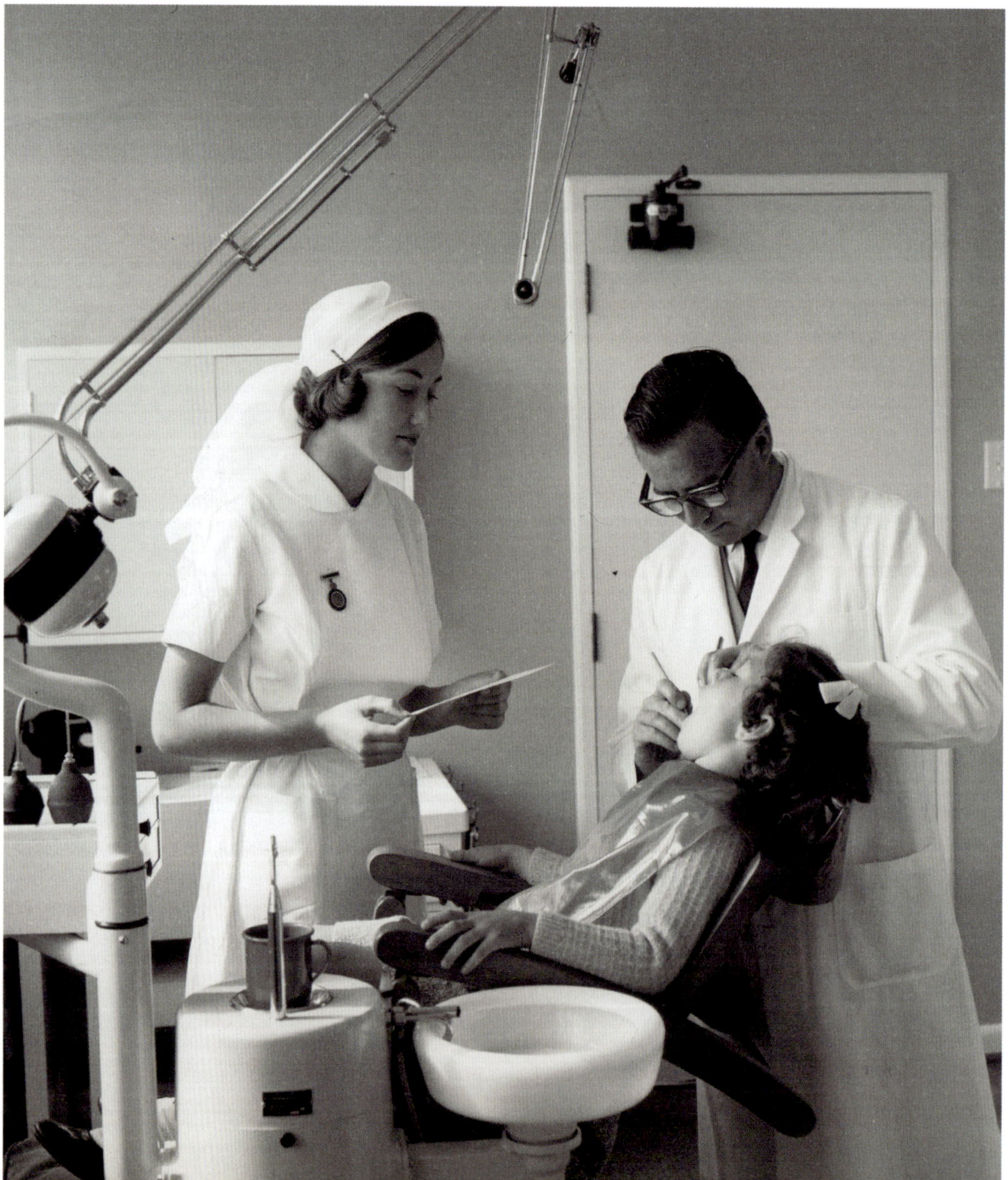

A dentist inspects a nurse's work. Dental nurses were required to drill and fill, as they had been instructed, and keep detailed records of all work done on children's teeth. They had no say in policy.

supervising dentists. In the 1940s and '50s that included filling teeth as a preventative measure. Susan Moffat, in her thesis on the service, explains:

> As well as 'extension for prevention', the dental nurses practised prophylactic odontotomy, first introduced into the dental profession in the United States, and which involved filling the deep fissures of permanent molars in order to prevent decay of those fissures. While the result was a filled tooth, the restoration was very narrow and less extensive than had the tooth had been left to decay. The SDS found that this practice decreased the number of extractions and large silver amalgams needed. The fact that some teeth were being filled that may never have decayed did not appear to be an issue. Teeth were selected on the basis that they were newly-erupted and had deep fissures in which a dental explorer would stick. Prior to the introduction of fluoride, it was more likely than not that the fissures of these teeth would decay, particularly the fissures of permanent six-year-old molars.[7]

Pain, discomfort and sometimes unnecessary fillings — it's easy to point to the failings of the School Dental Service. But what was the alternative? No treatment at all. Many families, particularly in the early years of the service, did not take their children to a dentist. Dental care was as unaffordable for the poor as it is now. Children had to endure toothaches and abscesses that made their young lives a misery, putting their general health in danger and affecting their ability to learn in school. Schoolteachers kept a jar of cloves in the classroom to hand out to pupils obviously troubled by toothache. Cocaine Drops, another all-natural remedy, promised 'Instantaneous cure!' for toothache. They were popular at the turn of the twentieth century but proved so moreish that they were banned.

Bad experiences in the chair need to be seen in the context of the time. Dental technology was slow to advance and the School Dental Service was even slower to install up-to-date equipment and implement new techniques. For many decades a visit to the dentist was just as likely to be painful as treatment from a dental nurse. But whatever the shortcomings of the School Dental Service, it remains a legacy to be proud of.

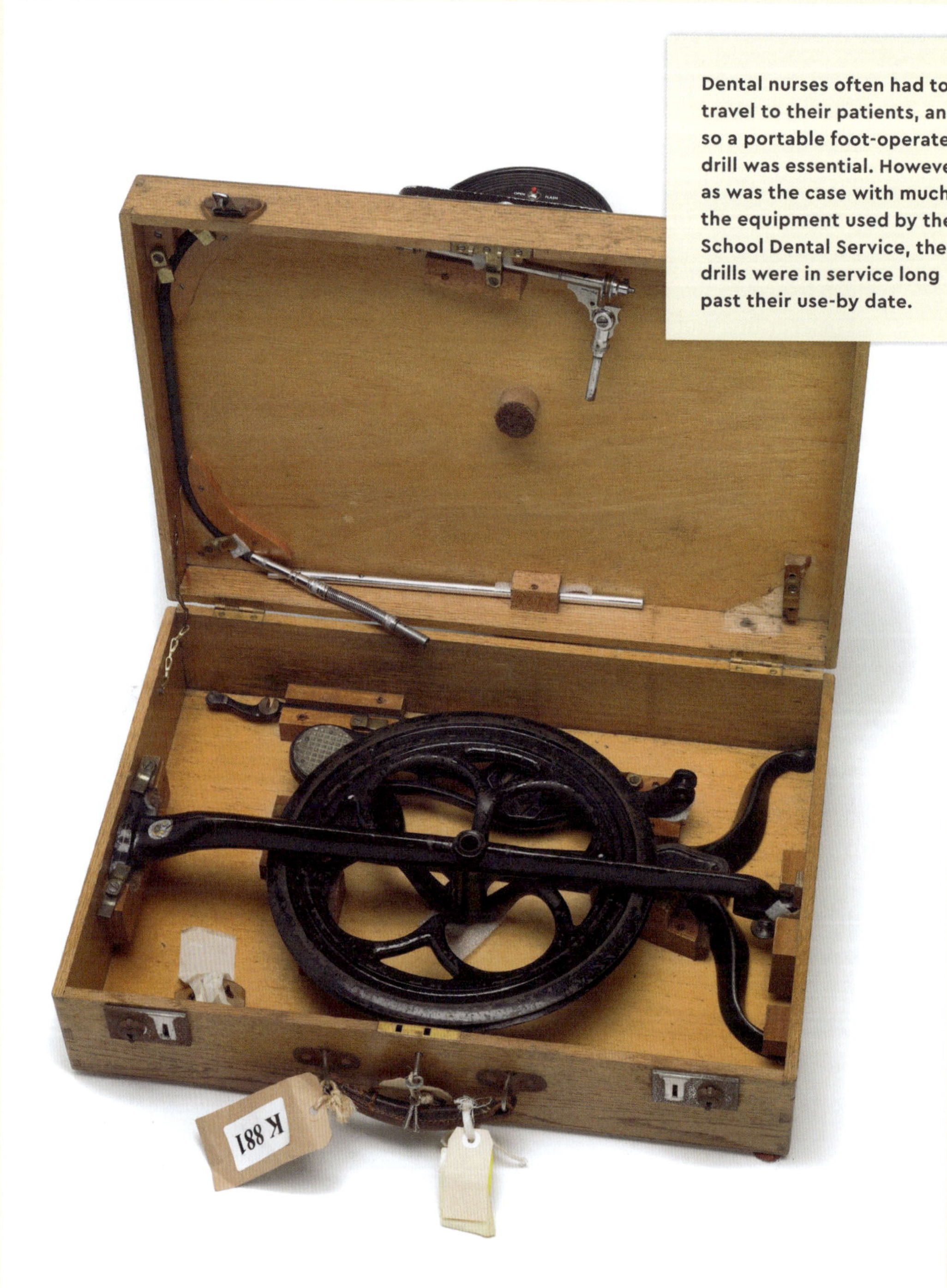

Dental nurses often had to travel to their patients, and so a portable foot-operated drill was essential. However, as was the case with much of the equipment used by the School Dental Service, these drills were in service long past their use-by date.

THIS MAY HURT A LITTLE: DENTISTRY'S PAINFUL PAST

Teeth have troubled both animals and humankind since they first sprouted in ancient gums. The earliest evidence of dental caries has been found in herbivorous dinosaurs of the Cretaceous period. Mastodons, camels, cave bears and sabre-toothed cats were also prone to dental caries. Their diet was so coarse that teeth were worn down until the pulp — and nerves — were exposed. The same applied to the paleo diet of early cave-dwellers. Later the grit in stone-ground bread, a big part of the diet in the Middle Ages, had the same effect on teeth, which eventually required extraction.

Evidence of dental caries and abscesses has been found in Egyptian mummies, and the dental 'profession' flourished in ancient Egypt. In ancient Greece, the philosopher Celsus wrote that 'toothache may be just ranked even among the greatest torments'. There was no shortage, though, of touted cures. Frankincense and myrrh, *de rigueur* gifts when visiting baby gods, were highly valued for easing toothache, but these resin gums from Arabian trees were not always to hand. A standby remedy, water in which a penis had been washed, was deemed to be just as effective.

The ancient Chinese believed 'excessive sexual intercourse' caused dental decay; and of the 388 pin sites in acupuncture, 26 are for toothache.

A common belief for many centuries was that tooth decay and toothache were caused by tooth worms. Hippocrates was closer to the mark, suggesting that food and debris caused decay in weakened teeth. Like Aristotle, however, he obviously spent little time peering into mouths, as he was convinced that men had more teeth than women.

With so little reliable knowledge of tooth decay and its causes, people were at the mercy of every charlatan and quack touting a cure. When the cures failed to work, the only option left was extraction. In his book *The Excruciating History of Dentistry* James Wynbrandt paints a colourful picture of the itinerant tooth-drawers, called 'toothers', 'toothis', or grossly misnamed 'kindhearts', who plied their trade in medieval Europe, inflicting agony on their customers. Wearing a necklace of extracted teeth, they promised painless dentistry. Tooth extraction was often a spectator sport, performed on stage at a fair. After demonstrating how easy and painless an extraction could be by pretending to extract the tooth of an associate, the tooth-puller would invite customers onto the stage where their troublesome tooth would be extracted, accompanied by loud drumming and horns to drown out their screams. A painting by Dutch artist Lucas van Leyden in 1523 depicts a tooth-puller extracting a patient's tooth while a female assistant extracts the patient's purse from his pocket. (A scene, perhaps, that the modern dental patient can identify with.)

Itinerant tooth-pullers may have been part of the fun of the fair, but barber-surgeons did most of the dental work in towns: besides trimming locks, barbers did bloodletting, minor surgery and teeth extractions. Bloodletting was considered good for all that ails you and drawing blood from an arm was a routine part of the barber's treatment for toothache.

Right up until the 1850s dentists were still drawing blood from their patients. Poor people, however, could not afford the services of barber-surgeons; instead they visited the local blacksmith to have their problem teeth extracted with pliers or simply knocked out. The tool of choice for anyone who fancied themselves as a tooth-puller was an instrument called the pelican. A claw that resembled the beak of a pelican, it was placed over the crown of a tooth to lever it out, usually with gum tissue as well. The pelican was superseded by the dental key, which fitted around the tooth and was then rotated, often causing the tooth to break and the jaw to fracture. The dental key evolved into the forceps, still used today.

William Addis, the first person to mass-produce the toothbrush, in the late eighteenth century, made a fortune, but his invention wasn't enough to arrest the decline of dental health. A tsunami of decay was on the way. In 1874, the punitive tax on sugar in Britain was repealed and sugar became affordable for people of every class. By the time of the Boer War in 1899, tooth decay among the masses was so bad that mincing machines were needed to enable soldiers to eat.

Dental treatment had not advanced. By the turn of the twentieth century, barbers were still bloodletting and extracting teeth. Self-styled dentists needed only a brass plate and a strong wrist to set up shop. Since only the desperate were inclined to visit, early dentists combined their trade with occupations such as chemists. Some drapers, booksellers, storekeepers and jewellers also extracted teeth as a sideline. 'Perhaps most notorious of all were the "bush" dentists,' writes Tom Brooking. 'One noted exponent of this form of torture was "Rack-a-Rock Bill" Christie who served the needs of railway construction workers in the Catlins area. He claimed to carry out extractions "where is, as is" and on the basis of all care but no responsibility. After removing every fragment, Christie would replace his pliers in their hygienic container, his bush shirt!'[1]

Filling was an alternative to extraction, but it was a difficult operation. First, the dentist chipped away the overlying enamel with a chisel to get at the decay, which was then removed with excavators. A hand-held drill twisted between finger and thumb was used to cut a cavity suitable for filling.

By the time the School Dental Service began in 1921, foot-operated treadle drills had speeded up dental treatment, but extractions and fillings were still painful experiences.

NOTES

Notes have intentionally been kept to a minimum. The reminiscences of each dental nurse can be ascribed to a single listed source, unless otherwise stated, and any unattributed quotation can be ascribed to the last-named source above it in the text.

INTRODUCTION

1 *Evening Post*, 29 March, 1974.

2 Annette King, interviewed by Noel O'Hare, 14 December 2015.

1: RAISED IN THE TOMATO HOUSE

1 Shirley Smith, *Memories of Early Days at the Tomato House: Dental nurses' personal accounts 1921–1941*, 1983. This cyclostyled booklet is the main source for the reminiscences of early days in the School Dental Service.

2 Marian Edith Burgoyne (Meba) Foxon (née Armstrong), interviewed by Hugo Manson, 19 April 1985. NZOHA NZ State Dental Nurses Institute Fiftieth Jubilee Oral History Project, held in Alexander Turnbull Library.

3 Elsie Mary Haines, interviewed by Hugo Manson, 9 March 1985. NZOHA NZ Fiftieth Jubilee Oral History Project.

4 For a full account of the opposition to the School Dental Service, see T. W. H. Brooking, *A History of Dentistry in New Zealand* (Dunedin: New Zealand Dental Association, 1980), p. 94.

5 Handwritten recollections of Sir Thomas Hunter, Hocken Library, MS-1146/3, folder 1.

6 Kath Young, *Colonel, Sir Thomas Anderson Hunter, K.B.E: A family history* (Wellington: 2007).

7 *Punch*, vol. 147 (19 August 1914), p. 166.

8 *Otago Daily Times*, 20 November 1920, p. 7.

9 Smith, *Memories of Early Days at the Tomato House.*

10 *Otago Daily Times*, 23 November 1920, p. 4.

11 *Niho Pai* (NZ School Dental School Dental Nurses' Journal), November 1933.

12 Frederick Truby King, *The Story of the Teeth and How to Save Them* (1917; Auckland: Whitcombe & Tombs, 1935).

13 Lloyd Chapman, *In a Strange Garden: The life and times of Truby King* (Auckland: Penguin, 2003), http://nzetc.victoria.ac.nz/tm/scholarly/tei-ChaStra-t1-body-d20.html

14 Haines, interview.

15 Frederick Truby King, *The Evils of Cram*, Robert Stout Collection, vol. 78, http://nzetc.victoria.ac.nz/tm/scholarly/tei-Stout78-t9-body-d1.html

16 *New Zealand Dental Journal*, no. 123, September 1931.

17 Erik Olssen, 'Truby King and the Plunket Society: An analysis of a prescriptive ideology', *New Zealand Journal of History*, vol. 15, no. 1 (1981), pp. 3–23, www.nzjh.auckland.ac.nz/docs/1981/NZJH_15_1_02.pdf

18 Smith, *Memories of Early Days at the Tomato House.*

19 *New Zealand Dental Journal*, July 1921.

20 Ibid.

21 John Llewellyn Saunders, *The New Zealand School Dental Service: Its initiation and development 1920–1960* (Wellington: Government Printer, 1964).

22 Smith, *Memories of Early Days at the Tomato House.*

23 The BBC documentary *Drills, Dentures and Dentistry: An oral history* gives a good account of the gruesome development of dentistry and the use of 'Waterloo teeth'; youtu.be/WPgLZtgClWY

24 Smith, *Memories of Early Days at the Tomato House.*

25 Ibid.

2: THE COLONELS TAKE CHARGE

1 Unpublished biographical notes by John Llewellyn Saunders, supplied to the author by his daughter Christine Kershaw.

2 'Into the Storm', editorial notes, *New Zealand School Dental Service Gazette*, vol. IX, no. 3 (1949).

3 Saunders, biographical notes.

4 Elsie Mary Haines, interviewed by Hugo Manson, 9 March 1985. NZOHA NZ State Dental Nurses Institute Fiftieth Jubilee Oral History Project, held in Alexander Turnbull Library.

5 Ibid.

6 Cecily Marguerite Montefiore, interviewed by Hugo Manson, 20 April 1985. NZOHA Fiftieth Jubilee Oral History Project.

7 Shirley Smith, *Memories of Early Days at the Tomato House: Dental nurses' personal accounts 1921–1941*, 1983.

8 Charles Truax, *The Mechanics of Surgery* (Chicago: C. Truax, 1899).

9 *Evening Post*, 19 October 1929, p. 10.

10 Elsie Mary Haines, interviewed by Hugo Manson, 9 March 1985.

11 Smith, *Memories of Early Days at the Tomato House.*

12 Ibid.

13 K. N. McCormick, 'First Impressions of Central Otago', *Niho Pai* (New Zealand School Dental Nurses' Journal), vol. II, no. 2 (1927), p. 39.

14 'I Start My Clinic', by a Sister of the Order of St Apollonia, *Niho Pai*, vol. II, no. 2 (1927).

15 Ibid.

16 Smith, *Memories of Early Days at the Tomato House.*

17 Ibid.

18 Michael Smythe, 'Industrial design — Protectionism, 1938 to 1988', Te Ara — the Encyclopedia of New Zealand, www.TeAra.govt.nz/en/zoomify/41850/wooden-dental-chair

19 Ngaire Mune, 'The Life of a Dental Nurse', part 3, unpublished reminiscences.

20 Ibid.

21 *Spectator*, 10 September 1927.

22 *Evening Post*, 30 December 1929, p. 1.

3: SURVIVING THE DEPRESSION

1 Shirley Smith, *Memories of Early Days at the Tomato House: Dental nurses' personal accounts 1921–1941*, 1983.

2 *Niho Pai*, March 1932.

3 Ibid.

4 Smith, *Memories of Early Days at the Tomato House.*

5 Tony Simpson, *The Sugarbag Years* (Auckland: Godwit, 1997).

6 *Disputed Ground: Robin Hyde, journalist*, introduced and selected by Gillian Boddy and Jacqueline Matthews (Wellington: Victoria University Press, 1991).

7 John Llewellyn Saunders, *The New Zealand School Dental Service: Its initiation and development 1920–1960* (Wellington: Government Printer, 1964).

8 *Evening Post*, 16 April 1932, p. 10.

9 'Unemployed riot rocks Queen St', https://nzhistory.govt.nz/queen-st-riot-auckland (Ministry for Culture and Heritage).

10 Smith, *Memories of Early Days at the Tomato House.*

11 Margaret Jepson, *Via Panama* (London: Hamish Hamilton, 1934).

12 Stephen Barnett, *Those Were the Days: A nostalgic look at the 1930s from the pages of the* Weekly News (Auckland: Moa, 1987).

13 Smith, *Memories of Early Days at the Tomato House.*

14 Ibid.

15 Ibid.

16 Ibid.

17 Kath Salter, interviewed by Judith Fyfe, 12 April 1985. NZOHA NZ State Dental Nurses Institute Fiftieth Jubilee Oral History Project, held in Alexander Turnbull Library.

18 Labour Party film, 1938, duration 0:23:36, F4372, Ngā Taonga Sound and Vision Television Archive, https://www.ngataonga.org.nz/collections/catalogue/catalogue-item?record_id=65294

19 Saunders, *The New Zealand School Dental Service.*

20 Elsie Mary Haines, interviewed by Hugo Manson, 9 March 1985. NZOHA NZ State Dental Nurses Institute Fiftieth Jubilee Oral History Project.

21 Saunders, *The New Zealand School Dental Service.*

22 Cecily Marguerite Montefiore, interviewed by Hugo Manson, 20 April 1985. NZOHA NZ Fiftieth Jubilee Oral History Project.

23 Alfreda Mary Patterson, Pai, July 1936, interviewed by Judith Fyle, 12 March 1985. NZOHA NZ Fiftieth Jubilee Oral History Project.

24 Megan Hutching, 'Hallam, Clara Evelyn', Dictionary of New Zealand Biography, first published in 1998, updated December, 2013. Te Ara – the Encyclopedia of New Zealand, https://teara.govt.nz/en/biographies/4h8/hallam-clara-evelyn

4: KEEP DRILLING AND CARRY ON

1 'The Dominion Training School for Dental Nurses, by Dr J. B. Bibby, Principal', *School Dental Service Gazette*, October 1941.

2 Margaret Sybil McLean, interviewed by Hugh Manson, 13 March 1985. NZOHA NZ State Dental Nurses Institute Fiftieth Jubilee Oral History Project, held in the Alexander Turnbull Library.

3 Frances Porter, *Away From Home: The story of Victoria House* (Wellington: Bridget Williams Books, 2002).

4 Marjorie Orchiston, interviewed by Noel O'Hare, 28 April 2016.

5 Shirley Smith, *Memories of Early Days at the Tomato House: Dental nurses' personal accounts 1921–1941*, 1983.

6 Ibid.

7 *Evening Post*, 8 December 1941, p. 6.

8 *Women at War* (National Film Unit, 1941) was a promotional film about New Zealand women's contribution to the war effort; youtu.be/__JIkmQ3lZI

9 Orchiston, interview.

10 Nancy Taylor, *The Home Front*, vol. 1 (Wellington: Historical Publications Branch, 1986), ch. 14 — 'The American Invasion', http://nzetc.victoria.ac.nz/tm/scholarly/tei-WH2-1Hom-c14.html

11 Lauris Edmond (ed.), with Carolyn Milward, *Women in Wartime: New Zealand women tell their story* (Wellington: Government Printing Office, 1986).

12 'A Pair of Silk Stockings', *National Weekly Review*, 1942, www.youtube.com/watch?v=OgwBnRCno7g&t=14s

13 Dame Enid Lyons, quoted in *The Home Front*, vol. 2, by Nancy Taylor (Wellington: Historical Publications Branch, 1986), ch. 16 — 'The Shoe Pinches', http://nzetc.victoria.ac.nz/tm/scholarly/tei-WH2-2Hom-c16.html

14 NZ History, 'Battle of Manners Street', https://nzhistory.govt.nz/battle-of-manners-street (Ministry for Culture and Heritage), updated 9 December 2016.

15 *Dominion*, 24 November 1941.

16 Kath Salter, interviewed by Judith Fyfe, 12 April 1985. NZOHA NZ State Dental Nurses Institute Fiftieth Jubilee Oral History Project.

17 Ibid.

18 *School Dental Service Gazette*, October 1941.

19 *Evening Post*, 15 August 1945, p. 7.

20 Ibid., p. 8.

21 Edmond, *Women in Wartime*.

5: THE BABY BOOM YEARS

1 Pauline White, interviewed by Noel O'Hare, 30 June 2017.

2 *The School Dental Nurse* (brochure, New Zealand Department of Health, 1950).

3 James A. Michener, *Return to Paradise* (New York: Random House, 1951).

4 Jenny Carlyon and Diana Morrow, *Changing Times: New Zealand since 1945* (Auckland: Auckland University Press, 2013).

5 National Film Unit for the Department of Health, *A Friendly Career* (or *The Story of the Training and Life of the New Zealand School Dental Nurse*), www.nzonscreen.com/title/a-friendly-career-1953

6 Martin Edmond, *The Dreaming Land* (Wellington: Bridget Williams Books, 2015).

7 NZ History, 'The royal visit, 1953–54', https://nzhistory.govt.nz/culture/royal-visit-of-1953-54, (Ministry for Culture and Heritage).

8 John Llewellyn Saunders, *The New Zealand School Dental Service: Its initiation and development 1920–1960* (Wellington: Government Printer, 1964).

9 Allen O. Gruebbel, 'Report on the Study of Dental Public Health Services in New Zealand', *Journal of the American Dental Association*, September/October/November 1950.

10 Ibid.

11 'School Dental Nurses, Fifth Draft – Auckland 1955–57', reminiscences compiled by Yvonne Wilkie, 2012.

12 National Institute of Dental and Craniofacial Research, 'The Story of Fluoridation', www.nidcr.nih.gov/health-info/fluoride/the-story-of-fluoridation

13 J. Colquhoun, 'Why I changed my mind about fluoridation', *Perspectives in Biology & Medicine*, vol. 41, no. 1 (1997), pp. 29–44.

14 John Colquhoun and Bill Wilson, 'The Lost Control and Other Mysteries: Further revelations on New Zealand's fluoridation trial', *Accountability in Research*, vol. 6, no. 4 (1999), pp. 373–394.

15 John Colquhoun, interviewed by Paul Connett, 1 May 1998, https://youtube/e8th-BbboLQ

16 *School Dental Service Gazette*, editorial, August 1963.

17 It is outside the scope of this book and the competence of the author to examine the pros and cons of water fluoridation. Fluoridationists argue that it is a false controversy, and they have the weight of scientific opinion on their side. The Cochrane Collaboration, regarded as the gold standard for its rigorous review of research literature and evidence-based medicine, recently found that: 'The introduction of water fluoridation resulted in children having 35 per cent fewer decayed, missing and filled baby teeth and 26 per cent fewer decayed, missing and filled permanent teeth'. But they added the rider: 'Our confidence in the size of the effect estimates is limited by the observational nature of the study designs, the high risk of bias within the studies and, importantly, the applicability of the evidence to current lifestyles.' A 2014 review of the medical literature by the Royal Society of New Zealand and the Department of Health found no evidence of ill effects to health from water fluoridation.

18 Kath Salter, 'The Beginning of a Colombo Plan Project', *Dental Nurses Journal* (New Zealand State Dental Nurses Institute, 1985), p. 2.

19 Jackie Humm, interviewed by Emma Dewson, 10 June 2005, Dental Therapists Association oral history project.

20 Maurice Gee, *Hostel Girl* (Auckland: Puffin Books, 1999).

21 Humm, interview.

22 Ngaire Mune, interviewed by Noel O'Hare, 26 April 2016.

23 Ibid.

24 Ngaire Mune, 'The Life of a Student Dental Nurse in the Late 1950s', unpublished biographical notes, part 1.

25 *School Dental Service Gazette*, March 1956.

26 *School Dental Service Gazette*, 1956.

6: 'WE WERE COOKIE-CUTTER PEOPLE, REALLY'

1 *Department of Health School Dental Service Standing Instructions*, 1966.

2 Pam Horncy, interviewed by Noel O'Hare, 25 January 2016.

3 Maggie Morgan, interviewed by Noel O'Hare, 23 April 2016.

4 Hazel Phillips, *Wild Westie: The incredible life of Bob Harvey* (Auckland: Penguin Books, 2014).

5 Jenny Carlyon and Diana Morrow, *Changing Times: New Zealand since 1945* (Auckland: Auckland University Press, 2013).

6 'The Progressive Youth Movement', https://mackievietnamwarprotestnz.weebly.com/pym.html

7 *School Dental Service Gazette*, December 1966.

8 Stephanie Johnson, *Music from a Distant Room* (Auckland: Vintage, 2004). Courtesy of Penguin.

9 Annette King, interviewed by Noel O'Hare, 14 December 2015.

10 Rosemary Kennedy, interviewed by Noel O'Hare, 14 April 2016.

11 King, interview.

12 Margaret Clarkson, interviewed by Noel O'Hare, 21 September 2016.

7: DISSENSION IN THE RANKS

1 G. H. Leslie, *School Dental Service New Zealand 1921–1971* (Wellington: Government Printer, 1971).

2 Wellington branch of the New Zealand School Dental Nurses Institute, minute book 19 June 1950 to 20 April 1968.

3 Administration — School Dental Service — School Dental Nurses Institute, 1967–1975, Archives New Zealand

4 Ibid.

5 Ibid.

6 Ibid.

7 Alfreda Mary Patterson, interviewed by Judith Fyfe, 12 March 1985. NZOHA NZ State Dental Nurses Institute Fiftieth Jubilee Oral History Project, held in the Alexander Turnbull Library.

8 Pam Horncy, interviewed by Noel O'Hare, 25 January 2016.

9 Paul Little, 'Cold Shivers: An ode to New Zealand's own Cold Duck wine', *North & South*, 8 December 2016, www.noted.co.nz/distractions/humour/cold-shivers-an-ode-to-new-zealands-own-cold-duck-wine/

10 NZ History, '"Join together" song, 1974 Commonwealth Games', https://nzhistory.govt.nz/media/photo/%26%23039%3Bjoin-together%26%23039%3B-song%2C-1974-commonwealth-games (Ministry for Culture and Heritage).

11 Betty Friedan, *The Feminine Mystique* (New York: W. W. Norton, 1963).

12 Germaine Greer, *The Female Eunuch* (London: Paladin, 1970).

13 *Craccum* (Auckland University Students Association magazine), vol. 46, no. 3 (16 March 1972), p. 8.

14 Ngaire Mune, interviewed by Noel O'Hare, 9 February 2016.

15 Pam Horncy, interviewed by Noel O'Hare, 25 January 2016.

16 *School Dental Service Gazette*, June 1974.

17 *Dominion*, 4 March 1974.

18 Ian Baldrick, interviewed by Noel O'Hare, 2 February 2016.

19 Jackie Humm, interviewed by Noel O'Hare, 21 September 2016.

20 Margaret Clarkson, interviewed by Noel O'Hare, 21 September 2016.

21 *Made in Dagenham*, dir. Nigel Cole, Paramount Pictures, 2010.

22 *PSA Journal*, vol. 29, no. 2 (March 1992), p. 9, https://psa.recollect.co.nz/nodes/view/537#idx12785

23 Ibid.

8: THE MARCH THAT CHANGED EVERYTHING

1 Margaret Hayward, *Diary of the Kirk Years* (Queen Charlotte Sound: Cape Catley & Reed, 1981), 15 March 1974 entry.

2 *PSA Newsletter*, 12 April 1974.

3 Mark Derby, *White-collar Radical: Dan Long and the rise of the white-collar unions* (Nelson: Craig Potton Publishing, 2013).

4 *PSA Newsletter*, 12 April 1974.

5 R. K. Logan, letter to Professor E. E. J. Kirk, 19 February 1975, Archives New Zealand.

6 Horncy, interviewed by Noel O'Hare, 25 January 2016.

7 Maggie Morgan, interviewed by Noel O'Hare, 23 April 2016.

8 *New Zealand Herald*, 22 March 1974.

9 Jack Batt's diary entries are courtesy of his daughter, Marg Walmsley.

10 Margaret Hayward, *Diary of the Kirk Years*, 25 March 1974 entry.

11 Ibid., 27 March 1974 entry.

12 Ibid., 18 February 1974 entry.

13 *Nationwide*, 28 March 1974, Ngā Taonga Sound and Vision Television Archive,_ catalogue nos ZNWI-74/012 Items 1 and 2.

14 David Grant, *The Mighty Totara: The life and times of Norman Kirk* (Auckland: Random House, 2014), p. 245.

15 *Dominion*, 29 March 1974.

16 Parliamentary Debates, Standing Order 88, 29 March 1974.

17 Margaret Clarkson, interviewed by Noel O'Hare, 21 September 2016.

18 Dave Morgan, interviewed by Noel O'Hare, 23 April 2016.

19 Annette King, interviewed by Noel O'Hare, 14 December 2015.

20 *Evening Post*, 29 March 1974.

21 NZ History, 'Basil Spence's first pencil impression of the Beehive', https://nzhistory.govt.nz/media/photo/beehive-drawing-basil-spence (Ministry for Culture and Heritage).

22 Tom Scott, Parliament, *NZ Listener*, 20 April 1974.

23 Jack Batt's diary entry.

24 Michael Bassett: *The Third Labour Government: A personal history* (Palmerston North: Dunmore Press, 1976).

25 *PSA Journal*, March 1992.

9: DECLINE AND FALL

1 Annette King, interviewed by Noel O'Hare, 14 December 2015.

2 Maynie Thompson, interviewed by Noel O'Hare, 10 February 2016.

3 Pam Horncy, interviewed by Noel O'Hare, 25 January 2016.

4 Marjorie Orchiston, interviewed by Noel O'Hare, 28 April 2016.

5 *Department of Health School Dental Service Standing Instructions*, 1966.

6 *School Dental Service Gazette*, vol. 34, no. 4 (October 1974).

7 '"Odes" and "Modes"', *School Dental Service Gazette*, vol. 32, no. 4 (August 1972), p. 52.

8 Review of career structure for New Zealand school dental nurses occupational class; School dental nurses, by the Public Service Association, 1977.

9 R. K. Logan, letter to Professor E. E. J. Kirk, 19 February 1975, Archives New Zealand.

10 Administration — School Dental Service — School Dental Nurses Institute, 1967–1975, Archives New Zealand.

11 Letter to the Ladies of the National Executive, 25 October 1974, Archives New Zealand.

12 *PSA Journal*, November 1980.

13 International Collaborative Study of Dental Manpower Systems. The Canterbury Study, 1974.

14 Susan M. Moffat, Lyndie A. Foster Page and W. Murray Thomson, 'New Zealand's School Dental Service over the Decades: Its response to social, political, and economic influences, and the effect on oral health inequalities', 2017, https://www.ncbi.nlm.nih.gov/pmc/articles/PMC5534465/

15 Susan Moffat, 'From Innovative to Outdated? New Zealand School Dental Service 1921–1989', DPhil thesis, University of Otago, 2015.

16 'Review of Career Structure for New Zealand School Dental Nurses Occupational Class: School dental nurses', Public Service Association, 1977.

17 'Dental Nurses Fight for Survival', *PSA Journal*, November 1980.

18 Ibid.

19 *PSA Journal*, July 1981.

20 Noel O'Hare, 'Janet Quigley: The restructuring of the School Dental Service', *PSA*, 2013, www.psa100.org.nz/stories/people/l-z/janet-quigley/

21 King, interview.

22 Abby Gillies, 'New Zealand Children's Dental Health Still Among Worst', *New Zealand Herald*, 6 March 2011, www.nzherald.co.nz/nz/news/article.cfm?c_id=1&objectid=10710408

23 Lydia Anderson, 'Children Forced to Wait More Than a Year for Dental Check-up', Radio New Zealand, 29 May 2017, www.radionz.co.nz/news/national/331868/children-forced-to-wait-more-than-a-year-for-dental-check-up

24 New Zealand Dental Association, 'Dental Association Conference: President calls out school dental service', media release, www.nzda.org.nz/assets/files/Public/Media/NZDA_Media__Release_20_August_2018.pdf

25 Moffat, 'From Innovative to Outdated?'.

26 Angela Fitchett, '"Murder House" was Pain and Gain', *Nelson Mail*, 18 October 2013.

10: EVERYDAY MERCURY POISONING

1 *New Zealand Herald*, 7 March 2017.

2 Julie Sloane, 'Mercury: Element of the ancients', Dartmouth Toxic Metals Superfund Research Programme, Trustees of Dartmouth College, 26 July 1016, https://sites.dartmouth.edu/toxmetal/mercury/mercury-element-of-the-ancients/

3 New England Historical Society, 'The Mad Hatters of Danbury, Conn.', www.newenglandhistoricalsociety.com/mad-hatters-danbury-conn/

4 'The History of American Amalgam Use', Dental Amalgam Mercury Solutions, http://amalgam.org/education/history-american-amalgam-use/

5 Alfred Stock, 'The Dangerousness of Mercury Vapor and of Amalgam Fillings', trans. Birgit Calhoun; orig. pub. 'Die Gefährlichkeit des Quecksilbers und der Amalgam-Zahnfüllungen', *Angewandte Chemie*, vol. 41, issue 24 (16 June 1928), pp. 663–85.

6 *School Dental Service Gazette*, October 1971.

7 'Health Effects Associated with Mercury Exposure', Ministry for the Environment, www.mfe.govt.nz/publications/waste/mercury-inventory-new-zealand-2008-section-iii-%E2%80%93-risk-assessment-1-introduction/2

8 Stock, 'The Dangerousness of Mercury Vapor'.

9 *Otago Daily Times*, 7 September 1927, p. 9.

10 *Evening Post*, 8 September 1927.

11 Margaret Clarkson, interviewed by Noel O'Hare, 21 September 2016.

12 *PSA Journal*, November/December 1974.

13 Margaret Sybil McLean, interviewed by Hugo Manson, 13 March 1985. NZOHA NZ State Dental Nurses Institute Fiftieth Jubilee Oral History Project, held in the Alexander Turnbull Library.

14 Ngaire Mune, interviewed by Noel O'Hare, 26 April 2016.

15 Maggie Morgan, interviewed by Noel O'Hare, 23 April 2016.

16 Pam Horncy, interviewed by Noel O'Hare, 25 January 2016.

17 *School Dental Service Gazette*, August 1975.

18 Linda M. Jones, 'The Quicksilver Quest: Two psychological studies investigating the effects of mercury in dentistry', DPhil thesis, Massey University, 2005.

19 Ibid.

20 Linda M. Jones, '"We Gave Good Patients Mercury in Burr Boxes": A view of mercury from its earlier use in the School Dental Service to contemporary dental practice', *New Zealand Dental Journal*, vol. 105, no. 3 (September 2009), pp. 96–100.

21 Linda Jones, Julie Bunnell and Jennifer Stillman, 'A 30-year Follow-up of Residual Effects on New Zealand School Dental Nurses, from Occupational Mercury Exposure', *Human & Experimental Toxicology*, vol. 26, no. 4 (April 2007), pp. 367–375.

22 Jones, 'The Quicksilver Quest'.

23 Ibid.

24 Reported in Michael Bender, 'Neurotoxic Effects of Mercury in Dental Nurses', FDA public hearing, Gaithersburg, MD, 7 September 2006, https://wayback.archive-it.org/7993/20170405065234/https://www.fda.gov/ohrms/dockets/ac/06/slides/2006-4218s2-04.pdf

25 WHO, 'Mercury in Health Care', policy paper, www.who.int/water_sanitation_health/medicalwaste/mercurypolpap230506.pdf

26 Caroline Cassels, 'Mercury Exposure May Contribute to Alzheimer's Risk', *Medscape*, 2 December 2010, www.medscape.com/viewarticle/733465

11: PAIN AND POLICY

1 Caitlyn Salter, 'Memories of Dental Nurses and the "Murder House"', *Stuff*, 16 February 2016, www.stuff.co.nz/national/health/76918041/null

2 Susan Cartwright, 'The Murder House Case Studies: An education in dental anxiety', MEd thesis, Auckland University of Technology, 2010.

3 Joanna Bourke, *Fear: A cultural history* (Emeryville, CA: Shoemaker & Hoard, 2005).

4 Helen Thomson: 'Study of Holocaust Survivors Finds Trauma Passed on to Childrens' Genes', *The Guardian*, 21 August 2015.

5 Kath Salter, interviewed by Judith Fyfe, 12 April 1985. NZOHA NZ Fiftieth Jubilee Oral History Project.

6 Susan Moffat, 'From Innovative to Outdated? New Zealand School Dental Service 1921–1989, DPhil thesis, University of Otago, 2015.

7 Ibid.

DENTISTRY'S PAINFUL PAST

1 T. W. H. Brooking, *A History of Dentistry in New Zealand* (Dunedin: New Zealand Dental Association, 1980).

ABOUT THE AUTHOR

Noel O'Hare is a freelance journalist and author. As senior writer and health columnist for the *New Zealand Listener* he won numerous awards, including Qantas senior magazine feature writer of the year. He is committed to social justice, and has worked for the New Zealand Educational Institute and Public Service Association unions.

ACKNOWLEDGEMENTS

This book was made possible only because of those who shared their stories and gave generously of their time. Sincere thanks to Margaret Clarkson, Pam Horncy, Jackie Humm, Rosemary Kennedy, Annette King, Maggie Morgan, Ngaire Mune, the late Marjorie Orchiston, the late Maynie Thompson, and Pauline White.

For the early chapters I was fortunate to be able to draw on the oral histories of Marian Edith Burgoyne Foxon, Elsie Mary Haines, Cecily Marguerite Montefiore, Margaret Sybil McLean, Alfreda Mary Patterson and Kath Salter. My thanks to the New Zealand Dental and Oral Health Therapists Association for allowing me to access and use this valuable oral history archive lodged in the Alexander Turnbull Library, and to Arish Naresh, Trish Delamore and Pitchin Ng for their help and encouragement.

I am indebted to Susan Moffat, whose thesis on the School Dental Service is thorough and comprehensive and was my principal source. Thanks to Andrea Jarrold, who provided me with information and useful contacts, and to Ian Baldrick and John Shennan for insights into politics of the Public Service Association. My thanks also to Mark Derby, biographer of Dan Long, for sharing information and advice, and to Yvonne Wilkie, who had collected dental nurses' 1950s reminiscences. I am grateful to Christine Kershaw for providing me with autobiographical notes by Colonel John Llewellyn Saunders, to Marg Walmsley for extracts from the diary of Jack Batt, and to Pamela Crump for the material on her late mother, Beryl Dickson.

My thanks to Linda Evans and other staff of the Alexander Turnbull Library, Debbie Gale of the Hocken Collections Uare Taoka o Hākena and the staff of Archives New Zealand.

Many former dental nurses contacted me during the course of writing this book. I would like to thank all of them for their interest in the project and regret that time and space constraints prevented me from following up on their offers of help.

This book was longer in the making for a variety of reasons than I had anticipated and I thank Paul Little for his encouragement and support to finish it.

Finally, I would like to thank my publisher, Nicola Legat, who enthusiastically embraced the book, and the team who worked on it. A special thanks to Matt Turner, whose editing was both rigorous and respectful of the text.

IMAGE CREDITS

Archives New Zealand Te Rua Mahara o te Kāwanatanga

Page 15: ABKI 667/1; page 19: ABKI 672/4; page 22 (and cover): ABKI 667/1; page 25: ABKI 672/4; page 30: ABKI 667/1; page 31: ABKI 667/1; page 33: ABKI 667/1; page 39: ABKI 672/1 [YQ256]; page 40: ABKI 667/1; page 41: ABKI 667/3; page 44: ABKI 672/2; page 48: ABKI 672/2; page 64 (and cover): ABKI 672/3; page 65: page 66: ABKI 667/3; page 77: ABKI 667/4; page 88: AAFB W2555 24223; page 91: ABKI 667/3; page 93: ABKI 667/4; page 94: ABKI 667/3; page 106: ABKI 673/1; page 111: ABKI 667/3; page 128: ABKI 667/3; page 133: ABKI 667/2; page 138 (and cover): ABKI 667/3; pages 144–46: R21081016; page 149 (and cover): ABKI 667/3; page 154: ABKI 667/3; page 155 (and cover): ABKI 667/3; page 192 (and cover): ABKI 667/3; page 203: ABKI 667/2; page 212: ABKI 667/3; page 227: ABKI 672/4; page 229: ABKI 667/3; page 230: ABKI 667/3; page 255 (and cover): ABKI 667/3

Hocken Collections Uare Taoka o Hākena

Page 35: AG-589-01, Nurse May Falconer and Nurse M. M. Anderson, 1926

Museum of New Zealand Te Papa Tongarewa

Page 2: PC004178, Shoes, woman's (School Dental Nurse's); page 42: GH004152/1; page 116 (top): GH004149; page 116 (lower left): GH004020; page 232: GH004148

MTG Hawke's Bay Tai Ahuriri

Page 49: 19959, *Post*, 3 Feb 1931, Richard Savage, Gifted by Charlotte Maxwell

National Library of New Zealand Te Puna Mātauranga o Aotearoa

Page 16: 1/1-014109-G, S. P. Andrew Collection (PAColl-3739); page 46: Eph-D-DENTAL-1940s-02, courtesy of the Ministry of Health; page 57: OHInt-0054/22; page 65: EP-Health-Hospitals-Dental-01; page 69: 1/2-106538-F; page 79: PAColl-7112-02; page 83: OHInt-0054/22; page 86 (and cover): ISSN 0110-5515, *School Dental Service Gazette*, May 1946, courtesy of the Ministry of Health; page 101 (top): Eph-A-DENTAL-1950s, courtesy of the Ministry of Health; page 101 (lower left): Eph-A-DENTAL-1950s, courtesy of the Ministry of Health; page 101 (lower right): Eph-A-DENTAL-1975/1979, courtesy of the Ministry of Health; page 103: 114/130/12-G; page 122: Eph-A-DENTAL-1960s, courtesy of the Ministry of Health; page 135: PAColl-5936-53; page 156: Eph-A-DENTAL-1970/1974 (Courtesy of PSA); page 208: Eph-C-DENTAL-1950s-04, courtesy of the Ministry of Health

Public Service Association

Pages 9; 10; 125; 153; 159; 171; 174; 175; 176; 179; 183 (and cover); 185; 191; 199; 200 (and cover)

Puke Ariki

Page 1: PA2004.093; badge awarded to Elaine Soothill on 17 August 1961 after two years of study at the Dental Nurses School at Wellington; page 6 (and cover): A58.333; page 12; A62.751; page 28: A62.754; page 64: A57.663; page 120: A58.332; page 140: A62.756; page 162 (and cover): A58.317; page 188: A62.757; page 224: A58.328

Private collections

Page 38 (and cover): Courtesy of Pamela Crump; page 59: Courtesy of Pamela Crump; page 73: Courtesy of Marjorie Orchiston; page 80: Courtesy of Marjorie Orchiston; page 108: Courtesy of Pauline White; page 109: Courtesy of Pauline White; page 113: Courtesy of Ngaire Mune; page 116 (lower right): Courtesy of Ngaire Mune; page 122: Collection of the author; page 131: Courtesy of Annette King; page 136: Courtesy of Rosemary Kennedy; page 205: Collection of the author; page 211: Collection of the author; page 220: Collection of the author

INDEX

Page numbers in **bold** indicate illustrations

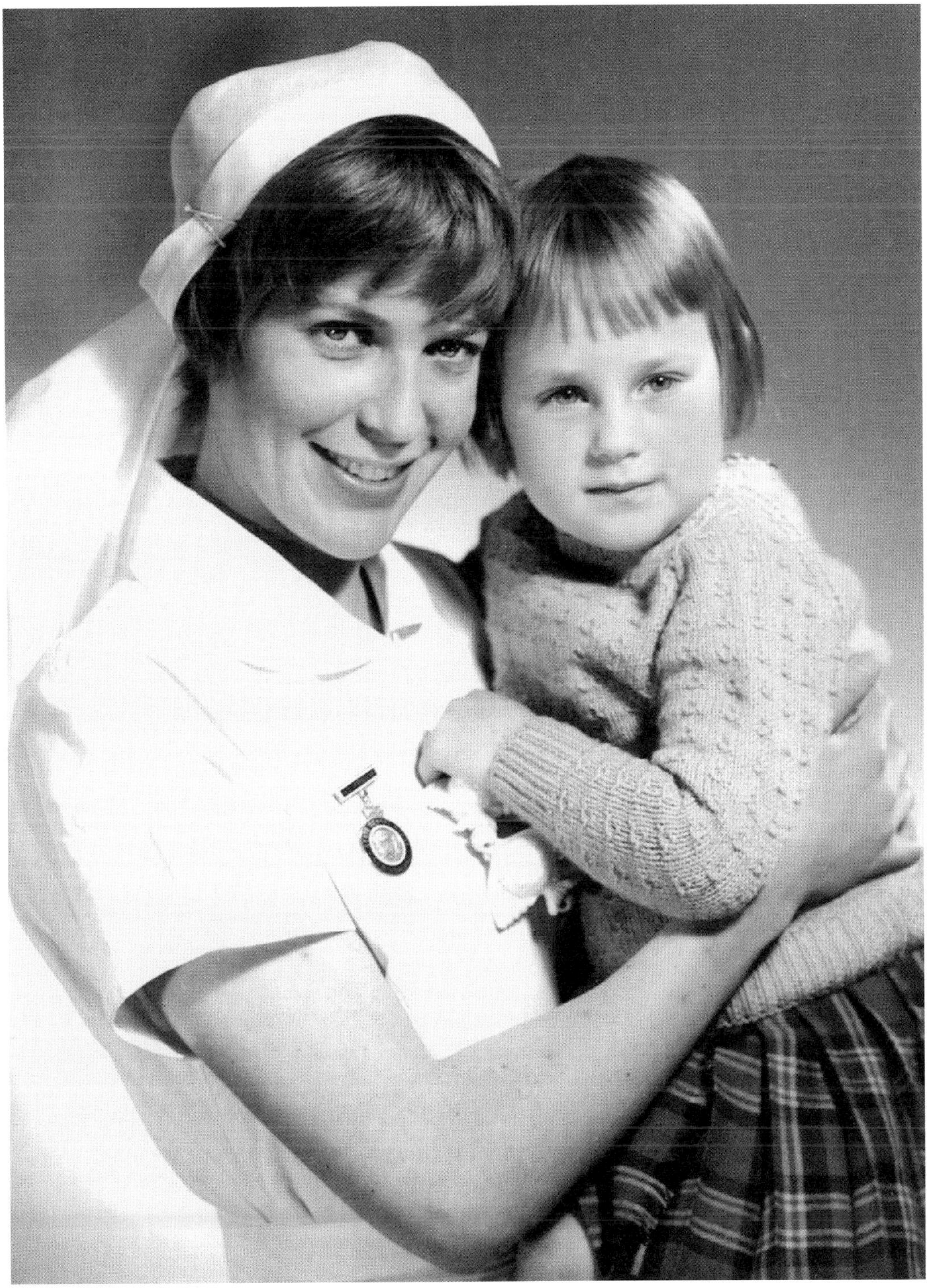

MASSEY UNIVERSITY PRESS

First published in 2020 by Massey University Press
Private Bag 102904, North Shore Mail Centre
Auckland 0745, New Zealand
www.masseypress.ac.nz

Design by Alice Bell
Front cover images: Archives New Zealand, ABKI 667/3, ABKI 672/3 (top) and Public Service Association (below); front flap: National Library of New Zealand, ISSN 0110-5515, School Dental Service Gazette, May 1946 (top), Archives New Zealand, ABKI 667/3 (middle) and Public Service Association (below); back cover: Archives New Zealand, ABKI 667/1 (top), ABKI 667/3 (middle) and Puke Ariki, A58.333 (below); back flap: Puke Ariki, A58.317 (top), courtesy of Pamela Crump (middle) and Archives New Zealand, ABKI 667/3 (below)

A catalogue record for this book is available from the National Library of New Zealand

Printed and bound in China by Everbest Printing Investment Ltd.

ISBN: 978-0-9951229-6-3